A PRACTICAL MANUAL OF LAPAROSCOPY:

A CLINICAL COOKBOOK

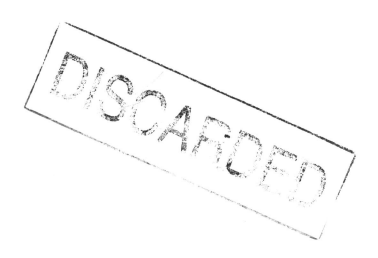

A PRACTICAL MANUAL OF LAPAROSCOPY:

A CLINICAL COOKBOOK

RESAD PASIC, M.D., PH.D.

Assistant Professor of Obstetrics, Gynecology & Women's Health
University of Louisville School of Medicine
Louisville, Kentucky

RONALD L. LEVINE, M.D.

Professor of Obstetrics, Gynecology & Women's Health
Director, Section of Operative Gynecologic Endoscopy
University of Louisville School of Medicine
Louisville, Kentucky

The Parthenon Publishing Group
International Publishers in Medicine, Science & Technology

A CRC PRESS COMPANY

BOCA RATON   LONDON   NEW YORK   WASHINGTON, D.C.

Library of Congress Cataloging-in-Publication Data
Data available on request

British Library Cataloguing in Publication Data
Data available on request

ISBN 1-84214-077-9

Published in the USA by
The Parthenon Publishing Group
345 Park Avenue South, 10th Floor
New York
NY 10010
USA

Published in the UK by
The Parthenon Publishing Group
23–25 Blades Court
Deodar Road
London SW15 2NU
UK

Printed and bound by Antony Rowe Ltd, Chippenham, Wiltshire

We would like to dedicate this book primarily to our families. To our wives, Djenita and Sonia, and to our children who have taught us the meaning of unconditional love and support.

We also owe great debts of gratitude and thus this dedication, to our teachers and colleagues who taught us the art of surgery and to our patients who ultimately taught us not only the art of medicine, but the art of caring.

CONTRIBUTING AUTHORS

LEILA ADAMYAN, M.D.
Professor of Operative Gynecology
Scientific Ctr for OB/GYN & Perinatology
Moscow, Russia

JEFF W. ALLEN, M.D.
Assistant Professor of Surgery
University of Louisville School of Medicine
Louisville, Kentucky

BERND BOJAHR, M.D.
Department for Gynaecology and Obstetrics
University of Greifswald, Germany

ANDREW I. BRILL, M.D.
Professor and Chief, General Obstetrics and Gynecology
Department of Obstetrics and Gynecology
The University of Illinois at Chicago
College of Medicine
Chicago, Illinois

LAURA CLARK, M.D.
Associate Professor of Anesthesiology
University of Louisville School of Medicine
Louisville, Kentucky

EKATERINA L. IAROTSKAIA, M.D.
Scientific Center for Obstetrics & Gynecology
Moscow, Russia

MIROSLAV KOPJAR, M.D.
Department for Gynaecology and Obstetrics
General Hospital Zabok, Croatia

DANIEL KRUSCHINSKI, M.D.
Institute for Endoscopic Gynaecology
University of Witten/Herdecke, Germany

RONALD L. LEVINE, M.D.
Professor of Obstetrics, Gynecology & Women's Health
University of Louisville School of Medicine
Director, Section of Operative Gynecologic Endoscopy
Louisville, Kentucky

BARBARA LEVY, M.D., P.S.
Assistant Clinical Professor of Obstetrics & Gynecology
Yale University School of Medicine
University of Washington School of Medicine
Seattle, Washington

C.Y. LIU, M.D.
Director of Chattanooga Women's Laser Center
and Advanced Laparoscopic Surgeons of New York
Chattanooga, Tennessee

ANTHONY LUCIANO, M.D.
Professor of Obstetrics and Gynecology
University of Connecticut School of Medicine
Director, Center for Fertility & Reproductive
Endocrinology
New Britain General Hospital
New Britain, Connecticut

THOMAS L. LYONS, M.D.
Director of Health South Surgery Center
Center for Women's Care & Reproductive Surgery
Atlanta, Georgia

DAN MARTIN, M.D.
Associate Clinical Professor of Obstetrics and
Gynecology
University of Tennessee
Memphis, Tennessee

TIMOTHY B. McKINNEY, M.D.
Clinical Associate Professor
University of Medicine and Dentistry of New Jersey-
SOM and University of Pennsylvania
Director of Urogynecology at Athena Women's Medical
Chief of Urogynecology and Pelvic Reconstructive
Surgery
Stratford, New Jersey

JOHN R. MIKLOS, M.D.
Director of Urogynecology
Atlanta Center for Laparoscopic Urogynecology &
Reconstructive Vaginal Surgery
Clinical Instructor
Medical College of Georgia
Atlanta, Georgia

CEANA NEZHAT, M.D.
Department of Obstetrics & Gynecology
Center for Special Pelvic Surgery
Atlanta, Georgia

FARR NEZHAT, M.D.
Director of Gynecologic Minimally Invasive Surgery
Department of Gynecologic Oncology
Mount Sinai School of Medicine
New York, NY

DAVID L. OLIVE, M.D.
Professor of Obstetrics and Gynecology
Director of Reproductive Endocrinology and Infertility
University of Wisconsin-Madison School of Medicine
Madison, Wisconsin

RESAD PASIC, M.D., PH.D.
Assistant Professor of Obstetrics, Gynecology &
Women's Health
University of Louisville School of Medicine
Louisville, Kentucky

TANJA PEJOVIC, M.D.
Department of Gynecologic Oncology
Yale University School of Medicine
New Haven, Connecticut

JOHN Y. PHELPS, M.D.

Assistant Clinical Professor of Obstetrics & Gynecology
Division of Reproductive Endocrinology & Infertility
University of Texas Medical Branch

JAY REDAN, M.D.
Attending Physician
St. Vincent's Hospital and Medical Center of New York
Community Medical Center
Scranton, Pennsylvania

HARRY REICH, M.D.
Attending Physician, Wyoming Valley Health Care
System
Wilkes-Barre, Pennsylvania
Community Medical Center, Scranton, Pennsylvania
St. Vincent's Hospital and Medical Center of New York
Lenox Hill, New York, NY

LISA M. ROBERTS, M.D.
Fellow
Advanced Gynecologic Endoscopic Surgery
Wilkes-Barre, Pennsylvania

ROBERT ROGERS, JR., M.D.
Attending Physician
The Reading Hospital & Medical Center
West Reading, Pennsylvania
Clinical Assistant Professor of Obstetrics and
Gynecology
University of Pennsylvania
Philadelphia, Pennsylvania

GERARD ROY, M.D.
Attending Physician
Clinical Instructor of Obstetrics and Gynecology
Center for Fertility and Women's Health
New Britain General Hospital
New Britain, Connecticut

BENJAMIN D. TANNER, M.D.
Surgical Resident
Department of Surgery
University of Louisville School of Medicine
Louisville, Kentucky

CLAIRE TEMPLEMAN, M.D.
Clinical Associate in Pediatric Gynecology & Endoscopy
Reproductive Specialty Center
Milwaukee, Wisconsin

PREFACE

Few fields in medicine have experienced as explosive an increase in knowledge and techniques as endoscopy, and, in particular, gynecologic laparoscopy. Just a few short years ago the formal teaching of laparoscopy in residency programs was virtually non-existent. Even today, the instruction in this modality of surgery is very inconsistent with the result that many gynecologists finish their training with only a minimal exposure to the multiple procedures that are not only acceptable now, but are rapidly becoming the standards of care. Indeed, many practicing gynecologists have had no additional training in current laparoscopic techniques.

As instructors in many postgraduate courses, both in the United States and in countries around the world, we have realized that, not only gynecologists in training, but also practicing physicians would benefit from an instructional book that utilized simplified illustrations to enhance their surgical knowledge. We believe that in combining the knowledge and experience of many of the leading laparoscopists with simplified, clear drawings to illustrate their written words, that we will add a significant contribution to the edification of both young and experienced gynecologic laparoscopists.

We wanted a book that was in the vein of a 'how to book' that would have material across the entire spectrum of operative laparoscopy. We thought that even the novice cook, to the most advanced gourmet chef, sometimes refer to a well written 'cook book'– hence the title.

With this in mind, we engaged the services of two graphic designers, Branko Modrakovic and Zvonimir Bebek to digitally create images that were submitted by the multiple authors, to a standard format used throughout the entire book. These digital drawings are clear and easily followed to supply the optimal information to the reader regarding the various procedures that are described. Mr. Modrakovic, a native of Sarajevo, is well qualified to produce these drawings as he was the leading designer for the Sarajevo Olympics in 1984 and presently works on various designing projects in Washington, D.C. where he currently resides (artico99@msn.com). Mr. Zvonimir Bebek, is also a graphic designer from Sarajevo, and he worked as the graphic designer and technical editor for the book.

FOREWORD

Another book on laparoscopy? Do we truly need it? What is new and advanced that warrants a new book?

The combination of Dr. Resad Pasic, a well experienced laparoscopist and Dr. Ronald Levine, the American father of operative gynecologic laparoscopy, and teacher extraordinaire ensures a worthwhile book. They have produced a truly unique text.

They have brought together many of the leading laparoscopists in the world with a truly capable graphic artist to present to the reader an easily understandable series of chapters on the relevant significant endoscopic state of the art that are easily digestible.

The artist has taken many of the photographs from the contributors and has a continuous understandable sequence of techniques. The authors have produced the text that goes with the art. This proximity of subject to pictures makes it both easy to follow and to comprehend.

'University of Louisville duo' Drs. Pasic and Levine have certainly fulfilled the requirements for a new book.

Every active gynecologic endoscopist must have this book in his library available for references.

Jordan M. Phillips, M.D.

Founder

Emeritus Chairman of the AAGL

ACKNOWLEDGEMENTS

When planning this book, we assembled some of the most outstanding laparoscopists to contribute their expertise. We are extremely grateful for the time and energy expended by all of our chapter contributors, for without their dedication, knowledge and skill, this book would not have come to fruition.

This book would not be possible without the financial support and encouragement from some of the leaders in producing new and innovative instrumentation in the field of operative laparoscopy. Our sincere thanks go to:

ACMI Circon Corporation
Cook OB/GYN
Ethicon Endosurgery
Gynecare, A Division of Ethicon, Inc.
Karl Storz Endoscopy
Lexion Medical

We also have to thank our University and the Department of Obstetrics, Gynecology and Women's Health for their support and encouragement, for without an environment that provides an exceptional milieu for teaching, writing and research, this book would not be possible.

Last, but certainly not least, we must thank Ms. Leta Weedman who was our editorial assistant and Ms. Laura Lukat-Coffman who was our secretarial support, for their enthusiasm, patience and ideas in order to bring this book to its completion.

CONTENTS

PATIENT PREPARATION

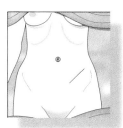

Ronald L. Levine, M.D.

Laparoscopic surgery, although minimally invasive, is and must always be considered as major surgery. Therefore, it is important to carefully prepare the patient for surgery, psychologically as well as physically. The surgeon must also be prepared by adequate training and practice in the techniques that will be necessary to complete the procedure in a safe and efficient manner. Patient preparation begins with the initial decision to perform laparoscopic surgery. Although it is tempting to convert most procedures to a minimally invasive route, the surgeon must consider if the particular pathology should be approached in this manner and is in the best interest of the patient. The surgeon must honestly evaluate his/her own ability and training.

PATIENT EVALUATION

The initial steps in the evaluation are considerations of the indications and contraindications of laparoscopic surgery. There are no hard and fast rules and even the term 'Absolute Contraindication' must be considered as a guideline, rather than a final decree.

ABSOLUTE CONTRAINDICATIONS

There are very few absolute contraindications as previously noted. With increased anesthesia ability, even some of these may not be considered absolute.

1. Severe cardiac disease: (Class IV) these patients will not tolerate the deep Trendelenburg positions necessary for most operative laparoscopy. These patients may also not tolerate an adequate pneumoperitoneum that may be necessary for satisfactory vision and instrument movement (See Chapter 4).

2. A hemodynamically unstable patient with the need to control bleeding probably should be approached by laparotomy. However, many surgeons believe that they can laparoscopically, rapidly enter an abdomen safely, even in the face of a ruptured ectopic.

3. Intestinal obstruction with distended bowel is best approached by laparotomy, however, with some of the techniques of open laparoscopy it may be possible to utilize laparoscopy even in these conditions.

RELATIVE CONTRAINDICATIONS

1. Multiple previous major surgeries must be considered as a possible contraindication, depending upon both the entry technique and the skill of the operating surgeon. Utilization of left upper quadrant insufflation techniques or open laparoscopy may afford safe entry even in the event of multiple previous surgeries (See Chapter 5).

2. Morbid obesity may be daunting to the inexperienced laparoscopist, however, with the use of operative techniques described in Chapter 5, patients as heavy as 350 to 400 lbs may be candidates for laparoscopy.

3. Pregnancy beyond five months gestation must be approached with a great deal of caution as the pelvis is almost completely filled with the enlarged uterus. Some surgeons

have used gasless laparoscopy in more advanced pregnancies. However, some studies have shown that the CO_2 gas of the pneumoperitoneum does not harm the fetus.

4. Severe chronically ill patients may present anesthesia problems, but still may be approached with caution with laparoscopic surgery. It is important not to compromise the respirations with the use of too large a pneumoperitoneum.

5. The patient should not be compromised by laparoscopic surgery if malignancy is a possibility. If a mass is known to be malignant and the surgeon does not have the skills necessary for complete removal without rupture of the mass, then laparoscopy is not the operation of choice. Some gynecologic oncologists have the skills not only to remove a mass, but also to perform lymph node dissections. In the hands of those surgeons, laparoscopy is then acceptable.

INFORMED CONSENT

Good informed consent actually provides much more than just a legal requirement. The patient who has a full understanding of the surgical procedure is much less anxious than one who is fearful because of lack of knowledge. We highly recommend the use of videotapes or movies to explain the surgery. Plastic models or pictures may also be used so that the patient has a full comprehension of her pathology and of the proposed operation. The patient should be given time to ask any questions that may be of concern to her. It is always best, if possible, to have a member of the family or a close friend present during these discussions. Because of nervousness and apprehension, patients frequently forget the information that has been explained to them and the support person will be able to 'fill in the blanks'.

The patient should be honestly informed of the alternative procedures. She should be told that general anesthesia is usually required and this will necessitate the use of a tube being placed into her throat. This may give her a slight sore throat. She should be seen preoperatively by the anesthesiologist who will explain the procedure and risks to her. She should be told of her position during surgery and of the method used to create a pneumoperitoneum. She should also understand about the placement of trocars and the possibility of injury to bowel or urinary tract. She must be apprised of the risks of injury up to and including death. It is advisable to design an informed consent sheet that is specific for laparoscopy. This should be written in layman's language. Never promise that the surgery will be accomplished by laparoscopy. It is best to say that if surgery can be performed by laparoscopy, then the patient will usually have certain advantages: quicker recovery time, less pain and less scarring. The patient should be informed at this time regarding her expected postoperative course. She should be advised of the degree of pain that may or may not be expected. She should be encouraged to call regarding any pain that is present for more than 48 hours postoperative.

PREOPERATIVE ROUTINE

The patient should be seen within 1–2 weeks of the surgery at which time a review of the history and a physical exam should be conducted that at least covers the following:

1. Weight;

2. Blood pressure and pulse;

3. Auscultation of the lungs and heart;

4. Palpation of the abdomen for organomegaly and hernias.

Many hospitals require laboratory tests within one or two weeks of the surgical procedure. Most laparoscopy requires a minimum of laboratory tests on the average patient: hemoglobin and hematocrit, and urine analysis is all that is usually necessary. A patient that has a history of bleeding problems should have a coagulation profile. The patient who has other medical problems may also need further evaluation by their general medical doctor who may require other laboratory testing such as a multi-panel test.

Patients who are over 40 years old often benefit from a chest X-ray if one has not been obtained for more than 2 years. It is important to review her medicines and to be sure to ask about the use of aspirin. Many patients do not consider aspirin a drug and neglect to inform the doctor of its chronic use. If the patient has been taking aspirin it should be discontinued for 3 or 4 days prior to surgery.

We recommend that all patients eat lightly for 24 hours and to be NPO at least 12 hours prior to surgery. It is very helpful for the patient to have a Fleet enema the night before most laparoscopic surgery and if extensive dissection is anticipated an oral preparation such as Golytely™ (Braintree Laboratories, Braintree, MA) is recommended the afternoon before. If the bowel is empty it permits better visualization during surgery, and in the event of a bowel injury it decreases the possibility of complications.

DAY OF SURGERY

Since most laparoscopic surgery is performed on an outpatient basis, it is recommended that surgery be started in the morning if possible. The patient is instructed to arrive at least 1.5 hours prior to surgery. This allows adequate time to have the patient seen by the anesthesiologist, and for all laboratory results to be checked. Before the patient receives any medication for anesthesia, it is helpful to review the anticipated surgery with her and to again allow opportunity for any questions.

When the surgery is completed and the patient is awake, she is given written instructions as to when to be seen for follow up and how to take care of herself. The instructions should cover when she should bath (anytime), begin to drive (after 24 hours), perform household duties, and when she may return to work. It should be carefully worded to explain expected postoperative discomfort and to differentiate it from severe pain that should require her to contact either the surgeon or a designated contact person with a telephone number that is answered 24 hours a day.

Patients should be discharged with all the appropriate instructions and medication or a prescription for pain relief.

SUGGESTED READING:

Pasic R, Levine R, Wolfe W. Laparoscopy in morbidly obese patients. J AAGL
1999;6:307-312

Laparoscopic Surgery. Editors: Ballantyne, Leahy & Modlin. W.B. Saunders Co. 1994

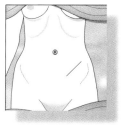

PELVIC ANATOMY SEEN THROUGH THE LAPAROSCOPE

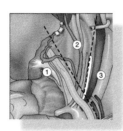

Robert M. Rogers, Jr., M.D.

For laparoscopists, female pelvic anatomy is that of surfaces and underlying abdominal and retroperitoneal structures. Surface landmarks on the anterior abdominal wall locate safe areas in which to pass laparoscopic trocars to establish ports through which laparoscopic instruments can be passed into the pelvic cavity to perform the planned surgery. Superficial peritoneal landmarks within the pelvis alert the operator to key anatomic structures in the retroperitoneal spaces. A sure knowledge of surgical and laparoscopic anatomy is a requisite for performing laparoscopic procedures that are safe for the patient and achieve the desired goal of the surgery. The three-dimensional field of pelvic anatomy as seen through the two-dimensional plane of the laparoscope is a difficult challenge to master. The diligent laparoscopic gynecologist must always study and then observe carefully in order to gain this sure, working knowledge. Just as technical

Chapter 2

8 | PELVIC ANATOMY SEEN THROUGH THE LAPAROSCOPE ·

skills can be consistently improved through frequent and proper practice, so can one's working knowledge of gynecologic surgical pelvic anatomy.

The following will be discussed: the anterior abdominal wall; the presacral space; the area of the pelvic brim; the sidewall of the pelvis; the area at the base of the broad ligament; the various spaces within the pelvis; and the anatomy of the retropubic space (space of Retzius).

THE ANTERIOR ABDOMINAL WALL

The various ports needed to perform laparoscopic surgery must traverse the anterior abdominal wall, thus knowledge of this anatomy is important to avoid a primary complication of injury to the arteries and veins contained therein. Landmarks of interest are the umbilicus, the anterior superior iliac spines, and pubic symphysis. In addition, landmarks on the interior abdominal wall will assist the laparoscopist in safely placing trocars in order to avoid injuring deeper vascular structures such as the aorta, common iliac vessels, and the external iliac vessels.

Depending upon the habitus and weight of the patient, the umbilicus may lie slightly above, at, or below the bifurcation of the aorta. In all patients, the left common iliac vein crosses the midline approximately 3-6 cm inferior to the

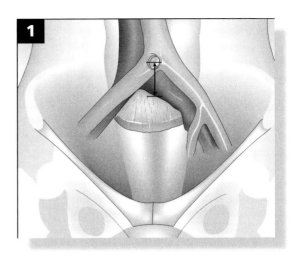

Left common iliac vein crosses the midline approximately 3-6 cm inferior to the level of the umbilicus.

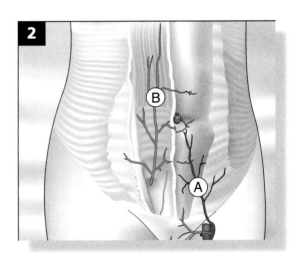

A SUPERFICIAL EPIGASTRIC ARTERY

B INFERIOR EPIGASTRIC ARTERY

bifurcation of the aorta and, therefore, inferior to the level of the umbilicus (Figure 1). In the thinner patient especially, the surface of the anterior abdominal wall is significantly closer to these great vessels.

In placement of lower lateral abdominal trocars, the surgeon must avoid lacerating the inferior and/or superficial epigastric arteries and veins and their branches. The inferior epigastric artery and vein travel on the posterior surface of the rectus abdominis muscle on its lateral third, particularly in the lower quadrants of the abdomen (Figure 2). The superficial epigastric arteries and veins travel within the subcutaneous tissue of the anterior abdominal wall in variable locations lateral to the umbilicus. The superficial vessels can be seen by transillumination of the anterior abdominal wall, while the inferior epigastric vessels cannot be seen due to shadowing from the rectus abdominis muscles. These latter vessels must be seen directly through the laparoscope.

Most injuries to these vessels within the abdominal wall itself can be avoided by placing the lateral ports approximately 8 cm from the midline and 8 cm superior to the pubic symphysis. This area also happens to be known as McBurney's point, which is anatomically located at one-third of the distance from the anterior superior iliac spine along the line from that spine to the umbilicus (Figure 3).

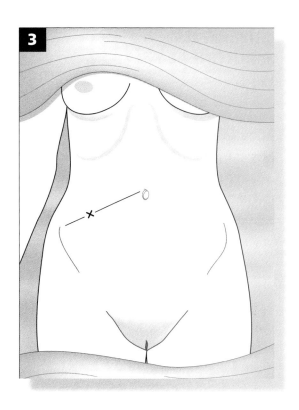

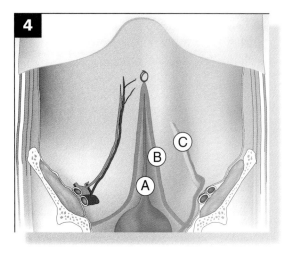

A MEDIAN UMBILICAL FOLD
 - obliterated urachus

B MEDIAL UMBILICAL FOLD
 - obliterated umbilical arteries

C LATERAL UMBILICAL FOLD
 - inferior epigastric vessels

SUPERFICIAL PERITONEAL ANATOMY

All laparoscopic procedures must begin with a systematic inspection of the surface areas of both the pelvis and upper abdomen. Such examinations should not only visually document the condition of the pelvic viscera and the surfaces within the pelvis, but also include inspection of the appendix, ascending colon, falciform ligament, liver and gall bladder, omentum, transverse colon, stomach, right and left hemidiaphragms, and the descending colon. The operating laparoscopist must visually search for evidence of adhesions, inflammation, endometriosis, cul-de-sac fluid, peritoneal studding, tumors or distortion of any pelvic or abdominal anatomy and structures. All laparoscopic procedures must begin with a systematic inspection of the surface areas of both the pelvis and upper abdomen.

Only through the laparoscope can the operating surgeon appreciate the structures on the undersurface of the anterior abdominal wall. Running from the dome of the bladder underneath a peritoneal fold is the obliterated urachus, known as the median umbilical fold. Just lateral to the median umbilical fold are the medial umbilical folds (Figure 4). These are formed by the peritoneum covering the obliterated umbilical arteries. Each obliterated umbilical artery, when fol-

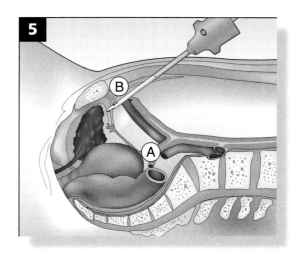

Pulling on the obliterated umbilical artery allows laparoscopic surgeon to locate the internal iliac artery and the origin of the uterine artery.

lowed back underneath the round ligament, into the broad ligament, will lead the surgeon to the superior vesicle artery and then back to the terminus of the internal iliac artery (Figure 5). Lateral to the medial umbilical fold is the lateral umbilical fold, which is formed by the tenting of the peritoneum over the inferior epigastric artery and vein. These latter vessels exit the external iliac artery and vein just medial to the exit of the round ligament from the body through the internal inguinal ring. Direct identification through the umbilical laparoscope will allow the laparoscopist to place lateral trocars through the anterior abdominal wall well lateral of these epigastric vessels.

Anterior traction on the uterus will place the uterosacral ligaments on tension and lead the surgeon to visualization of the ureters in the pelvic sidewall. The dome of the bladder is a semilunar outline overlying the pubic symphysis (Figure 6).

PRESACRAL SPACE

The presacral space is important to laparoscopic surgeons performing 'presacral neurectomies' for the hopeful alleviation of central and chronic pelvic pain. At this time, presacral neurectomy is considered a controversial procedure. The space is bounded anteriorly by the parietal peritoneum. Posteriorly it is bounded by the periosteum and anterior longitudinal ligament over the lower two lumbar vertebrae and the promontory of the sacrum. The middle sacral artery and a plexus of veins are attached to the posterior boundary of the space. The superior extension of the visceral endopelvic fascia in this area embeds fatty areolar tissue, presacral lymph nodes and tissue, and visceral nerves (Figure 7). There is not one presacral nerve but a multitude of finer visceral nerves that have great variability in their course and distribution within this space. These 'presacral nerves' are simply the multiple afferent and efferent visceral nerve fibers of the superior hypogastric plexus. The right

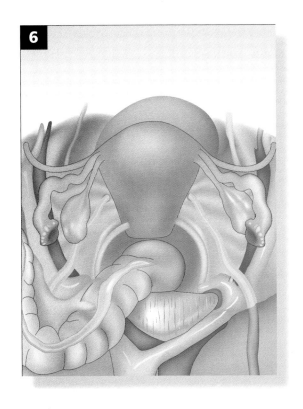

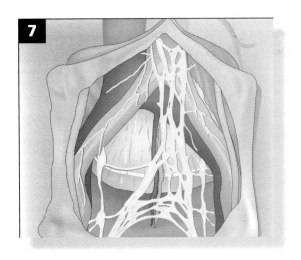

lateral boundary of this space is the right common iliac artery and ureter. The left lateral border is the left common iliac vein and left ureter, as well as the inferior mesenteric artery and vein traversing the mesentery of the sigmoid colon. Great care must be taken by even experienced laparoscopic surgeons in order to dissect safely within this space. Great damage to the ureter and the possibility of massive hemorrhage exist here.

PELVIC BRIM

The pelvic brim region at the location over the sacroiliac joint is the important location for the entry of multiple structures into the pelvic cavity. These structures course over the pelvic brim in a vertical manner and then will rotate in a 90° fashion to form the structures of the pelvic sidewall. From the peritoneal surface working posteriorly to the sacroiliac joint, the following structures are found coursing one over the other: the peritoneum; the ovarian vessels in the infundibulopelvic ligament; the ureter traversing over the bifurcation of the common iliac artery; the common iliac vein; the medial edge of the psoas muscle and, in the same plane, the obturator nerve overlying the parietal fascia just over the capsule of the sacroiliac joint (Figure 8). In the same plane as the obturator nerve, but more medial, the lumbosacral trunk is found coursing from the lumbar plexus of nerves to the sacral plexus of nerves that are found overlying the piriformis muscle in the pelvis. When ligating the

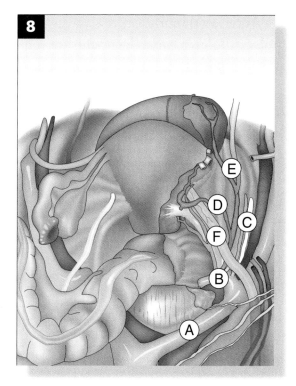

A COMMON ILIAC ARTERY
B INTERNAL ILIAC ARTERY
C OBTURATOR VESSELS AND NERVE
D UTERINE ARTERY
E SUPERIOR VESICAL ARTERY
  Obliterated umbilical artery
F URETER

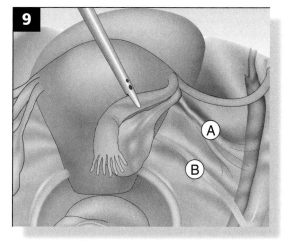

A INFUNDIBULOPELVIC LIGAMENT
B URETER

ovarian vessels in the infundibulopelvic ligament, the surgeon must lift the infundibulopelvic ligament well away from the course of the ureter in order to avoid injuring it (Figure 9).

THE PELVIC SIDEWALL REGION

Based on avascular planes, the pelvic sidewall consists of three surgical layers. Medially, the first layer is the parietal peritoneum with the attached ureter in its own visceral fascial capsule. When this peritoneum is incised and retracted medially the ureter comes with it (Figure 10).

The second surgical layer consists of the internal iliac artery and vein and their visceral anterior branches, all enveloped within the surrounding visceral fascia containing the lymph

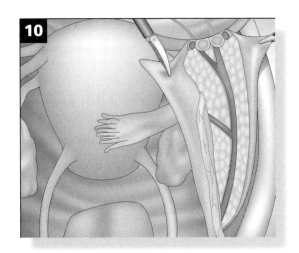

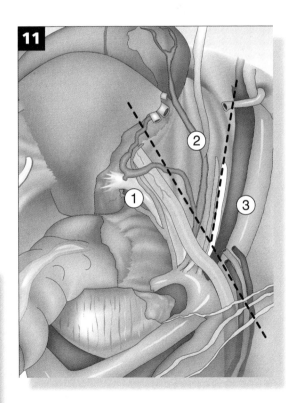

FIRST LAYER OF PELVIC SIDEWALL

Parietal peritoneum and ureter

SECOND LAYER OF PELVIC SIDEWALL

Internal iliac vessels and their tributaries: uterine, superior vesical, inferior vesical, vaginal, internal pudendal, and inferior gluteal artery and vein

THIRD LAYER OF PELVIC SIDEWALL

Obturator internus muscle

Obturator nerve, artery and vein

External iliac artery and vein

1 FIRST LAYER OF PELVIC SIDEWALL
2 SECOND LAYER OF PELVIC SIDEWALL
3 THIRD LAYER OF PELVIC SIDEWALL

tissue and the visceral hypogastric nerves.

The third surgical layer consists of the parietal fascia over the obturator internus muscle with the obturator artery, nerve and vein allowed to remain on this muscle. However, during obturator space dissections, the nerve can be retracted safely medially. In addition, the third layer consists of the external iliac artery and vein on the medial aspect of the psoas muscle at the bony arcuate line of the ileum or linea terminalis (Figure 11).

Blunt dissection by the laparoscopic surgeon easily separates the first surgical layer from the second surgical layer, and the second surgical layer from the third surgical layer. The second surgical layer of the pelvic sidewall can also easily be found by tracing the course of the obliterated umbilical artery back to the superior vesical artery within the broad ligament, back to the terminal root of the internal iliac artery. The medial offshoot at this junction is the uterine artery.

THE BASE OF THE BROAD LIGAMENT

The base of the broad ligament is that anatomic region where the cardinal ligament inserts into the pericervical ring of endopelvic fascia for upper vaginal

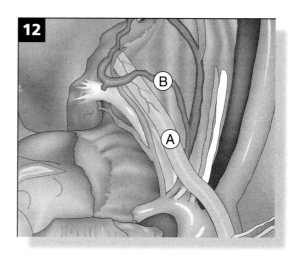

A URETER
B UTERINE ARTERY

support. It contains the ureter traveling underneath the uterine artery in an oblique fashion, approximately 1.5 cm lateral to the side of the cervix. This region is an important anatomic area where the ureter makes a 'knee-bend' in order to turn anteriorly and medially across the anterolateral fornix of the vagina to enter the bladder. It is approximately 2 cm medial and anterior from the ischial spine. It is also called the parametrium. The area located lateral to the vagina is called the upper paracolpium (Figure 12).

Posterior to the base of the broad ligament is the pararectal space, which is easily developed by dissecting the ureter medially toward the rectum, away from the internal iliac artery and vein, posterior to the origin of the uterine artery.

The anterior border of this space is the base of the broad ligament. The lateral and medial borders are the internal iliac artery and the ureter, respectively. This space also contains the uterosacral ligament laterally as it passes posteriorly toward the sacrum (Figure 13).

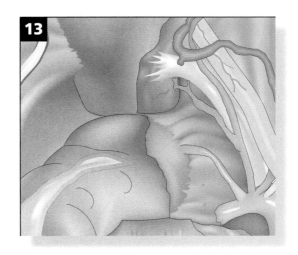

The paravesical space is found anterior to the base of the broad ligament and is bounded medially by the bladder and laterally by the obturator internus muscle fascia. The paravesical space simply leads into the lateral space of Retzius. The space within the paravesical space lateral to the obturator nerve is known as the obturator space (Figure 14). From this region above the level of the obturator nerve, the operating laparoscopic gynecologist will harvest the obturator lymph nodes.

SPACE OF RETZIUS

The space of Retzius or retropubic space is a potential space containing much areolar tissue between the back of the pubic bone and the anterior portion of the bladder. Surrounding the bladder is a visceral bladder capsule that contains the rich network of perivesical venous sinuses that are very fragile and bleed easily when surgery is performed in this space. Centrally over the urethra is the deep dorsal vein of the clitoris that feeds into these venous channels. The lateral border of the space of Retzius is the

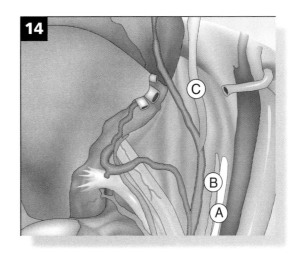

A Obturator nerve
B Obturator artery and vein
C Obliterated umbilical artery

obturator internus muscle and its parietal fascia, with the obturator nerve, artery, and vein just beneath the bony ridge of the ilium on its anterior border. The posterior border (toward the sacrum) is a visceral fascial sheath surrounding the internal iliac artery and vein and their anterior branches. Remember in the standing female patient, the internal iliac artery starts at the bifurcation at the pelvic brim over the sacroiliac joint and travels in a vertical direction along the anterior border of the greater sciatic foramen down towards the ischial spine (Figure 15).

The floor of the space of Retzius is simply the pubocervical fascia inserting into the lateral fascial white line. The fascial white line (arcus tendineus fasciae pelvis) is a thickening of the parietal fascia overlying the levator ani muscles and travels from the pubic arch straight back to the ischial spine. Just anterior to this fascial white line is a more variable and thinner thickening of the parietal fascia overlying the obturator internus muscle called the muscle white line (arcus tendineus levator ani). The muscle white line is the origin of the levator ani muscles from the lateral and posterior aspects of the pubic bone in a curvilinear fashion back toward the ischial spine that meets with the fascial white line (Figure 16).

When working in this space and performing a paravaginal defect repair or a Burch retropubic colposcopic suspension through the laparoscope, the surgeon must clear the areolar tissue off the white glistening pubocervical fascia before placing sutures directly into its thickness, which is attached to the underlying vaginal epithelium.

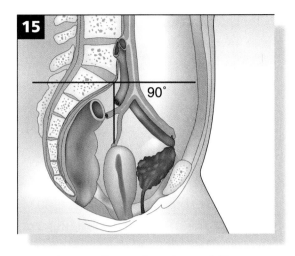

In the standing patient, internal iliac artery travels in a vertical direction over the sacroiliac joint toward the ischial spine.

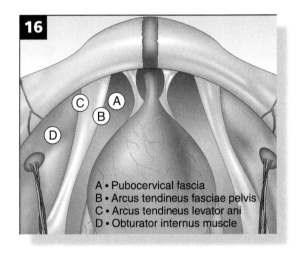

A • Pubocervical fascia
B • Arcus tendineus fasciae pelvis
C • Arcus tendineus levator ani
D • Obturator internus muscle

THE VESICOVAGINAL SPACE

The vesicovaginal space is found between the anterior surface of the vagina and the posterior aspect of the bladder down to the trigone. This space is bordered laterally by the bladder 'pillars', that allow for the passage of the inferior vesical arteries, veins, and ureter to the bladder (Figure 17). This space is important to the surgeon performing a hysterectomy since he/she must incise through the vesicouterine peritoneal fold. This potential space is created by dissecting between the visceral fascial coat around the bladder and the pubo-cervical fascia, found on top of the cervix and anterior vaginal wall, down to the level of the trigone. Care must be taken not to dissect too vigorously and laterally to avoid injury to the ureter and vasculature found within the bladder pillars.

RECTOVAGINAL SPACE

The rectovaginal space is bounded superiorly by the cul-de-sac peritoneum and the uterosacral ligaments, laterally by the iliococcygeus muscles of the levator ani, posteriorly by the visceral fascial capsule surrounding the anterior surface of the rectum, and anteriorly by the visceral fascial capsule surrounding the posterior aspect of the vagina. The rectovaginal septum is found just behind the vagina, somewhat adherent to it and yet dissectable away from it (Figure 18). The rectovaginal fascia is more and more commonly being used for repair of rectoceles.

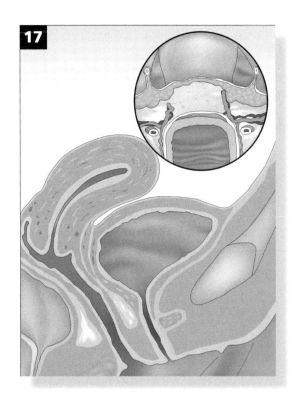

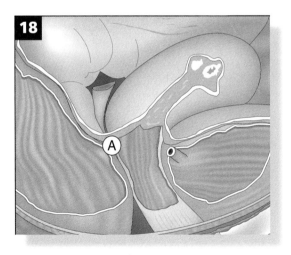

A Rectovaginal septum

Suggested Reading:

Atlas of Human Anatomy. Editor: Frank H. Netter. Publisher Ciba-Geigy, 1989

Hurd WW, Bude RO, DeLancey JOL, Newman JS. The location of abdominal wall blood vessels in relationship to abdominal landmarks apparent at laparoscopy. Am J Obstet Gynecol 1994;171:642-6

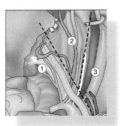

INSTRUMENTATION AND EQUIPMENT

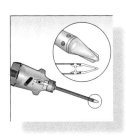

Ronald L. Levine, M.D.

Many modern operating rooms have been designed to accommodate operative endoscopies; however, there are many variations depending upon the individual requirements of the operating surgeon. Herein we describe the general requirements of both the setup and the basic equipment that is necessary to perform safe and efficient gynecologic endoscopic surgery.

GENERAL ROOM SETUP

The setup should be designed to optimize efficiency using the team concept. The team usually consists of the surgeon, a first assistant, a scrub nurse and a circulating nurse. The most recent addition to the traditional team is the biomedical technician. He/she may not be required for the entire case, but it is helpful if they are in attendance at the start, as well as intermittently, and at the end of the case. The technician should be trained and skilled in the use of all electronic equipment, the video camera, laser equipment, and other electronic supplies and be able to possess on-site trouble shooting skills. Since operative endoscopy is completely dependent on high tech equipment, all should be thoroughly checked prior to the start of each case.

The circulating nurse is the main coordinator of the team and he/she will be responsible during the procedure for running the video, checking suction and irrigation equipment, and generally providing support and maintaining the steady rhythm of the operating team.

ALWAYS CHECK THE INSTRUMENTS AND THE EQUIPMENT BEFORE EACH PROCEDURE

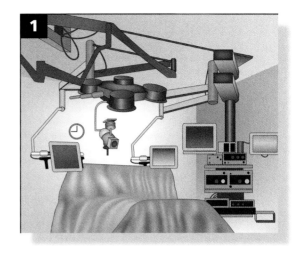

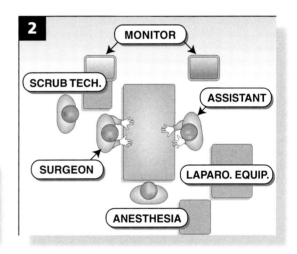

The operating room setup requires an operating table that can be placed in deep Trendelenburg position. It must have rails that will accommodate the stirrups, shoulder braces and other possible equipment. Most gynecologic surgeons perform laparoscopy from the left side; however, this is an individual idiosyncrasy. In the ideal OR, to decrease the floor clutter and to allow more room for lasers, fluid monitors and other large equipment, monitors and most electronic equipment may be suspended from the ceiling along with all gas lines and electric outlets (Figure 1). Many of the commands in the modern futuristic operating rooms can be voice operated and controlled by the surgeon's voice with the help of the Hermes™ system (Striker Endoscopy, Santa Clara, CA). Hermes provides digital control over various functions including insufflation pressure, light intensity, zoom on the camera, and power settings on the generator, video imaging and even the telephone in the operating room.

The operating room setup is seen in Figure 2. Ideally, two monitors would be available with one to each side of the legs; however, if only one monitor is available it should be between the legs.

The back table should hold all of the hand-held instruments that may be needed during the case. They should be grouped in an orderly manner just as the back table is arranged during open surgery. A Mayo stand can either be placed between the legs or adjacent to a leg with the equipment that will be frequently exchanged during the case, i.e. suction irrigator, scissors and several different types of graspers.

VIDEO IMAGING

Modern video cameras are based on the solid-state microprocessor chip. There are one- or three-chip cameras with a head that attaches to the eyepiece of the laparoscope and connects to the camera controller by a cable (Figure 3). The signal is then fed into the monitor to display the image.

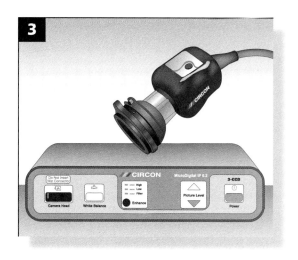

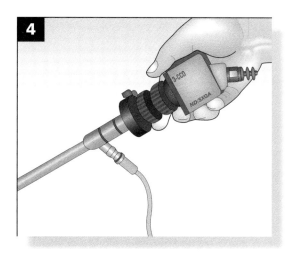

As technology advances, so does the quality of the video display. It is important to realize that the image as seen on the monitor is related to the resolution of the camera and the monitor. If one has a resolution capability of 750 lines and the other 500 lines, you will only be able to visualize at the lower level. High definition endoscopic cameras are also available (Figure 4). The HDTV camera and monitor have more than twice the number of scanning lines than the frame of the conventional videos, making the images more clear. Those high-definition systems may prove quite useful in diagnosing endometriosis and early metastatic spread.

After the patient is positioned on the table, anesthetized, prepped and draped she is then catheterized. The multiple instruments that are necessary for safe and efficient endoscopic surgery are now described.

UTERINE MOBILIZATION

Most laparoscopic surgery is expedited by the use of a good uterine manipulator. This device should be able to antevert the uterus, as well as position the uterus as needed depending upon the procedure. If a standard uterine manipulator is not available, one may insert a uterine sound high into the fundus and attach it with tape or rubber bands to a tenaculum previously placed on the anterior lip of the cervix. There are many types of commercial manipulators that are reusable such as the Semm vacuum cannula, Hulka Uterine Elevator™ (Richard Wolf Medical Instruments, Vernon Hills, VT), Pelosi (Apple Medical Corp., Bolton, MA) and the Valtchev Uterine Mobilizer™ (Konkin Surgical Instru-

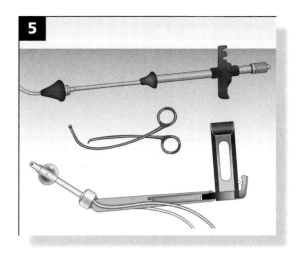

ments, Toronto, Canada). Partially disposable manipulators, such as the Rumi™ (Cooper Surgical, Shelton, CT), have disposable tips that are available in different lengths from 6 cm to 10 cm (Figure 5). Completely disposable manipulators, such as the Vcare™ (ConMed Corp, Utica, NY) can also be adjusted for the length of the tip. Ideally the manipulator should also have the ability to chromopertubate. The tip of the manipulator is usually held in place by a small balloon that may be inflated with a few milliliters of sterile water.

INSUFFLATION INSTRUMENTS

The various techniques of insufflation are addressed in Chapter 5. Most techniques utilize the Veress needle. These spring-loaded needles are available as reusable instruments, partially disposable or completely disposable. It is a delicate instrument that has a sharp outer sleeve and contains an inner sleeve with a dull tip on a spring mechanism that retracts back when a resistance is encountered. When the resistance is gone, the dull tip springs forward to protect intraabdominal structures from the sharp tip (Figure 6). If the reusable needle is sharpened frequently it is as functional and certainly less expensive than the disposable type. The disposable Veress needle has an advantage in always being sharp which enhances its use. The spring mechanism should be checked prior to insertion, even with the disposable instruments.

INSUFFLATORS

There are multiple insufflators on the market (Figure 7). The ideal insufflator

THE BASIC INFORMATION THAT SHOULD BE SUPPLIED BY THE READOUT OF THE INSUFFLATOR IS:

1. INSUFFLATION PRESSURE

2. INTRAABDOMINAL PRESSURE

3. INSUFFLATION VOLUME PER MINUTE

4. (The least important) TOTAL AMOUNT OF GAS USED

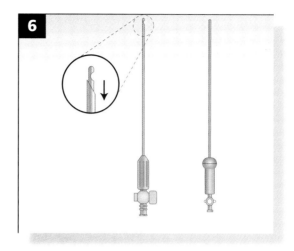

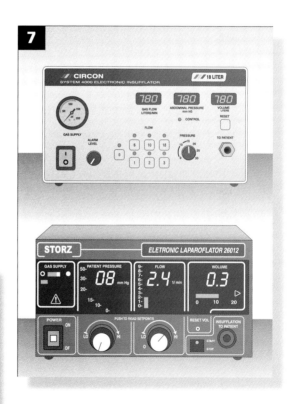

can deliver rapid, accurate flow rates up to 15 L/min. However, it is obvious that the gas flow supplied at the outlet of the machine is not what is delivered intraabdominally owing to the diameter and the distance of the connecting tube. In actual measurements, the true amount delivered at the end of the tube may be only 60-70% of the capable flow rate of the insufflator. Some insufflators have heating capability to warm the gas, thus decreasing the intraabdominal hypothermic effect of cold CO_2 gas and decreasing fogging of the distal lens of the laparoscope. The Insuflow® device (Lexion Medical, St. Paul, MN) is relatively inexpensive equipment that can be attached to the machine that will both hydrate and warm the gas (Figure 8).

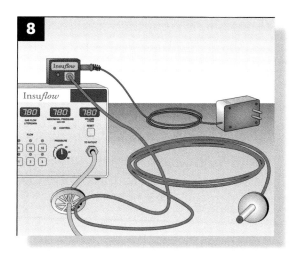

ABDOMINAL ACCESS INSTRUMENTS

An entire chapter could be used to address this highly debated issue. There are several categories in which all of the instruments may be grouped.

1. Disposable or reusable;

2. Open or closed technique;

3. Mini entry techniques or direct view.

The argument of disposable versus reusable equipment may be focused on trocars and sheaths (Figure 9). The traditional disposable trocars have become popular mainly because the tips are always sharp, thus requiring a much smaller force to achieve penetra-

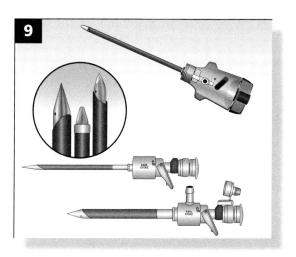

tion than the reusable instruments. The shield that springs out over the tip after entry into the abdominal cavity plays little, if any, role in safety. There has been a continuing area of contention regarding the style of the trocar tip in reusable instruments. Some surgeons favor the pyramidal tip while others extol the virtues of the conical tip. Most trocars today use the pyramidal style tip. There are advantages to each, but sharpness is of most importance in the closed technique.

Trocars are available in many sizes, from 3 mm up to 12 mm and even larger. Most standard laparoscopy is performed using a 10- or 12-mm umbilical port for the laparoscope and 5-mm lower abdominal ports for the secondary instruments. There are even smaller trocars that may be used for 3-mm instruments.

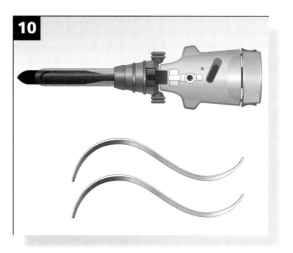

Closed technique instruments have sharp tips, which may have a potential to injure bowel or large blood vessels. One alternative is to use the open technique invented by Dr. Harrith Hasson (See Chapter 5). This instrument requires opening into the peritoneal cavity prior to the insertion of the sheath and does not develop a pneumoperitoneum prior to its use (Figure 10). The use of vision directed trocars such as the Endopath™ bladeless trocar by Ethicon Endosurgery (Cincinnati, OH) (Figure 11) produces a hybrid that combines a bit of each technique. Expandable sheath technology InnerDyne Medical™ (Sunnyvale, CA) permits the passage of a Veress needle type instrument that has a sheath, which can then be expanded allowing passage of larger sheaths without potential damage, particularly to major vessels (Figure 12).

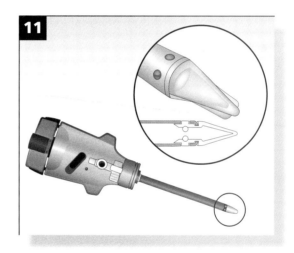

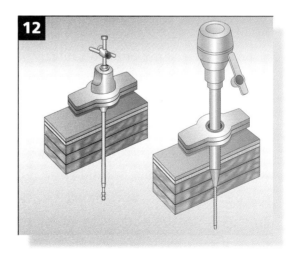

LIGHT SOURCE

An adequate light source is absolutely necessary for performing laparoscopic surgery, as it is important to have good illumination in order to obtain image clarity and true colors. A 250 W halogen or xenon light source provides excellent light intensity. The temperature of 6000°K obtained from xenon provides true white light that enhances visualization to permit recognition of pathological changes (Figure 13). A fluid light cable that connects the light source with the laparoscope may provide optimal light transmission. The fiberoptic light cord should be handled with care, since the fibers within the housing may be broken if the cord is kinked or dropped. If there is a decreased light transmission, one end of the light cord can be held up to a room light and by looking at the other end it is possible to assess whether a significant number of fibers are broken. Due to the concentrated light intensity at the end of the light cable, a significant amount of heat is produced. Therefore, the end of the light cable should not be placed on drapes nor allowed skin contact with the patient in order to prevent possible burns.

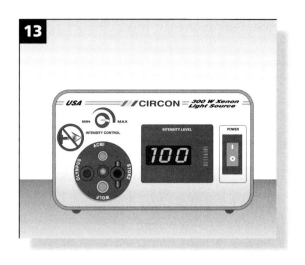

OPTICS (LAPAROSCOPES)

It is important to obtain as panoramic view as possible, allowing the operator to coordinate proper placement of the instruments. Often the surgeons do not realize the magnification afforded by laparoscopy. Indeed, the magnification is one of the many advantages of this technique. The lenses in the scope enable magnification up to 6 times depending upon the distance between the end of the scope and the object. At 3 cm from the tip to the object, the magnification is 4× and at 4 cm it is 6×.

Laparoscopes may be considered by several categories: function, size and angle of view.

Function: Although most laparoscopic procedures begin with a 10-mm scope, many surgeons prefer operating laparoscopes to be used in the entire case. Scopes may be either diagnostic only or they may be operative. Most operative scopes have a channel that will allow at least the passage of a 5-mm diameter, 44-cm long instrument. Some scopes have a channel that will allow the passage of 8-mm diameter instruments that can be used in sterilization procedures. These are large diameter scopes that require a 12-mm trocar sheath. The larger diameter scopes may also be utilized for either connecting to a CO_2 laser or permitting the passage of a fiber for a YAG laser.

Size: The optimal diagnostic scope is a 10-mm diameter instrument. However, as fiber optics have improved through the years, the ability to decrease the size of scopes while enhancing the objective view has increased. Frequently a 5-mm scope is utilized for diagnostics as well as directing the use of 3-mm instruments (Figure 14).

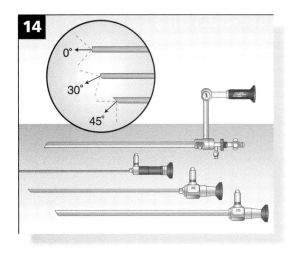

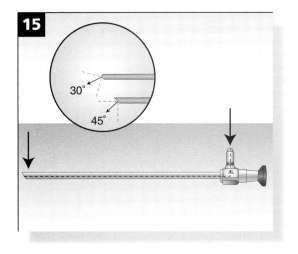

Angle of view: When using a 10-mm scope as the viewing instrument during operative procedures, it is optimal to have a zero degree vision (i.e. looking straight ahead). If a scope is used just for diagnostics, it may be advantageous to have an increased angle of vision to observe a more panoramic view of the pelvis. Operative laparoscopes may have a 6°

viewing angle. Other scopes may have viewing angles up to 50°. It is important to mention that on every scope there is the engraved number by the eyepiece that specifies the angle of view. If the scope has an angled view, the direction of vision is always pointing away from the light source attachment (Figure 15).

ELECTROSURGICAL GENERATORS

Electrosurgical generators are designed to produce a high frequency electric energy in either a monopolar or bipolar format (see Chapter 6). Generators have the ability to deliver the energy in either a coagulation (modulated/interrupted) or cutting (non-modulated/continuous) waveform. Many generators have some style of ammeter to permit either visually, or by sound, the monitoring of the current flow. This is important in informing the surgeon of the complete desiccation of the tissue, either when coagulating a blood vessel or when sealing a Fallopian tube during sterilization (see Chapters 6 and 8). Some instruments have built-in circuitry to detect insulation failure or capacitative coupling. The generator may be connected to various instruments including scissors, graspers, needles and bipolar forceps (Figure 16).

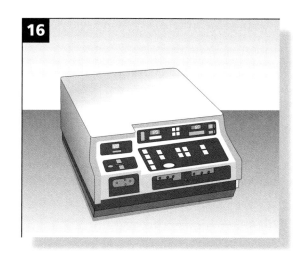

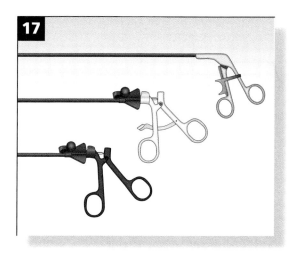

OPERATIVE INSTRUMENTS

The instruments used during operative laparoscopy may be divided into the following groups.

1. Graspers – traumatic or atraumatic;

2. Cutting instruments;

3. Coagulating instruments (bleeding control) (staplers, bipolar graspers, harmonic energy instruments, ligation and suturing equipment);

4. Morcellating and retrieval instruments;

5. Irrigation suction instruments;

6. Lasers;

7. Specialty instruments (sterilization and mini–instruments).

A complete book would be needed
to describe all of the various instruments produced by a myriad number
of companies. Therefore, only examples of instruments will be described.

1. All graspers, whether atraumatic or
traumatic may be found in a variety of
diameters and lengths. They usually
range from 3 mm to 11 mm, however
the most commonly used graspers are
5 mm in diameter and 33 cm long.
Longer instruments (44 cm) are
designed to pass down the channel of
operating scopes. Handles are generally
of two basic types – those that will lock
(box lock type) and handles that are
not locked. The non-locking handles
are best used on dissecting type instruments (Figure 17). The tips vary in
design depending upon their use.
Some have very rounded tips that are
extremely dull and the inside of the
jaws are also blunt with rounded
ridges. This style of instrument is best
used for mobilization of bowel and the
Fallopian tubes (Figure 18) and may be
referred to as atraumatic. The best way
to determine whether an instrument is
atraumatic or not is to grasp the web
space between the thumb and forefinger. If absolutely pain free it may be
considered atraumatic (Figure 19). The
more pronounced and sharp the ridges

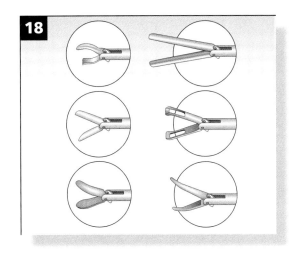

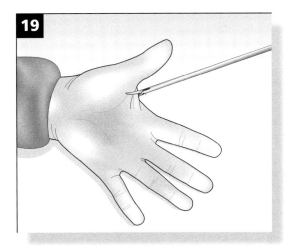

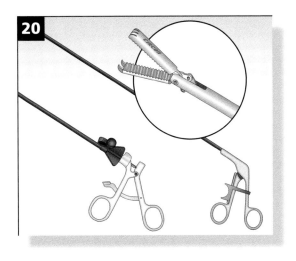

in the jaw, the more traumatic the instrument. This type of instrument should only be used on tissue that will be removed or on tissue not expected to bleed (Figure 20). It does afford a stronger hold on tissue than the atraumatic type.

2. Cutting instruments are usually scissors, however, lasers, harmonic energy and electrical energy may also be used to incise tissue. Scissors may be found in a multitude of forms. Straight or curved or hooked and may be reusable or disposable. Some are designed with semi-disposable tips that may be replaced after a number of uses or if they become dull (Figure 21). No matter which scissor is used, the most important aspect is having a sharp instrument. Monopolar electrical energy may be used with the scissor for simultaneous coagulation and tissue cutting. Harmonic energy may be used either in the form of a cutting instrument alone, or in the form of a combination grasper/cutting instrument that not only cuts the tissue, but also coagulates (Figure 22). It also can be used as a blunt, ball-shaped instrument to control bleeding or for ablating endometrial lesions.

3. The control of bleeding is the most crucial element in all surgery. For hemostasis, the most commonly used instrument in laparoscopy is the

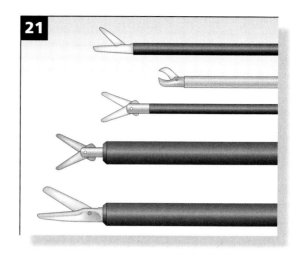

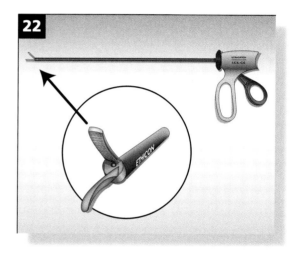

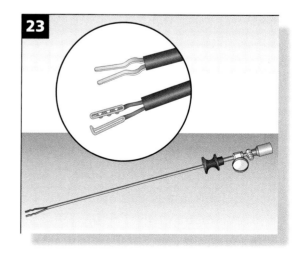

bipolar forceps. Dr. Richard Kleppinger invented this type of forceps and most surgeons refer to this type of instrument as Kleppingers, even though they may not be in the classic form. The use of bipolar, high frequency electrical energy is a safe, inexpensive and reliable type of laparoscopic control of bleeding (Figure 23). As stated previously, the harmonic energy instruments may also be used to perform this task, however, larger vessels are better controlled either with bipolar electrical energy or with ligation, clips or staples. The use of linear stapler/cutter instruments became popular in the early 90s. They may now be found in a variety of styles and are extremely useful for a rapid cutting of tissue while simultaneously firing double rows of titanium staples for the control of bleeding (Figure 24).

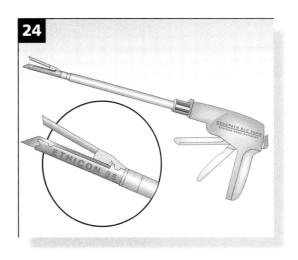

The traditional surgical use of suturing and ligation requires some special materials and equipment. Simple ligation is possible through the use of loop ligation as introduced by Dr. Kurt Semm. This requires an Endoloop™ (Ethicon Endosurgery Inc., Cincinnati, OH) that is a preformed, looped slipknot available in a variety of suture materials and suture sizes (Figure 25). This loop can be placed around tissue pedicles and blood vessels. The loop is introduced

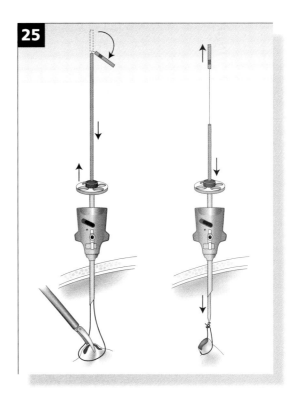

into the abdomen by using a 3-mm suture applicator. Endoscopic suturing can be accomplished using a variety of needles and suture materials. The techniques will not be addressed in this chapter, however, some of the instruments that may be required are needle drivers and knot pushers. There are many different types and sizes of needle drivers. Basically, differences are either in the type of handle or tips. A large number of laparoscopic surgeons prefer the bayonet type of handles (Figure 26), however, the classic Cook needle driver Talon™ (Cook, OB/GYN Spencer, IN) remains a favorite of many. The Cook instrument will self-right a curved needle, but has a spring loaded handle (Figure 27). It is also available in versions that will hold the needle at a 45° angle.

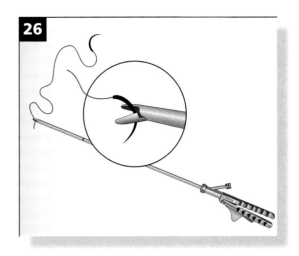

4. An effective method for removing tissue from the body has been called the 'Holy Grail' of laparoscopy. Presently the two methods of tissue removal are either through morcellation or by use of a sack or some combination of both. The ideal method has to be safe, efficient and prevent spillage within the abdomen. A retrieval system plays a vital role in laparoscopic surgery. To supply this system it may be necessary to use some type of extraction sack. The specimen bag must be used in the removal of ovarian tissue that has a possibility of neoplasia in order to obviate the dissemination of possible malignant cells and prevent spillage during removal of a benign teratoma. It is necessary that a removal bag be very strong

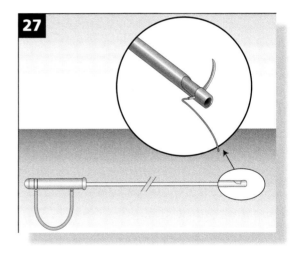

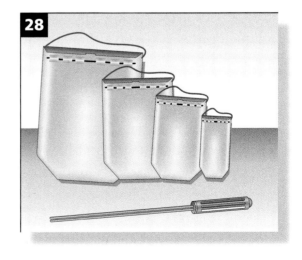

so that it may resist breakage in the face of a large force in pulling it through a small opening. The sack also should be easily deployed within the abdomen and be capable of holding a mass larger than 7 cm such as a Cook sac (Figure 28). Newer bags are equipped with a self-opening and closing mechanism that facilitates easy removal of tissue (Figure 29).

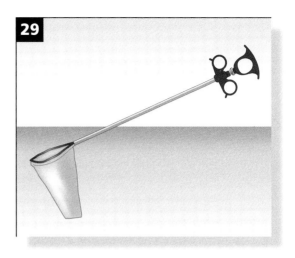

There are several motorized morcellators that answer many of the problems of morcellation (Figures 30 and 31). The existing morcellators require a large trocar sheath (12-15 mm). Steiner™ Electromechanical Morcellator (Karl Storz Endoscopy, Tuttlingen, Germany) (Figure 30) can be applied through a 12-mm trocar sheath. The Gynecare Morcellator Diva™ (Gynecare, Johnson and Johnson Corp. Somerville, NJ) (Figure 31) uses disposable handle and blades and does not require a trocar sheath.

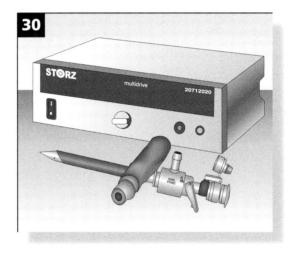

5. Irrigation and aspiration are necessary for operative laparoscopy because without a clear surgical field the surgeon is blind. Irrigation is used to clear away debris, blood, blood clots and char that may be produced by electrosurgery or laser treatment. The ideal irrigator must produce enough hydraulic pressure to disrupt clots and assist in aqua dissection. The hand-controlled valve should be easy to operate

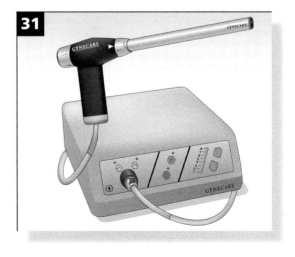

both the suction and irrigation. It is important that it be usable with a large enough channel so that large clots may be removed rapidly without clogging the instrument. If the probe tip is to be used for suctioning near bowel, small holes near the tip are useful to avoid pulling bowel into the probe. There are several different types of instruments with varied pumps to deliver the fluid for irrigation (Figure 32). The disposable suction/irrigator made by Striker Endoscopy is gaining in popularity. It uses a battery operated disposable pump that is attached to the irrigation fluid bag, and provides excellent fluid pressure (Figure 33).

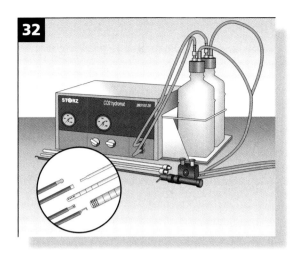

6. The major types of lasers that are currently used for gynecologic surgery are the CO_2, argon, KTP-532 and the Nd–YAG (neodymium: yttrium, aluminum garnet). Each of these has various indications that are not within the purview of this chapter. The basic instruments that supply these different energy sources are fairly large, expensive and require specific training in their use (Figure 34).

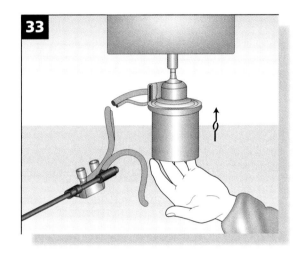

7. As the interest in laparoscopy performed under local anesthesia for pain mapping has expanded, the demand for small instruments has subsequently increased. Pediatric laparoscopy has also necessitated a need for smaller instruments. Small trocar sheaths for 3-mm

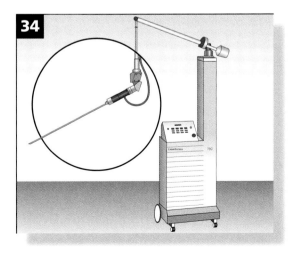

instruments may be used, but there are even smaller instruments such as the mini-retractor set and grasping instruments (Figure 35).

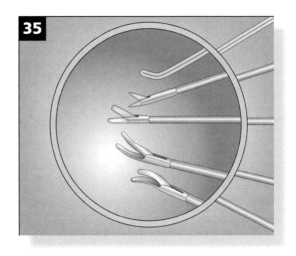

Instruments that are unique to sterilization may be used either through secondary trocars or through the 8-mm channel of an operating laparoscope. The three most commonly used instruments are the Hulka Clip Applicator™ (Richard Wolf Medical Instruments, Vernon Hills, IL), the Filshie Clip Applicator™ (Avalon Medical Corp., Williston, VT) or the Fallope Ring Applicator™ (Circon Corp., Santa Barbara, CA). Their use will be described in Chapter 8 (Figure 36).

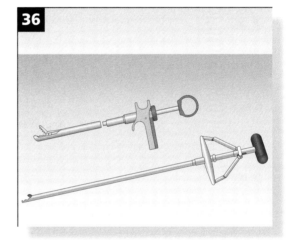

It is impossible to describe every instrument available for use in laparoscopy. Literally new instruments are being invented every day, but it is important for the surgeon to be aware of the basic instruments that are currently available and be familiar not only with their function, but how to assemble and trouble shoot their use.

SUGGESTED READING:

Operative Laparoscopy: The Masters' Techniques in Gynecologic Surgery. Editor: Richard Soderstrom. 2nd Edition. Publisher: Lippincott-Raven, 1998

Textbook of Laparoscopy. Hulka and Reich. 2nd Edition. Publisher: W.B. Saunders, 1994

Manual of Gynecological Laparoscopic Surgery. Luca Mencaglia and Arnaud Wattiez. Publisher Endo-Press – Tuttlinger, Germany, 2000

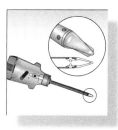

ANESTHESIA IN LAPAROSCOPY

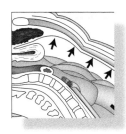

Laura Clark, M.D.

Many surgical procedures dictate the management of anesthesia. For example, in an abdominal aortic aneurysm repair, clamping of the aorta creates a significant impact on the inherent physiology of the individual patient in addition to their particular medical factors. The procedure of laparoscopy also creates its own subset of factors unique to the procedure itself. The impact of laparoscopy on the human body went relatively unnoticed in its infancy because the majority of cases initially were laparoscopic tubal sterilizations on young, healthy individuals.

Barring complications, these individuals could adjust quite well to the changes that occur during laparoscopy. Only when the technique expanded, both in use and type of operations, was the full impact apparent. Now laparoscopic operations are longer and the population has many ongoing disease processes, and may be older or even elderly. This subset of patients has not been able to compensate as well as young healthy patients and the true impact of these physiologic changes is being delineated. This expansion has been a useful and productive development but as shown later in this chapter, the choice of laparoscopy versus an open procedure will be made considering the physiologic impact of the laparoscopy on the individual patient during the operative procedure and not just the physical factor of surgery without a major incision.

PHYSIOLOGIC CHANGES

The patient responses resulting during laparoscopy can be divided into mechanical and physiologic. Mechanical changes are a result of the physical pressure of superinflating the abdominal cavity and the challenges to the system from being placed in steep Trendelenburg position. Physiologic changes are a result of the absorption of CO_2 and the neurohormonal response to the procedure.

The respiratory and cardiovascular are the primary systems involved. However, hepatic, gastrointestinal, renal, and cerebral changes have been described. These changes can range in severity from

LAPAROSCOPY CAN BE BENEFICIAL:

- LESS PAIN
- EARLY MOBILIZATION
- SHORT TO NO HOSPITALIZATION

CHANGES

1. MECHANICAL

2. PHYSIOLOGICAL

Cardiovascular and respiratory systems are the most involved.

VERY SICK PATIENTS MAY NOT BE CANDIDATES

- cannot compensate for changes that occur during laparoscopy

unnoticed to severe depending on the initial condition of the patient. A detailed preoperative assessment is imperative in the compromised patient when laparoscopic surgery is an option. Some severely ill patients for this reason are not candidates for laparoscopy even though the operation is possible by this method.

MECHANICAL EFFECTS

CARDIOVASCULAR

Pneumoperitoneum

There is a mechanical pressure effect from pneumoperitoneum on the large vessels just as one might expect. Aortic compression will increase systemic vascular resistance coupled with inferior vena cava and intraabdominal vessel compression causing an initial brief increase in preload. This is short lived, however, with the main result being a decrease in preload. This most often results in a decrease in cardiac output. The greater the intra-

affecting operating conditions. The act of inflating the abdomen and the ensuing distension may stimulate the vagus nerve resulting in marked brady-cardia requiring vagolytic drugs.

PATIENT POSITION

Most gynecologic operations are accomplished in steep Trendelenburg. This causes an initial drain of the elevated lower limbs' venous volume with an increase in preload.

For the compromised patient, this could present an overload to the heart. Swan-Ganz numbers should be interpreted with caution and may not be reliable in this position.

IVC AND AORTIC COMPRESSION

INCREASED SVR

INCREASED PRELOAD FOLLOWED BY

- Decreased Preload
- Decreased CO
- Increased or no change HR

A SMALL DECREASE IN

INTRAABDOMINAL PRESSURE MAY

BE ALL THAT IS NEEDED TO

IMPROVE HEMODYNAMICS.

---

abdominal pressure the more pronounced these effects become on the patient.

If deterioration is seen, it is prudent to communicate with the anesthesiologist and decrease the insufflation. Often, improvement is achieved with a small decrease in pressure without

---

TRY TO AVOID

UNNECESSARY

TRENDELENBURG.

Chapter 4

40 ANESTHESIA IN LAPAROSCOPY . . . .

PULMONARY

The effects of laparoscopy in the supine position are limited to a decrease in compliance and a possible increase in peak airway pressure. These are usually not a problem except in the obese patient. The effects of Trendelenburg on the respiratory system can be severe in all patients, but the possibility of serious compromise is magnified in the obese or those with asthma or other pulmonary

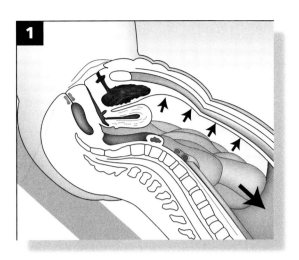

PULMONARY EFFECTS INCLUDE:

↓ COMPLIANCE

↑ AIRWAY PRESSURE

↓ FRC

↓ VC

disease. These effects may be so critical that the patient cannot be adequately ventilated in this position.

The compression of the viscera in the Trendelenburg position can cause the diaphragm to move cephalad (Figure 1). This may increase the work of ventilation resulting in increased airway pressure, decreased compliance, decreased vital capacity, and decreased functional residual capacity. Even in healthy patients, these can be changed by as much as 50%.

The endotracheal tube may become endobronchial with the Trendelenburg position. The endotracheal tube does not actually move, but the movement of the abdominal contents forward may cause the tube to favor one bronchus or actually enter the bronchus creating a one-lung ventilation scenario. This also causes an increase in the peak airway pressure and a picture similar to Trendelenburg itself. One should not assume the position is responsible, but should listen to both lungs once the position is assumed and at any time during the operation that a drop in oxygen saturation occurs. Once two-lung ventilation is assured and barring other physiologic effects then a decrease in intraabdominal pressure and a decrease in severity of Trendelenburg may result in improvement.

BE ALERT FOR

ENDOBRONCHIAL INHALATION

PHYSIOLOGIC CHANGES

PULMONARY

Carbon dioxide is absorbed into the bloodstream in a variable manner. Hypercapnea may increase moderately or profoundly and is thought to be due primarily to the absorption of CO_2 rather than decreased mechanical ventilation. The increase may occur early and become fairly steady state in most patients with an increase in minute ventilation of 30%. If compensatory mechanisms are not available to the patient because of other organ system disease, a significant acidosis can develop.

This trend can be observed to some degree from end-tidal CO_2 monitoring, but is not reliable. There can be a significant difference in the end-tidal and arterial value. Arterial trends should be monitored with frequent arterial samples from an arterial line in long cases or medically compromised patients. The ability to eliminate CO_2 varies widely and may persist for several hours. It is not uncommon to see elevated hemidiaphragm in a postoperative X-ray. The absorption is greater if the insufflation has occurred in the subcutaneous or extraperitoneal tissue. So if that has occurred, expect a larger increase in CO_2 in the arterial system.

> NEED TO INCREASE MINUTE VENTILATION BY 30% OR MORE.
>
> Arterial line may be necessary to monitor pH in patients who would not need one in an open procedure.
>
> ↓ pH COULD BE SEVERE

The anesthesiologist will increase the minute ventilation to help compensate for this change. But they are limited as to that increase and may not be successful in ill patients. The patient could be placed in a severely acidotic state. Since this is temporary, bicarbonate use would outlast the operation and usually is not considered an option. This possibility must be considered, as some patient's conditions may not tolerate this situation even on a temporary basis. Respiratory status should also be considered. One study suggests a forced expiratory volume of less than 70% or a diffusion defect less than 80% would identify patients at risk.

> IF FEV IS < 70% OR DIFFUSION CAPACITY IS < 80%, THE PATIENT MAY NOT BE A CANDIDATE FOR LAPAROSCOPY.

CARDIOVASCULAR

Cardiovascular effects that are visible to the available monitors are variable depending on the patient's inherent condition. Initial changes in cardiac function depend on the ability of the patient to compensate. Also to be considered, are the patient's pre-existing condition of volume status and medications. Arterial blood pressure may increase or decrease and is not an indication of cardiac output. An increase in dead space may lead to an increased pulmonary vascular resistance, mean arterial pressure and myocardial filling pressure with a decrease in cardiac output. As compensation occurs the output will gradually increase if the patient is capable.

CARDIOVASCULAR

↑ SVR

↑ SHUNT

↓ OR ↑ MAP

↑ OR NO CHANGE HR

↓ CO

Hypercapnea usually results in sympathetic stimulation, however, the direct effect of CO_2 is myocardial depression and vasodilatation. One study comparing nitrogen to CO_2 insufflation found a decrease in stroke volume and tachycardia that did not occur with nitrogen. These direct effects of hypercapnea are felt to be factors in laparoscopy.

Measuring cardiac output and filling pressures may not be accurate in the face of increased intrathoracic and intraabdominal pressure. Although the ability of the ventricle to contract is not affected by laparoscopy, general anesthesia in addition to changes in resistance in the presence of acidosis may lead to a continuing decrease in cardiac output. A transesophageal echo (TEE) may be necessary to evaluate the actual ability of the heart to contract under these circumstances and to observe for adequate filling pressure. It may also be of use if CO_2 embolus is suspected.

Changes to other systems result from a decreased blood flow to major organs

SWAN-GANZ IS NOT RELIABLE IN TRENDELENBURG.

MAY NEED TEE TO MONITOR COMPROMISED PATIENT.

due to the mechanical pressure and decreased cardiac output. Decreased flow is a risk factor for infection, increased gastric pH, and decreased urine output. There is one study of insufflation of warm versus cold CO_2 resulting in greater urine output due to less renal vasoconstriction. Intracranial pressure rises with insufflation regardless of CO_2 tension. This is further complicated with the Trendelenburg position.

ARRHYTHMIAS

Other systems such as the kidneys and gastrointestinal system have demonstrated effects of the pneumoperitoneum. The glomerular filtration rate is decreased. Gastric pH may increase and the splanchnic flow is reduced.

Arrhythmias usually occur early and therefore are not thought to be due to the presence of increased CO_2. Bradycardia most often occurs during insuf-

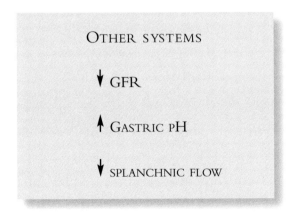

flation due to distension of the peritoneum. Ectopy can occur as well as asystole. Arrhythmias are usually treated easily by robinal, atropine, and slowing or stopping insufflation.

★ PREOP VISIT -

GOAL – TO OPTIMIZE THE MEDICAL CONDITION

– HISTORY AND PHYSICAL
– LAB TEST
– MODIFY TREATMENT REGIMENS
– IDENTIFY CARDIOVASCULAR DISEASE
– OPTIMIZE CONGESTIVE HEART FAILURE
– PULMONARY FUNCTION TESTS IF INDICATED

────────────

★ Consider holding ACE-inhibitors the day of surgery
 – continue other medications

PREOPERATIVE ASSESSMENT

The preoperative assessment of the patient is imperative for the successful outcome of any surgical procedure. In laparoscopy this is two-fold. Obviously, any patient will have a better outcome if their medical condition is optimized. The surgeon and the anesthesiologist should assess the patient's condition as soon as the operation is planned so the patient is referred to the proper channels in a timely manner, adjustments may be made to improve the patients condition and optimize their medical status prior to surgery. This is more important in the aging and elderly patient but cannot be overlooked in the younger patient as well. Asthma or uncontrolled hypertension may have ramifications that can be magnified by this procedure and should, therefore, be well controlled. Many more elderly patients are now being placed on ACE inhibitors to optimize their cardiac status. These drugs should be stopped the day before surgery to minimize hypertension at the time of induction of anesthesia. All other cardiac medication, other than diuretics, which can be administered at the discretion of the anesthesiologist during the procedure, should be maintained. All these issues should be addressed with a timely preoperative visit to the anesthesiologist.

gist need to communicate with each other about the acceptability of each patient for this method. Several conditions must be met for the procedure to be successful.

MONITORED ANESTHESIA CARE

Although not widely accepted as a common clinical practice, short procedures such as tubal sterilizations can be performed with a sedated but arousable patient with proper precautions.

Some anesthesiologists will not perform monitored anesthesia care for this procedure citing concern for the airway, patient comfort, and the ability to ensure adequate respiration in the

ANESTHETIC CHOICES
1. MONITORED ANESTHESIA
2. REGIONAL
3. GENERAL

SURGEON MUST BE REASONABLY EFFICIENT WITH SHORT DURATION OF OPERATIVE TIMES FOR MAC TO BE SUCCESSFUL.

The preoperative visit is vital to the success of a tubal sterilization in which the patient and her physicians have elected to accomplish with monitored anesthesia care, a sedated and conscious patient without general anesthesia. This is not a widely accepted method and the surgeon and the anesthesiolo-

Trendelenburg position. This also holds true for a regional technique, although spinal, epidural and monitored anesthesia care have been used in this procedure. Many general surgeons also have reservations in performing this procedure without general anesthesia.

The surgeon must be efficient and adept at handling tissue gently, and adequately anesthetize the tissue with local anesthesia. The anesthesiologist must be able to sedate the patient adequately without losing the patient's protective reflexes. Most important is an informed, motivated patient.

We have performed large numbers of these procedures in this manner with highly successful outcomes and pleased and satisfied patients. This method requires more work and preplanning on the part of the surgeons and anesthesiologists to be successful. The main factor that would exclude the patient as a candidate for this procedure is morbid obesity because of the technical difficulties involved in each aspect of the operation. In the preoperative clinic visit, each patient is shown a video detailing all aspects of the procedure. Such phrases as "when the gas enters your abdomen you will feel as if you are pregnant" and "when your head is lowered it feels like you are standing on your head" are included.

Trendelenburg position may be duplicated on the stretcher prior to surgery

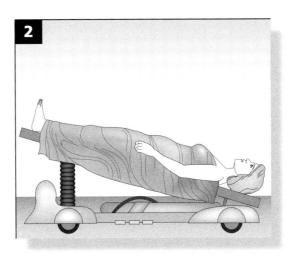

to make sure the patient is comfortable with that position (Figure 2). Some surgeons require more Trendelenburg than others, which may limit the possibility of this method for certain patients for whom the excessive position is uncomfortable. The ability to accept this position is usually the most common limiting factor for the patient.

The video of the procedure is extremely important because the patient becomes a participant in the procedure and her understanding of every aspect is vital to the successful outcome. The patient is instructed that she will receive sedation by the anesthesiologist as she wishes, but it is emphasized that there are aspects that they will be aware of but which should not be painful. The pressure of the gas in their abdomen and insertion of the trocar are the main stimulating events. If the sensation is disturbing, a small

> *A VIDEO OF PROCEDURE IS VERY IMPORTANT TO INFORM THE PATIENT OF WHAT TO EXPECT.

release in pressure usually brings acceptable conditions to the patient without compromising the visualization of the surgical field. During insertion of the Veress needle or trocar, the surgeon can time the insertion by observing the movement of the abdomen with respiration. No attempt is made to coerce the patient or give them unrealistic expectations, but if they are told of the awareness of these sensations ahead of time, the patient can make an informed decision which is much more acceptable to the patient during surgery.

An important adjunct to the clinic visit is the clinic nurse. She helps to explain the procedure in her own words and past experiences are shared. She often is quite adept at quickly establishing a rapport with the patient and is vital as an additional source of information for the patient. She will also accompany the physician to the operating room, which greatly enhances continuity of care and an atmosphere of trust for the patient.

Given a motivated, knowledgeable patient, a safe and successful operation will depend on the skills of the surgeon and anesthesiologist. Enough volume and proper deposition of local anesthetic must be utilized. The tenaculum placement on the cervix is facilitated by a paracervical block. A

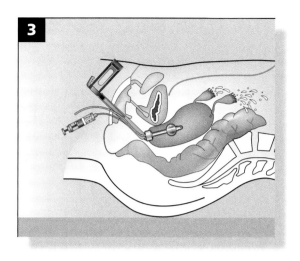

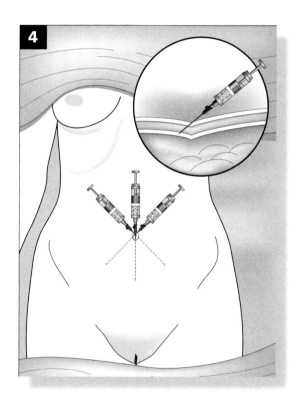

uterine manipulator that has the ability to perform transuterine hydrotubation is placed into the cervix (Figure 3). The skin of the abdomen is infiltrated with 1% lidocaine, usually with a small gauge needle initially followed by a 22-gauge spinal needle needed for its length in a four-quadrant pattern to anesthetize the skin and subcutaneous tissue (Figure 4). It takes at least 15–20 cc of lidocaine to be adequate. The 22-gauge spinal needle is then inserted into the fascia and approximately 10 cc of local anesthetic is deposited directly into the fascia. This should permit insertion of the Veress needle and trocar. At this stage, 20 cc of 0.5% xylocaine is infused through the uterine manipulator. After ensuring entry into the abdomen, lidocaine is dripped into each tube under direct visualization. This usually takes 10 cc per tube.

The anesthesiologist will provide sedation according to the patient's needs. Occasionally, some patients will watch the procedure on the monitors, although this is uncommon. Preoperative anxiolytics titrated with midazolam to effect is usually adequate. Speech may begin to slur or a slight disinhibition may be observed. Occasionally, 50 µg of fentanyl is needed to augment the sedation. While the monitors are being attached, a propofol drip is started at 25 µg/kg/min. This allows a blood level to be achieved gradually over time so that a bolus is not necessary prior to the beginning of surgery. It is important to maintain a level of sedation where patients are arousable but sedated. This is usually accomplished with a combination of midazolam, fentanyl and propofol. Usually a propofol drip is the primary sedating agent with fentanyl given only as necessary. One method is a combination of 50 mg (1 cc) of ketamine to 50 cc (500 mg) of propofol for the maintenance infusion. If this method is chosen, very little fentanyl is necessary. The amount of ketamine is so small that dysphoria is not encountered. The ketamine, however, provides some augmentation of analgesia

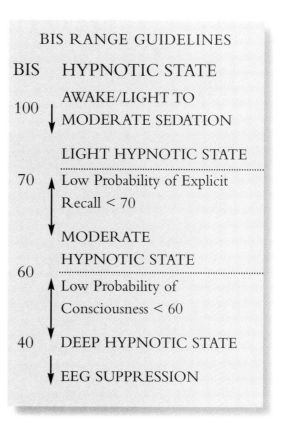

and sedation with no respiratory depression. In addition to the usual monitors for general anesthesia, end tidal CO_2 monitors as well as a BIS monitor are useful. This information will help monitor sedation levels and respiratory pattern without disturbing a sedated patient. It must be stressed that verbal communication should always be possible to assure the presence of adequate airway reflexes. The BIS levels for this type of anesthesia are somewhat patient variable, but are usually in the 75-85 ranges.

The anesthesiologist must be prepared at any time to intubate the patient and proceed with general anesthesia. This could be for surgical

- EKG, 3–5 LEAD DEPENDING ON THE PATIENT'S CONDITION

- BLOOD PRESSURE

- OXYGEN SATURATION

- END-TIDAL CO_2

- INSPIRATORY AND END-TIDAL ANESTHETIC AGENT CONCENTRATIONS

- BIS MONITOR

- ESOPHAGEAL STETHOSCOPE

- MUSCLE TWITCH MONITOR

or anesthetic reasons such as complications or discomfort. The continuing communication between the surgeon and the anesthesiologist will allow the optimum conditions to be achieved for all parties.

GENERAL ANESTHESIA

General anesthesia is by far the most common method of anesthesia for laparoscopy. In an adequately prepared patient, laparoscopy has greatly accelerated the recovery process. All of the routine monitors should be employed for this procedure.

In elderly patients, or during a prolonged procedure, an arterial line pressure monitor may be helpful to determine acid-base status. Other invasive monitors are used as the patient condition warrants.

General anesthesia for laparoscopy should always be accompanied by endotracheal intubation to ensure protection of the airway secondary to increased intraabdominal pressure and the Trendelenburg position.

NITROUS OXIDE CAN BE USED

FOR SHORTER PROCEDURES.

After the airway has been secured and the endotracheal tube position is confirmed, an oral gastric tube should be inserted for decompression of the stomach prior to instrumentation of the abdomen. This minimizes the risk of puncturing the stomach in addition to emptying it to help minimize nausea and vomiting during recovery.

General anesthesia can be accomplished by the intravenous or inhalation method. The use of N_2O varies by anesthesiologist. It is controversial as to its effects on nausea and possible increased bowel distension. It has been reported that if the procedure lasts longer than 30 minutes, there is enough N_2O to support combustion.

If the patient gives a positive history of nausea, elimination of N_2O may be

A HIGH CONCENTRATION OF OXYGEN HAS BEEN SHOWN TO DECREASE THE INCIDENCE OF NAUSEA AND VOMITING.

• • • • • • •

PROPOFOL HAS ALSO BEEN SHOWN TO DECREASE NAUSEA AND VOMITING.

of some benefit as well as the use of antiemetics. The use of 80% oxygen may also reduce nausea and vomiting and decrease the incidence of wound infections. Routine use of antiemetics is not indicated. The use of a muscle relaxant that does not require reversal may also improve the chances of

SUSPECT SUBCUTANEOUS INFILTRATIONS WITH LARGE INCREASES IN END-TIDAL CO_2.

eliminating nausea during recovery. The use of propofol for induction and as the primary anesthetic, or as an adjunct to decrease the amount of inhalation agent, will also help to prevent nausea and vomiting and provide a quick recovery.

The use of steroids in the recovery period may also be considered if nausea becomes a problem during that time.

POST-OPERATIVE VENTILATION MAY BE REQUIRED IN SEVERE CASES.

Chapter 4

50 | ANESTHESIA IN LAPAROSCOPY ....

COMPLICATIONS

SUBCUTANEOUS EMPHYSEMA

Any increase in end-tidal CO_2 after stabilization should be cause to suspect subcutaneous emphysema. If the CO_2 level does not respond to increased minute ventilation, subcutaneous emphysema should be suspected.

Subcutaneous emphysema should not cause an increase in airway pressure. The patient should be physically observed and examined and if crepitus and swelling of the tissue is seen, the case should be converted to open or aborted. Depending on the level of arterial CO_2, the patient will often need mechanical ventilation until the CO_2 levels return to normal. This usually occurs within 24 hours or less depending on the severity.

PNEUMOTHORAX, PNEUMOMEDIASTINUM, AND PNEUMOPERICARDIUM

Intraperitoneal gas may find its way through openings in the diaphragm at the aortic and esophageal hiatus. Opening of pleural peritoneal ducts, as in ascites, may also lead to the accumulation of gas in the mediastinum or to pneumothorax. Pneumothorax is the most common of the three and can also occur from positive pressure ventilation.

GAS FOLLOWS OPENINGS IN THE DIAPHRAGM AND ESOPHAGEAL HIATUS OR PNEUMOTHORAX.

·······

AN INCREASE IN AIRWAY PRESSURE WITH DECREASE IN CV STATUS.

·······

RESOLVES WITH RELEASE OF INTRAABDOMINAL GAS.

·······

LIMIT PRESSURE TO LOWEST POSSIBLE LEVELS.

Pleural tears may also occur iatrogenically. Whatever their origin, they must be recognized as quickly as possible. Airway pressure should increase and blood pressure may not decrease until some time has passed. End-tidal CO_2 will increase unless the pneumothorax is from a spontaneous cause. Tension pneumothorax is a possibility. However, spontaneous resolution may occur within 60 minutes of release of abdominal gas. If N_2O is used, it should be stopped and ventilator settings should be adjusted. Communication with the surgeon to reduce intraabdominal pressure as much as possible, and careful observation of the patient should correct the situation without thoracentesis.

Limiting the intraabdominal pressure to the lowest possible levels will decrease the incidence. The most helpful monitor in this situation is transesophageal echocardiography.

GAS EMBOLISM

Gas embolism may occur from direct insufflation into a vessel or organ from direct needle or trocar placement. There appears to be an increased incidence during hysteroscopy more than laparoscopy. The volume of gas necessary to produce symptoms is 25 mL/kg of CO_2 as opposed to 5 mL/kg of air. It usually occurs at the beginning of surgery so insufflation should be initiated at 1 L/min while the patient is watched carefully. Signs of embolism include tachycardia, arrhythmias, hypotension, millwheel murmur, and EKG signs of right heart strain. End-tidal CO_2 may be decreased due to the decrease in cardiac output. Aspiration of gas, foamy blood from a central venous line or air bubbles demonstrated on TEE will provide definitive diagnosis. To help

---

INCREASED INCIDENCE WITH HYSTEROSCOPY BUT CAN OCCUR WITH LAPAROSCOPY.

SIGNS INCLUDE:

↑ HR

↓ B/P

ARRHYTHMIAS

MILLWHEEL MURMUR

EKG SIGNS OF RIGHT HEART STRAIN

• • • • • • •

- MUST ACT QUICKLY TO AVOID SEVERE COMPLICATIONS OR DEATH
- HEAD DOWN
- LEFT LATERAL POSITION
- 100% O_2
- ASPIRATE GAS FROM CENTRAL LINE
- SUPPORT B/P WITH ISOTOPES

PROPHYLACTIC TREATMENT NOT INDICATED

POSITIVE HISTORY SHOULD REALIZE PROPHYLACTIC RX

MULTI-MODAL

- METODOPRAMIDE
- ANTI-EMETIC OF CHOICE
- PROMPT TX. IF OCCURS
- SMALL AMOUNTS OF STEROIDS AND BENADRYL MAY HELP
- ALLOW ENOUGH TIME TO EXPEL AS MUCH GAS AS POSSIBLE

reverse the symptoms, deflate the abdomen with the patient placed in the head down and left lateral position trying to keep as much CO_2 as possible in the right atrium, administer 100% oxygen, and aspirate as much gas as possible. Although gas embolism may be fatal, rapid diagnosis and treatment is highly successful as long as blood pressure is supported.

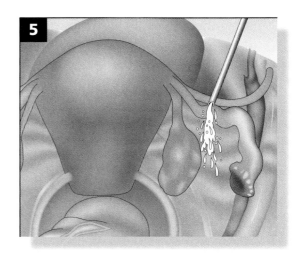

POSTOPERATIVE RECOVERY

Postoperative nausea and vomiting can be a significant problem. A positive history should be treated with preventive measures. Metoclopramide will help to empty the stomach preoperatively. Careful suctioning of the orogastric tube prior to emergence will relieve the stomach distension that may have occurred intraoperatively. For patients with a positive history, an antiemetic prior to emergence is indicated as well as a propofol-based anesthetic. Prompt treatment in the recovery room with antiemetics and a steroid will usually prevent a continuing problem. A multimodal treatment of pain will prevent the total dependence of opioids and thus lessen the propensity for nausea and vomiting. Allowing enough time for as much gas as possible to escape the abdomen is an important and often neglected step to provide patient comfort.

A lidocaine-ropivicaine drip on the Fallopian tubes will greatly decrease the pain of tubal ligation (Figure 5). Preemptive analgesia by local infiltration of the skin prior to instrumentation is a useful adjunct if done with a long-acting anesthetic in combination with lidocaine. Many maneuvers have attempted to decrease shoulder pain.

INFILTRATION OF SKIN
AND MESOSALPINX
WILL HELP WITH POSTOP PAIN

PAIN MEDICINE SHOULD INCLUDE
RETOROLZE

COX–2

Instillation of a long-acting anesthetic may help this condition in some patients. Some studies show that if the insufflation gas is heated and hydrated, the incidence of shoulder pain decreases.

Ketorolac and Cox-2 inhibitors are helpful adjuncts for the treatment of pain and will decrease the amount of opioids needed. Transdermal scopolamine and benadryl may also be of benefit. At the time of skin closure, 60–80 mg of toradol may avoid postoperative cramping.

SUMMARY

Laparoscopy has obvious benefits to the patient and will continue to develop as better instruments, greater experience, and more knowledge about the effects on the body are further elucidated. As this occurs, our ability to apply this technique with greater expertise will improve patient morbidity and provide anesthetic challenges to supply a physiologic milieu in the presence of a myriad of physiologic variations caused by this procedure.

SUGGESTED READING:

Goll V, Akca O, Greif R, et al. Ondansetron is no more effective than supplemental intra-operative oxygen for prevention of postoperative nausea and vomiting. Anes Analg 2001; 92:112-7

Greif R, Laciny S, et al. Anesthesiology 1999;V91, No. 5: 1246-1252

Howie MB, Kim MH. Gynecologic surgery in ambulatory anesthesia and surgery. White PF, 1997: 282-284

Jon's JL. Anesthesia for Laparoscopic Surgery - Anesthesia (5th Ed) Miller RD, (Ed) 2000: 2003-2023

Mortero R, Clark L, et al. The effects of small-dose ketamine on propofol sedation: respiration, postoperative mood, perception, cognition, and pain. Anesth Analg 2001; 92:1-5

Weingram J. Laparoscopic Surgery. In: Yao and Artusio. Anesthesiology: Problem Oriented Patient Management, 4th ed. 1998: 732-759

Bardoczky GI, Engleman E, Levarlet M, et al. Ventilatory effects of pneumoperitoneum monitored with continuous spirometry. Anesthesia 1993;8:309

Wittgen CM, Ngunhein KS, Andrus CH, et al. Preoperative pulmonary evaluation for laparoscopic cholestectomy. Arch Surg 1993;128:880

Ho HS, Saunders CJ, Gunther RI, et al. Effectors of hemodynamics during laparoscopy: CO_2 absorption or intra-abdominal pressure? J Surg Res 1995;59:497

Backlund M, Kellolumpu I, Scheimint, et al. Effect of temperature of insufflated CO_2 during and after prolonged laparoscopic surgery. Surg Endosc 1998;12:126

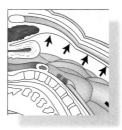

CREATION OF PNEUMOPERITONEUM AND TROCAR INSERTION TECHNIQUES

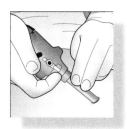

Resad Pasic M.D., Ph.D.

PATIENT POSITIONING AND PREPARATION

The patient is placed in a dorsolithotomy position with the buttocks extended over the end of the table. The thighs should be flexed (120°) to allow good instrument manipulation (Figure 1). Attention should be given to proper positioning of the patient's legs to avoid peroneal nerve injury during lengthy procedures. Shoulder braces may be used to make the steep Trendelenburg position possible during surgery. If shoulder braces are used they should be placed over the acromion to avoid possible brachial plexus injury. It is advisable that both arms should be tucked along the patient's body to prevent brachial plexus injury and provide more space for the surgeons. If electrosurgery is to be used during the procedure, a ground electrode for the unipolar instruments must be properly placed over the patient's thigh, and full surface contact of the electrode must be assured.

Straight bladder catheterization is performed for short laparoscopic procedures or a Foley catheter is placed in the bladder if prolonged surgery is anticipated. The bladder has to be emptied to minimize any potential injury during ancillary trocar placement.

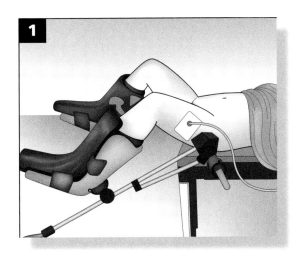

After placement of a cervical tenaculum a uterine manipulator is inserted into the cervix and uterine cavity to properly manipulate the uterus during the procedure (Figure 2). Manipulators with a capability for tubal lavage may be used, as well as dilute indigo carmine dye for chromopertubation. If the patient does not have a uterus, or is pregnant, a sponge stick is introduced into the vagina and the cul-de-sac is pushed upward. A rectal probe can also be introduced for manipulation and better visualization of the rectum and identification of the rectovaginal septum during extensive laparoscopic resections.

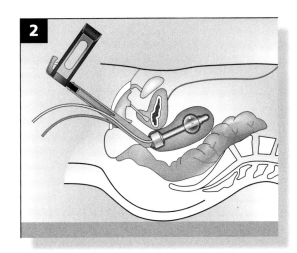

Povidone iodine is applied to the abdominal area and vagina extending from the nipple line to the inner thighs. The patient is draped with leggings and a laparoscopy sheet. If extensive surgery is likely to be performed, and bowel manipulation or injury anticipated, as in the case of extensive adhesions or endometriosis, it is advisable to administer a mechanical bowel preparation prior to surgery. The use

- LITHOTOMY POSITION WITH EXTENDED BUTTOCKS
- SHOULDER BRACES
- FOLEY CATHETER IN THE BLADDER
- UTERINE MANIPULATOR
- NASOGASTRIC TUBE
- RETURN ELECTRODE

of a nasogastric tube prior to the establishment of the pneumoperitoneum is suggested to minimize the risk of gastric injury. Prophylactic antibiotics are not routinely used but can be administered if an increased risk of infection appears possible.

CREATION OF PNEUMOPERITONEUM

Creation of a pneumoperitoneum and the insertion of a Veress needle and primary trocar are the most critical steps when performing laparoscopy. Common sites of Veress needle and trocar insertion are shown on Figure 3.

Extra-peritoneal insufflation is one of the most common complications of laparoscopy regardless of body weight

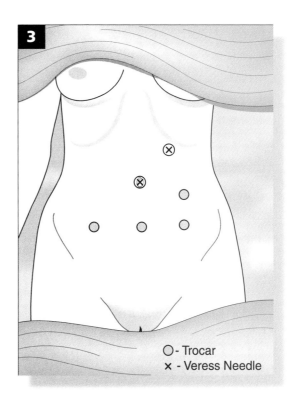

○ - Trocar
× - Veress Needle

VERESS NEEDLE TECHNIQUES

- TRANSUMBILICAL PLACEMENT
- LEFT UPPER QUADRANT PLACEMENT
- PALMER'S POINT
- 9TH INTERCOSTAL SPACE
- TRANSUTERINE PLACEMENT

OPEN LAPAROSCOPY

DIRECT TROCAR PLACEMENT

and is responsible for technical failures that frequently lead to the abandonment of the procedure.

There are three subgroups of patients who can present problems during the development of the pneumoperitoneum during laparoscopy:

1. Obese patients;

2. Patients with scars from previous abdominal surgeries;

3. Patients with failed insufflation;

The abundant abdominal wall and intraabdominal fat of obesity decreases tactile sensation and poses difficulty for the standard transumbilical Veress needle insertion and establishment of a pneumoperitoneum. Higher insufflation pressures may be encountered in these patients.

Presence of abdominal scars increases the possibility of omental or bowel adhesions to the abdominal wall, which may interfere with the successful development of the pneumoperitoneum, and may lead to bowel injury.

In patients with failed insufflation or preperitoneal insufflation it becomes difficult to enter the peritoneal cavity since the peritoneum is peeled off and an artificial space is created by trapped CO_2 gas that prevents re-entry of the Veress needle into the peritoneal cavity. Therefore, in these cases an alternative insufflation site should be chosen.

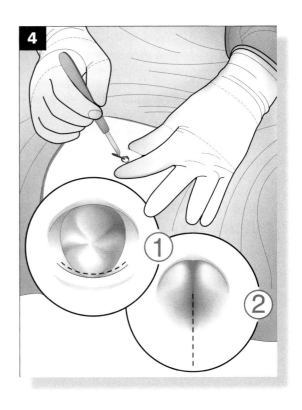

> CAREFUL SELECTION OF THE INSUFFLATION TECHNIQUE AND THE INSUFFLATION SITE SHOULD BE CHOSEN FOR EACH PATIENT.

TRANSUMBILICAL INSUFFLATION

The umbilical area is the most common site for Veress needle placement. Carbon dioxide or nitrous oxide (N_2O) are most often used for insufflation, since room air is not very soluble in blood and may cause embolism if it enters a blood vessel. CO_2 is preferred for laser surgery and N_2O is used for laparoscopy under local anesthesia.

A skin incision of about 1.5 cm may be made using a number 11 scalpel blade at the umbilical area (Figure 4). The Veress needle should be inspected and checked before insertion.

The operating table with the patient should be placed in the flat position (Figure 5). The needle is usually inserted at a 45° angle at the midline, and directed toward the uterine fundus.

Placing the patient in Trendelenburg position prior to the insertion of the Veress needle and primary trocar changes the position of the major retroperitoneal vessels, and places them in the path of the needle and the trocar, subsequently, placing the patient at greater risk of major vascular injury (Figure 6).

Lifting the abdominal wall prior to needle insertion is favored by many surgeons (Figure 7), but some insert the Veress needle directly into the abdomen using gentle traction without abdominal wall elevation. Some surgeons use towel clips to grab and lift the abdominal wall at the time of Veress needle insertion. Depending upon the abdominal wall thickness, the angle of insertion may vary from 45° to 90°. In obese patients, the angle of insertion is close to 90°. Bowel and other intraabdominal structures have great motility and are resistant to needle puncture unless they are fixed to the abdominal wall by some pathologic process. The needle valve should be placed in open position during insertions since it allows air to enter the abdominal cavity and help bowel drop back from the abdominal wall.

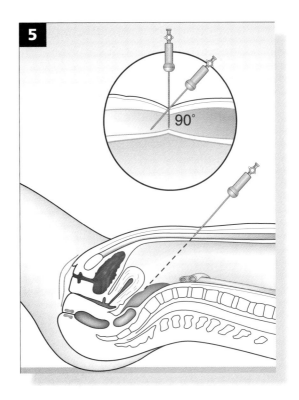

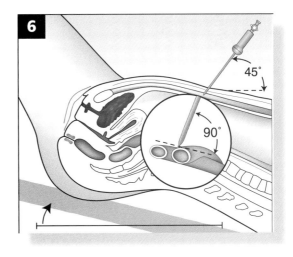

If proper intraperitoneal placement of the needle is not obtained, one more attempt should be considered before choosing an alternative site. There are a number of tests that may ensure proper needle placement and avoid possible complications during the insufflation procedure.

- Hanging drop test: attaching an open syringe filled with saline to the Veress needle and observing drop of saline while negative intra-abdominal pressure is created by lifting the anterior abdominal wall (Figure 8).

- Intraabdominal insufflation pressure (Figure 9)

- Aspiration and sounding test, using an aspiration needle on the syringe (Figure 10)

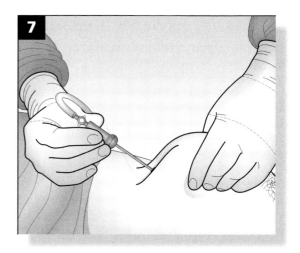

Although these tests might be of some value in determining proper needle placement, many operators rely primarily on the intraabdominal insufflation pressure and flow volume to ensure proper intraperitoneal needle placement.

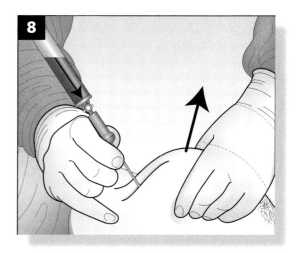

Initial intraabdominal insufflation pressure should not exceed 10 mmHg, and it is the most reliable parameter for monitoring of insufflation and proper needle placement. If the initial insufflation pressure exceeds 10 mmHg, the Veress needle is most likely in the preperitoneal space or has entered an intraabdominal viscus or omentum and it should be withdrawn. If the surgeon is uncertain that the needle is not placed intraperitoneally, the Veress needle should be withdrawn and re-inserted before too much preperitoneal emphysema has developed. During insufflation other clinical signs

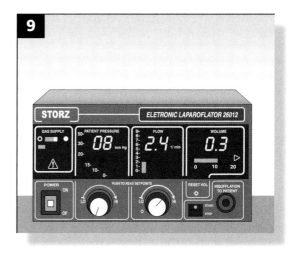

such as disappearance of liver dullness and symmetric distension of the lower abdomen can be observed. If the needle is properly placed, the peritoneal cavity is insufflated with 3-5 L of CO_2, depending upon the patients size, and the needle is withdrawn. After insufflating about 2 L of CO_2 intra-abdominal pressures will begin to rise.

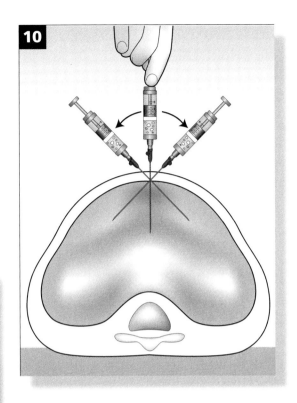

- CHECK THE VERESS NEEDLE BEFORE INSERTION

- CHECK THE STARTING PRESSURE IF MECHANICAL INSUFFLATORS ARE USED

- PLACE THE PATIENT IN FLAT POSITION

- MAKE THE SKIN INCISION OF ABOUT 1.5 CM

- INSERT THE NEEDLE IN MIDLINE POSITION AT A 45° ANGLE WHILE PULLING ON THE ABDOMINAL SKIN TO FORM A COUNTERTRACTION

- IF THE INSUFFLATION PRESSURE IS ABOVE 10 MMHG WITHDRAW THE NEEDLE AND REPEAT THE SAME PROCEDURE AT THE PROXIMAL END OF THE UMBILICAL INCISION

- IF HIGH PRESSURE IS OBTAINED AGAIN, WITHDRAW THE NEEDLE AND CONSIDER AN ALTERNATIVE PUNCTURE SITE

- IF DEALING WITH A MORBIDLY OBESE PATIENT OR PATIENTS WITH SCARS FROM PREVIOUS ABDOMINAL SURGERIES, AN ALTERNATE PRIMARY INSUFFLATION SITE MAY BE CONSIDERED

Insufflation should be continued until the pressures reach at least 20–25 mmHg. Since the abdominal cavity is a closed space and its volume varies from patient to patient, insufflation pressure is a better indicator of adequate peritoneal insufflation and distension than the volume of gas used. When the insufflation pressure reaches 20–25 mmHg, distension of the abdominal cavity should be adequate for safe insertion of the trocar. After the trocar is inserted the cut off insufflation pressure on the insufflator should be set at approximately 15–16 mmHg.

ALTERNATIVE SITES AND TECHNIQUES

An alternative site for needle placement can be selected if the umbilical area is deemed unsuitable for insertion.

SUBCOSTAL

INSUFFLATION TECHNIQUE

Insertion of the Veress needle through the subcostal space in the left midclavicular line is a safe alternative to transumbilical insufflation. A small stub skin incision is made in the left midclavicular line just underneath the rib cage. A Veress needle is placed at a 90° angle and pushed into the abdominal cavity. No abdominal wall elevation is performed. Three distinct pops of the needle can be felt as the needle advances toward the peritoneal cavity. The abdominal wall is usually thin in this area, no more than 3-4 cm (Figure 11).

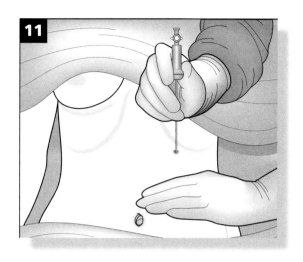

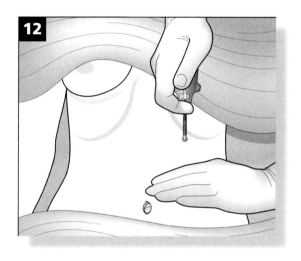

The left upper quadrant is easily accessible and is usually free of intraabdominal adhesions. This area is relatively safe for needle and trocar insertion because the rib cage provides adequate tension and prevents the downward displacement of the abdominal wall. This technique works well for patients with a failed transumbilical insufflation. It should be used as a primary route in obese patients, or patients who have had previous abdominal surgeries and have abdominal scars with suspected adhesions in the umbilical area regardless of if the scar is from a midline, Pfannenstiel, or any other incision.

Subcutaneous emphysema is rarely encountered when insufflating in this space. The spleen is unlikely to be injured when using the midclavicular subcostal space, although, very rarely the left lobe of the liver may be punctured with the Veress needle. To avoid liver injury, the Veress needle should be directed caudate, at an angle slightly less than 90°.

In a patient with suspected abdominal adhesions, upon successful insufflation, the Veress needle is withdrawn, and a 5-mm trocar is inserted through the same space (Figure 12). Through this trocar sleeve, a 5-mm scope is

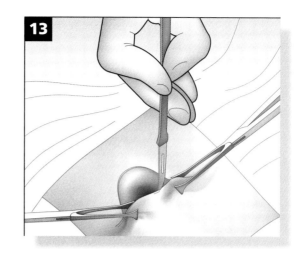

SUBCOSTAL APPROACH:

- MAKE A SMALL STAB INCISION IN THE MIDCLAVICULAR LINE, JUST BELOW THE COSTAL MARGIN, ON THE PATIENT'S LEFT SIDE

- INSERT THE VERESS NEEDLE AT A 90° ANGLE

- THREE POPS OF THE NEEDLE ARE USUALLY FELT

- IF INITIAL PRESSURES ARE TOO HIGH, PULL THE NEEDLE BACKWARD. IT MAY BE STUCK IN THE OMENTUM.

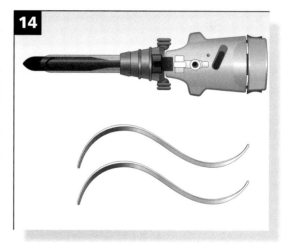

introduced, and the umbilical area is inspected for the absence of adhesions. If the umbilical area is free of adhesions, a 10-mm trocar is inserted into the peritoneal cavity under direct vision.

OPEN TECHNIQUE

Open laparoscopy (Hasson technique) is indispensable in some patients, especially those suspected of having adhesions from previous surgeries and abdominal scars. The open technique utilizes a small 2-3 cm umbilical skin incision (Figure 13). The dissection is performed into the abdomen with Kelly clamps and special 'S' shaped retractors. After the abdominal fascia is visualized and incised, two 0-Vicryl™ sutures are placed into the fascia to support and hold the blunt trocar that is inserted

Chapter 5

64 | CREATION OF PNEUMOPERITONEUM AND TROCAR INSERTION TECHNIQUES . . . .

into the abdominal cavity after the incision is carried through the peritoneum. The blunt trocar contains a conical obturator that plugs off the abdominal skin incision. Gas is insufflated directly through the cannula and an obturator is replaced with the laparoscope (Figures 14-16).

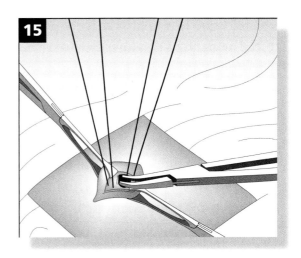

This technique may be safer than blind, Veress needle and trocar incision as noted by the lower rate of vascular injuries; however, its routine application may not be always warranted. Open laparoscopy is very difficult to perform in a morbidly obese patient, because one must penetrate 8 to 10 cm of adipose tissue before reaching the fascia and peritoneal cavity through a small skin incision. This technique, therefore, can be very impractical and time consuming. Some authors suggest that open techniques are suited for use in obese patients, especially to prevent vascular injuries. However, this technique does not seem very reliable in preventing bowel injuries.

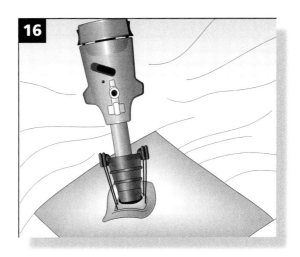

DIRECT TROCAR INSERTION

Direct trocar insertion is reserved mostly for thin patients with a flaccid anterior abdominal wall. In this technique, a small incision is made in the umbilical area, the abdominal wall is lifted with one hand, and a trocar is pushed with the dominant hand into the potential space of the abdominal cavity. Insufflation tubing is attached to the trocar, and the laparoscope is inserted (Figure 17).

This technique is fast and reliable in carefully chosen patients. Surgeons who routinely use the direct insertion technique consider it to be safer than using the Veress needle. Direct trocar insertion works well for multiparous, thin patients with a flaccid anterior abdominal wall, however, we find it impractical and hazardous in obese patients. In obese patients, it is difficult to grasp and elevate the abdominal wall sufficiently for safe placement of the trocar.

Direct trocar insertion may also present a problem for female surgeons because it requires significant strength and force to lift the abdominal wall and push the trocar into the peritoneal cavity.

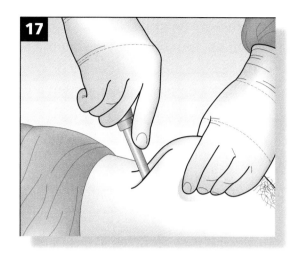

DIRECT TROCAR INSERTION:

- MAKE A 1.5 CM UMBILICAL INCISION
- LIFT THE ANTERIOR ABDOMINAL WALL WITH LEFT HAND
- INSERT THE TROCAR WITH THE RIGHT HAND AIMING TOWARD THE UTERUS
- CONNECT THE TUBING AND BEGIN THE INSUFFLATION

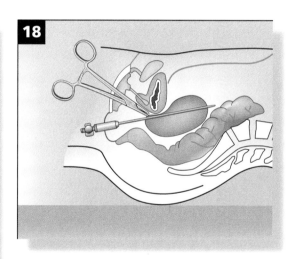

TRANSUTERINE INSUFFLATION

This method enables easy and safe access to the peritoneal cavity, bypassing transabdominal entry of the Veress needle in obese patients. Transuterine insufflation is a useful modality in patients with a large abdominal panniculus, because the peritoneal cavity can be easily entered with the Veress needle via the transcervical route and through the uterine fundus (Figure 18).

This technique is very simple and safe, it should not be considered in patients with large uterine fibroids and patients who are candidates for chromotubation, since the hole in the uterine wall created by the Veress needle may facilitate the escape of the dye.

With the patient in a moderate Trendelenburg position, a speculum is placed in the vagina. The anterior cervical lip is grasped with an atraumatic grasper and the uterus is pulled forward to straighten its axis. The uterine cavity is sounded to obtain information on the size and direction of the cavity. A long Veress needle is passed through the cervix into the uterine cavity until slight resistance is felt, when the needle reaches the fundus. The needle is then pushed through the uterine fundus until it reaches the peritoneal cavity, detected by a pop of the needle as it advances through the uterus. The peritoneal cavity is then insufflated with CO_2. Somewhat higher initial insufflation pressures, up to 20 mmHg, can be encountered initially with this method. As the abdominal cavity is being insufflated, the pressures begin to drop.

This technique should be considered in patients with abdominal scars, suspected adhesions, obese patients and patients with failed transabdominal insufflation where an artificial preperitoneal space is created.

TROCAR PLACEMENT

Extensive insufflation of the peritoneal cavity will create enough elevation and resistance against the peritoneum for safe insertion of the trocar.

The trocar and sheath are held between the middle and index finger with the hub of the trocar against the palm of the hand. With wrist motion, the trocar is usually advanced with the dominant hand at a 45° angle in midline position toward the hollow of the sacrum. The other hand rests on the abdomen holding the trocar sheath between the index finger and the middle finger to act as a safeguard to prevent excessive penetration of the trocar through the abdominal wall (Figure 19). The trocar sheath is slightly

---

TRANSUTERINE APPROACH:

- INSERT VAGINAL SPECULUM

- GRASP ANTERIOR CERVICAL LIP WITH THE TENACULUM AND PULL IT FORWARD

- SOUND UTERINE CAVITY USING UTERINE SOUND

- GRASP THE LONG VERESS NEEDLE WITH SPONGE FORCEPS AND INTRODUCE THE NEEDLE THROUGH THE CERVIX INTO THE UTERINE CAVITY. APPLY THE PRESSURE TO PERFORATE THE FUNDUS.

- CONNECT THE TUBING, AND TURN THE INSUFFLATION ON. THE HIGHER PRESSURE IN THE RANGE OF 15–20 MMHG IS EXPECTED.

- INSERT THE TROCAR AND REMOVE THE VERESS NEEDLE UNDER DIRECT LAPAROSCOPIC VISION.

wider than the trocar tip and it may get caught in the fascia. As the force is applied to the trocar, its tip may be pushed too far into the abdomen, as the trocar sheath passes the resistance of the fascia. Therefore, some type of safeguard mechanism should be applied on the trocar to avoid its excessive penetration. Another way to control the excessive penetration of the trocar is to hold the index finger extended along the shaft of the trocar (Figure 20). Depending upon the abdominal wall thickness the angle of insertion may vary from 45° to 90°. In obese patients, the angle of insertion is close to 90° (Figure 21).

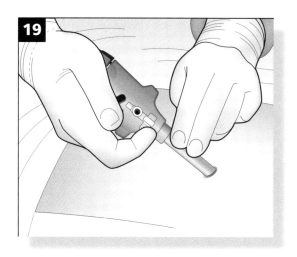

There is no need to lift the abdominal wall during the trocar insertion if the abdominal cavity is properly insufflated. If the abdominal cavity has been insufflated to the pressure of 20 mmHg, the cushion of gas in the abdominal cavity is sufficient to hold the abdominal wall elevated for safe insertion of the trocar. Once the trocar is safely inserted into the abdominal cavity, the obturator is removed and the trocar sheath is held in place. Hiss of escaping gas can be heard by depressing the flap valve. This is the most comforting sound as it assures the surgeon that the trocar is in the right place.

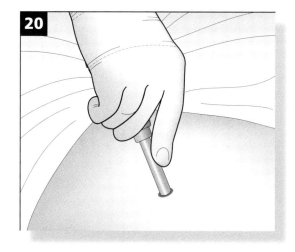

Ancillary trocars should be inserted under direct endoscopic control (Figure 22). The suprapubic midline

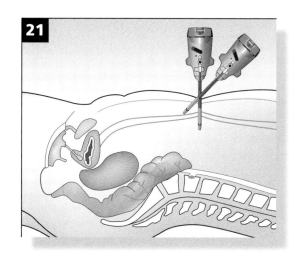

site is the most common, and two additional lower quadrant sites above the pubic hairline lateral to the deep epigastric vessels are recommended for performing operative laparoscopic

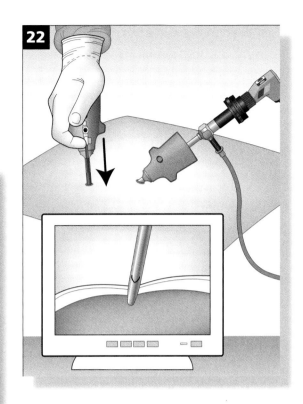

- EXTENSIVE INSUFFLATION OF THE PERITONEAL CAVITY. THE MORE THE BETTER

- ANGLE OF INSERTION USUALLY 45–60°

- SAFEGUARD MECHANISM DURING TROCAR PLACEMENT

- BEFORE PLACING ANCILLARY TRO- CARS, INSPECT THE INSIDE ABDOMI- NAL WALL FOR THE PRESENCE OF ADHESIONS.

- GENTLY TAP THE AREA WITH THE INDEX FINGER, WHERE THE PUNC- TURE IS PLANNED AND LOOK FOR THE INDENTATION OF THE ABDOMI- NAL WALL THROUGH THE LAPARO- SCOPE.

- TURN THE ROOM LIGHTS OFF, AND ILLUMINATE THE AREA ON THE ABDOMINAL WALL WITH THE LAPARO- SCOPE FROM INSIDE, LOOKING FOR BLOOD VESSELS.

- MAKE A SMALL 5-MM SKIN INCISION IN THE AREA CLEAR OF BLOOD VESSELS.

- INTRODUCE THE TROCAR SLEEVE UNDER LAPAROSCOPIC VISION, AIMING TOWARD THE POSTERIOR CUL–DE–SAC.

- REPEAT THE SAME PROCEDURE FOR EACH ANCILLARY PORT.

procedures. The abdominal wall may be transilluminated by the laparoscope at the site of the lateral secondary trocar placement in order to display and avoid deep epigastric blood vessels. This technique is useful, but cannot be relied upon to locate the deep vessels, especially in obese patients. Finger-tapping the skin from above can identify the area of trocar placement, and a small skin incision should be made before the trocar sleeve is inserted. The upper margin of the bladder should be identified, and a Foley catheter should help avoid accidental bladder perforation. Note the patient's position and anatomical landmarks when inserting the trocars. All ancillary trocars should be directed toward the posterior cul-de-sac. Both hands should be used for trocar insertion. If only one hand is used because the second hand is holding the camera and therefore cannot be used as a safe stop for the trocar, the index finger should be extended along the trocar shaft to be used as a safeguard against deep penetration of the trocar. Most laparoscopic surgeries can be performed using 5 mm trocar sleeves, but if a stapler or a laparoscopic morcellator are to be used, a 12-mm trocar is inserted usually in the midline position.

TERMINATION OF THE LAPAROSCOPIC PROCEDURE

At the end of the laparoscopic procedure, all ancillary trocars should be withdrawn under direct laparoscopic vision to ensure hemostasis. The patient is placed in a flat position and the laparoscope removed. Prior to the removal of the trocar, the abdominal cavity should be inspected for absence of bleeding or retroperitoneal hematoma (Figure 23).

Abdominal gas should be relieved by gentle pressure on the lower abdomen with the trumpet valve open to allow gas escape. The trocar sheath is removed with the valve open to prevent room air from entering the abdominal cavity. If any difficulties were encountered during needle or

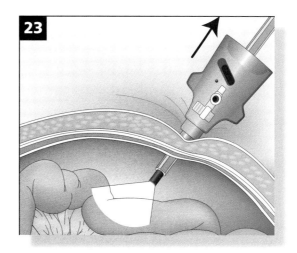

ALWAYS INSPECT THE ABDOMINAL CAVITY FOR ABSENCE OF BLEEDING, HEMATOMA OR BOWEL INJURY BEFORE WITHDRAWING THE LAPAROSCOPE.

trocar placement or if omental or bowel adhesions were seen during the laparoscopic procedure, the umbilical trocar should be withdrawn under laparoscopic guidance to make sure that no bowel adhesions were present in the umbilical area that might have been injured during trocar placement. Each fascial incision greater than 5 mm should be closed to prevent hernia formation. For incision closure, a 3-0 absorbable suture is used to approximate deep fascia and skin (Figure 24). Usually after laparoscopic procedures a certain amount of gas or irrigation fluid stays trapped in the peritoneal cavity. This gas may irritate the peritoneum, and patients may feel discomfort and minor pain referred to

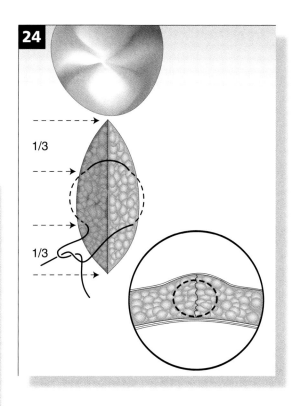

- CHECK FOR HEMOSTASIS BEFORE TERMINATING THE LAPAROSCOPIC PROCEDURE.

- WITHDRAW THE ANCILLARY TROCARS UNDER DIRECT LAPAROSCOPIC VISION TO CHECK FOR HEMOSTASIS.

- IF MORE ATTEMPTS WERE MADE BEFORE ESTABLISHING ADEQUATE PNEUMOPERITONEUM, OR IF UMBILICAL ADHESIONS ARE OBSERVED, WITHDRAW THE TROCAR SLOWLY BEFORE RELEASING THE PNEUMOPERITONEUM TO CHECK FOR POSSIBLE BOWEL INJURIES. IF NO ABNORMALITIES ARE OBSERVED REINSERT THE TROCAR SLEEVE, AND RELEASE THE PNEUMOPERITONEUM.

- CLOSE ALL FASCIAL INCISIONS OF 1 CM AND GREATER USING THE ABSORBABLE SUTURE.

- FOR 5-MM INCISIONS ONLY SKIN CLOSURE IS PERFORMED.

the shoulder area up to 2 weeks after the procedure.

After laparoscopic surgery, proper written documentation should be recorded. The advantage of the laparoscopic procedure is that each surgery can be videotaped, or color prints can be made, using a video printer. This visual documentation may be used for future reference.

SUGGESTED READING:

Mumford SD, Bhiwandiwala PP, Chi IC. Laparoscopic and minilaparotomy female sterilization compared in 15,167 cases. Lancet 1980;ii(8203):1066-70

Hasson HM. Open laparoscopy: a report of 150 cases. J Reprod Med 1974;12:234-8

Morgan HR. Laparoscopy: introduction of pneumoperitoneum via transfundal puncture. Obstet Gynecol 1979;54:260-1

Wolfe WM, Pasic R. Transuterine insertion of Veress needle in laparoscopy. Obstet Gynecol 1990;75:456-7

Palmer R. Safety in laparoscopy. J Reprod Med 1974;13(1):1-5

Childers JM, Brzechffa PR, Surwit EA. Laparoscopy using the left upper quadrant as the primary trocar site. Gynecol Oncol 1993;50:221-5

Reich H, Levie M, McGlynn F, Sekel L. Establishment of pneumoperitoneum through the left ninth intercostal space. Gynaecological Endoscopy 1995;4:141-3

Dingfelder JR. Direct laparoscope trocar insertion without prior pneumoperitoneum. J Reprod Med 1978;21:45-7

Mlyncek M, Truska A, Garay J. Laparoscopy without use of the Veress needle: results in a series of 1600 procedures. Mayo Clin Proc 1994;69:1146-8

Vakili C, Knight R. A technique for needle insufflation in obese patients. Surg Laparosc Endosc 1993;3:489-91

Ballem RV, Rudomanski J. Techniques of pneumoperitoneum. Surg Laparosc Endosc 1993;3:42-3

Penfield AJ. How to prevent complications of open laparoscopy. J Reprod Med 1985;30:660-3

Chapter 5

72 | **CREATION OF PNEUMOPERITONEUM AND TROCAR INSERTION TECHNIQUES** . . . .

A Consensus document concering laparoscopic entry techniques. Middlesbrough, March 19-20 1999 Gynecol Endoscopy 1999;8: 403-6

Byron JW, Fujiyoshi CA, Miyazawa K. Evaluation of the direct trocar insertion technique at laparoscopy. Obstet Gynecol 1989;74:423-5

Poindexter AN, Ritter M, Fahim A, Humprey H. Trocar introduction performed during laparoscopy of the obese patient. Surg Gynecol Obstet 1987;165:57-9

Hurd WW, Bude RO, Delancey JO, Pearl ML. The relationship of the umbilicus to the aortic bifurcation; implications for laparoscopic technique. Obstet Gynecol 1992;80:48-51

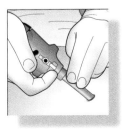

USING ELECTROSURGERY AND ULTRASONIC ENERGY DURING OPERATIVE LAPAROSCOPY

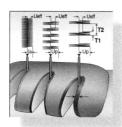

Andrew I. Brill, M.D.

FUNDAMENTALS OF ELECTRICITY

Electricity is produced when valence electrons are freed from atoms of conductive materials. When these electrons are set in motion in the same direction an electric current (I) is produced that is measured in amperes. Opposite charges on the ends of the conductor cause the electrons to flow in one direction toward the positive terminal. The difference in potential between the positive and negative poles provides the electromotive force (voltage) to drive the current through the conductor (Figure 1).

Current that flows in one direction through a circuit is called direct current (DC). When alternating current (AC) flows through a circuit, the movement of electrons reverses direction at regular intervals, which is expressed as cycles per second (Hertz). Since the effects of current on the load are all that is important, the periodic reversal of current flow does not undo its work.

The amount of current that flows through a circuit is determined by the electromotive force (voltage) across the circuit and the resistance that circuit provides to the current. Resistance (R) is the difficulty that a material presents to the flow of electrons and is measured in Ohms. Resistance of biologic tissues varies depending upon the water content. It is very high in desiccated tissue, moderate in lipid-rich adipose tissue, and very low in vascular tissue. Resistance for alternating current is expressed as impedance due to the induction of additional resistive phenomena (inductance) that include the effects of imploding electrostatic fields and the oppositional electromotive force of out-of-phase magnetic fields.

Current is directly proportional to the voltage and inversely proportional to the resistance, as expressed by Ohm's law:

$$I = V / R$$

Therefore, greater resistance requires greater voltage and, with a fixed resistance, greater voltage creates greater current. When the switch of an electrical circuit is left open (i.e., when the resistance is infinite) as when keying an electrosurgical electrode without tissue contact, it is logical that the energy

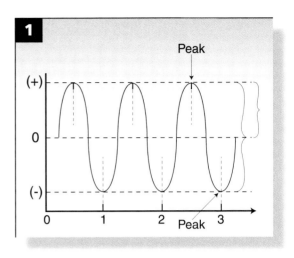

source will work at maximum voltage. This means that an electrosurgical generator produces the highest voltage across the electrode when it is activated remotely from the tissue surface without current flow.

Power is the rate of doing work and is expressed in watts (W). It represents the total quantity of electrons moved and the pressure gradient against which the movement occurred, as expressed by the equation.

$$W = I \times V$$
Inserting Ohm's Law:
$$W = I^2 \times R \text{ and } W = V^2 / R$$

Therefore, power to tissue increases as a function of both the square of the voltage and the square of the current.

The ratio of voltage to current is primarily responsible for the electrosurgical effects on tissue. Other important factors are time (duration of current application) and power density. The power density represents the amount of energy applied per unit of surface and time, and can be represented in the following way.

$$\text{Power density} = \frac{\text{Power output} / \text{Time}}{\text{Surface}}$$

This equation shows that if time is kept constant, power density depends upon the wattage and surface of the active electrode. Change in power density can be achieved by changing the power output, or by changing the contact area. Indeed to maximize power density we use higher energy output and a small contact electrode (Figure 2).

PRINCIPLES OF ELECTROSURGERY

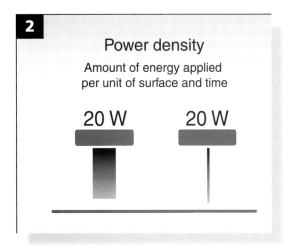

Power density
Amount of energy applied per unit of surface and time

20 W   20 W

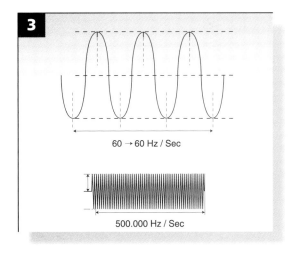

60 → 60 Hz / Sec

500.000 Hz / Sec

CURRENT

Using current that reverses its direction periodically, electrosurgery is exclusively performed with high frequency alternating current. The frequency with which current changes direction is measured in cycles per second or Hertz (Hz). Since electrosurgery only relies on the effects of current on the load (tissue), this periodic reversal does not undue the tissue effects. Normal household current has a frequency of 60 Hz (cycles per second). Low frequency alternating current causes tetanic neuromuscular activity by rapidly reversing depolarization of neuromuscular tissue (faradic effects). These effects do not occur at frequencies greater than 100,000 cycles per second (Hz), where the net positional change of cellular ions is minimal.

Justifiably then, electrosurgery is typically performed using alternating currents ranging between 500,000 and 3 million Hz (Figure 3).

BIPOLAR AND MONOPOLAR MODES

Bipolar electrosurgery utilizes two terminals of equal size that are extremely close by virtue of being situated across from one another at the end of an electrosurgical instrument. Rather than the patient being part of the electrical circuit, the current is only conducted by the tissue restricted between the distal electrodes (Figure 4). In monopolar electrosurgery, current is passed through the body by applying two differently shaped electrodes at distant locations of the body. Since the surgical electrode is much smaller than the return electrode, tissue effects are moderated by substantially different current densities (Figure 5).

WAVEFORMS

Although most contemporary electrosurgical generators have front panel controls that are labeled 'cut', 'blend', and 'coag', these terms are not necessarily related to actual tissue effects. The variety of choices simply reflect different degrees of waveform modulation (damping) that can be incre-

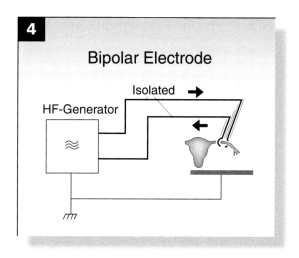

4

Bipolar Electrode

HF-Generator

Isolated

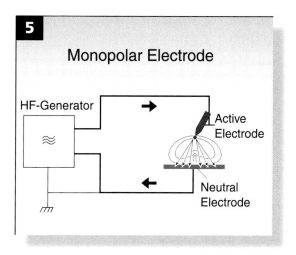

5

Monopolar Electrode

HF-Generator

Active Electrode

Neutral Electrode

mentally produced by the generator's solid state circuitry. Modulation is the periodic interruption of current flow (Figure 6). The 'cut' mode of the generator produces an unmodulated (undamped) pure sine wave with a relatively low peak voltage. The 'coag' mode produces the most modulated waveform that correspondingly has the highest peak voltage. Therefore, for equal power settings, increasing waveform modulation (i.e., switching from 'cut' to 'blend' to 'coag') causes the peak voltage to proportionally increase, i.e., energy must be conserved (Figure 7).

GROUNDING

A fundamental understanding of grounding is necessary to practice monopolar electrosurgery with safety. A ground is any form of conductive connection between an electrical circuit and earth. Since the earth has an infinite capacity to absorb electrical charges, any electrically charged object connected to earth will equalize its potential difference with the earth.

THE DISPERSIVE ELECTRODE PAD

Although the dispersive electrode pad provides a pathway of low impedance for returning current to the generator, its misapplication can result in catastrophic thermal insult that is usually undetected at the time of injury. The rules for proper usage seek to minimize impedance while providing the greatest surface area for current return. Impedance is primarily minimized by choosing a site with adequate water content for conduction. Areas of skin with hyperkeratosis or hair and those that overlie dense fat deposits

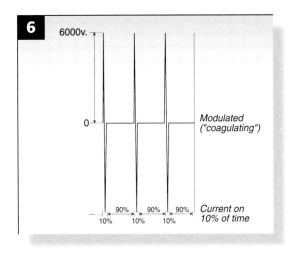

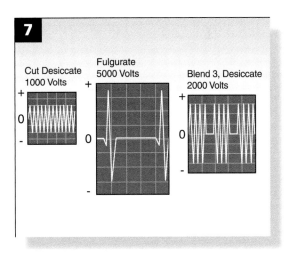

(e.g., buttocks) should be avoided, while hair-free or shaved skin over larger muscles is preferred (e.g., upper thigh). Impedance is further reduced by choosing a site as close as possible to the active electrode (Figure 8). The surface area of the return electrode must be large enough to permit the returning current to be widely dispersed. Tissue heating is intimately related to current density; current density is inversely related to the square of the surface area, and the rise in tissue temperature is directly proportional to the square of the current. Therefore, small decrements in the surface area between the dispersive pad and the skin can dramatically result in injurious thermal effects to the underlying tissues. A large surface area is guaranteed by a uniform and unalterable application. Areas with bony prominences are prone to movement on patient repositioning (such as the back and buttocks) and should be avoided. Since the edge of the dispersive electrode pad closest to the active electrode tends to concentrate the current, the longer edge of the pad should be placed toward the operative site.

ELECTRODE MONITORING SYSTEMS

Contemporary electrosurgical generators are equipped with an automatic alarm and shutdown mechanism that activates when the connection between the generator and the return electrode is not intact. However, this does not monitor the adequacy of contact between the surface of the grounding pad and the patient. Since the impedance to the flow of current via the dispersive electrode is quite

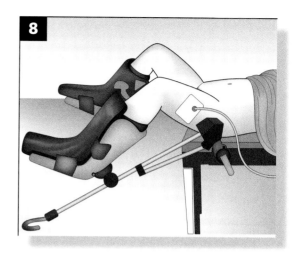

small until most of the pad has peeled away, any drop in electrosurgical effectiveness should alarm the surgeon to check the application of the dispersive electrode.

Valleylab (Boulder, CO) originally introduced a return electrode monitoring system (REM) that monitors the dispersive pad's connection to the generator and the degree of contact with the patient. The dispersive pad is split into two functional halves; a small current is generated to flow through the first half, through the contiguous skin and tissue, and then via the other half to return to the generator, which electronically monitors the local impedance. If the impedance is exceeded by separation from the skin, then the circuit is opened and an alarm is sounded (Figure 9). This innovation in dispersive pad technology completely eliminates the risk of thermal damage from an unpeeled electrode.

TISSUE EFFECTS OF ELECTROSURGERY

Electrical energy when applied to the tissue owing to the impedance is transferred to thermal energy, and the tissue effect of this thermal energy directly depends on the temperature inside of the tissue and the time required to reach that temperature (Figure 10). Electrosurgical energy produces three distinct effects on tissue, and they are cutting, fulguration and desiccation.

By varying the rate and extent of the thermodynamic effects of electric current in biological tissue, high frequency electrosurgery is used to cut and/or coagulate. Although the efficiency of hemostasis is related to the depth of coagulation, it is of paramount importance that no more tissue suffers thermal damage than is absolutely needed. The art of electrosurgery is balancing between the need for absolute hemostasis and the least amount of deep coagulative necrosis.

CUTTING (ELECTROSECTION)

The cutting of tissue occurs when there is sufficient voltage (at least

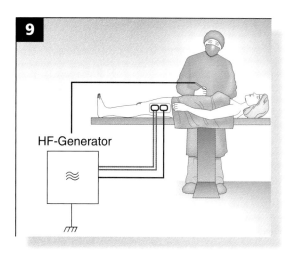

HF-Generator

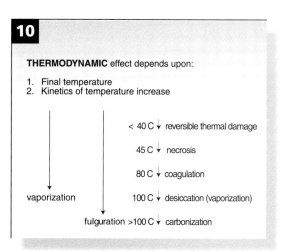

THERMODYNAMIC effect depends upon:

1. Final temperature
2. Kinetics of temperature increase

< 40 C reversible thermal damage
45 C necrosis
80 C coagulation
vaporization 100 C desiccation (vaporization)
fulguration >100 C carbonization

200 V) between the electrode and the tissue to produce an electric arc, which concentrates the current to specific points along the tissue surface. The open circuit creates an electric field that ionizes the intervening air. An avalanche of colliding and accelerating charged ions forms a plasma cloud that gives off light and sound as the ions pass to lower energy states to produce an electric arc (Figure 11). The

extremely high current density delivered by the arc rapidly superheats the cellular water to temperatures greater than 6000°C. Explosive cellular vaporization ensues secondary to the production of highly disruptive pressure (steam occupies 6 times the volume of liquid water!) and acoustic forces. Arcing is then enhanced by an envelope of steam vapor that becomes instantly ionized. The use of the unmodulated 'cut' waveform helps sustain this envelope by producing an uninterrupted current that continuously maintains the same pathways for arc formation. However, since the 'cut', 'blend' and 'coag' outputs all provide peak voltages greater than 200 V, any generator setting can be utilized to perform electrosection. In any case, tissue contact eliminates the steam envelope and abolishes the cutting arc.

In general, the depth of coagulation along the cut edges increases with increasing voltage and length or intensity of the electric arcs. Therefore, an unmodulated 'cut' waveform produces a cut with the least amount of coagulative necrosis, whereas waveforms with greater modulation and higher peak voltages (i.e., higher 'blend' and the 'coag' settings) result in substantially larger zones of coagulation (Figure 12).

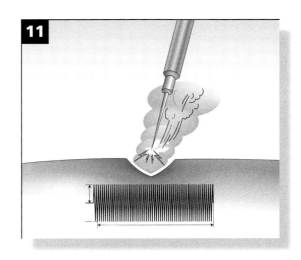

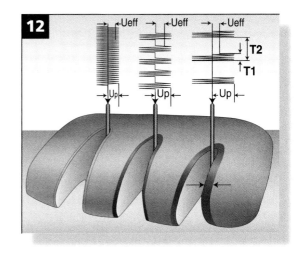

When using conventional electrosurgical generators, the smallest volume of coagulation during electrosection is assured by employing the thinnest possible electrodes (i.e., edge rather than surface), using the unmodulated 'cut' waveform with low peak voltage, and cutting as rapidly as possible using a single pass of the electrode. Deeper coagulation occurs when opposite parameters are applied. A higher 'blend' (i.e., blend 2 or 3) or the 'coag' waveform may be selectively employed during the electrosection of highly vascular tissues (e.g., leiomyoma) to provide a significant measure of hemostasis along the cut margins.

A new breed of electrosurgical generators incorporate automatic control circuits to ensure that the intensity of the electric arcs and the output voltage are kept constant (constant voltage generator). This makes the depth of coagulation relatively independent of the cutting rate and depth, as well as the magnitude of the output current. Thus, the distance of coagulation remains constant regardless of the magnitude of the output current. With this type of equipment, the operator can move the electrode as quickly or slowly as desired and at any angle without significantly affecting the depth of coagulation.

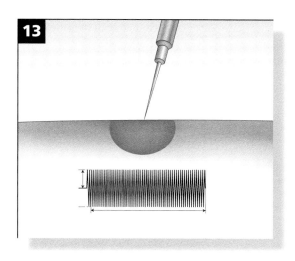

DESICCATION AND COAGULATION

Contact of tissue with the surface of an active electrode leads to conduction of current with a low current density (Figure 13). Resistive heating is produced by the high frequency agitation

of intracellular ionic polarities. As the tissue is slowly heated to temperatures above 50°C and maintained, irreversible cellular damage is initiated by deconfiguration of regulatory proteins followed by the denaturation of cellular proteins (white coagulation). Further heating to 100°C leads to complete evaporation of cellular water (desiccation), hemostasis secondary to the contraction of blood vessels and the surrounding tissues, and conversion of collagens to glucose that has an adhesive effect between the tissue and electrode. Temperatures above 200°C cause carbonization and charring. The prudent application of monopolar electrosurgery to tissue is continuously moderated by monitoring for the terminal evanescence of steam formation and tissue whitening; tissue charring and smoke are indicative of overzealous coagulation.

Until the tissue reaches a temperature of 100°C and is completely desiccated, the rise in tissue temperature is directly proportional to the tissue resistance (degree of desiccation), time of current flow, and the square of the current density. Therefore, temperature change is more rapid at superficial depths, and evolves more gradually with larger surface electrodes.

As the tissue is progressively desiccated, current flow is moderated by a zone of electrically insulated steam vapor that forms between the electrode and tissue. The flow of current will eventually cease based on the output voltage. At lower voltages using the unmodulated 'cut' waveform, the coagulative process continues until the tissue is entirely dried out (soft coagulation). Continued application of current after completion of the evaporative phase leads to tissue adherence. Therefore, soft coagulation should ideally be terminated at the time of vapor formation.

At higher voltages when using modulated waveforms (especially with smaller electrodes and higher current densities), the vapor layer and desiccated tissue are punctured by electric arcs (forced coagulation) causing further coagulation until the coagulum is

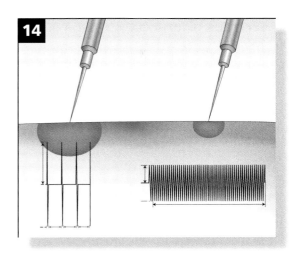

so thick it cannot be penetrated. Tissue becomes carbonized, sticky, and precariously unstable. This results in deeper coagulation at the expense of greater force, intense arcing, and increased temperature generation (Figure 14).

During soft coagulation, the lower voltage of the 'cut' waveform heats the tissue more slowly so heat can flow into deeper tissue layers. Hence, it can be said that soft coagulation is more effective coagulation. Since the reduction of abnormal uterine bleeding after endometrial ablation is related to the degree of destruction of the basalis layer and superficial myometrium, it can be formally argued that the unmodulated 'cut' waveform should be used during hysteroscopic electrocoagulation of the endometrium .

In consideration of all the physical parameters that govern the behavior and effects of high frequency alternating electric current in biological tissue, laparoscopic monopolar electrosurgery should ideally be performed using the unmodulated 'cut' waveform for cutting and deep coagulation of tissue. Any electrode configured with both a flat surface and an edge (e.g., spatula electrode, electrosurgical scissors) can be used as an all-purpose electrosurgical tool with this waveform. The concentration of current at the edge or tip of the electrode provides arcing and hemostatic cutting of tissue. Blunt dissection, tissue traction, coaptation of small blood vessels, and contact coagulation can all be effectively accomplished using the flat surface (Figure 15).

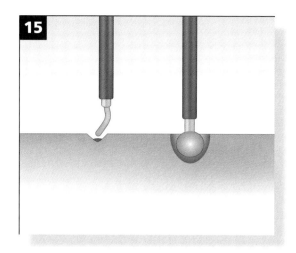

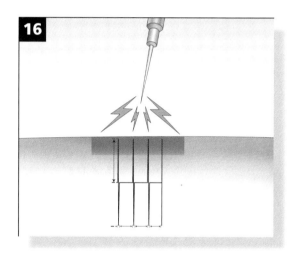

FULGURATION

Electric arcs generated by modulated waveforms with higher peak voltages (fulguration) can superficially coagulate a broad surface of tissue with open vessels as large as 2 mm (Figure 16). Current modulation allows the steam envelope to dissipate between the interruption of sparks, causing the electric arcs to strike the tissue surface in a widely dispersed and random fashion, thereby preventing tissue cutting. Although the higher voltage sparks are larger and create broad areas of charring (T0 > 500°C) and tissue destruction, current flow is limited to the superficial tissue layers due to rapid desiccation and the build-up of tissue resistance. Fulguration is relatively useless in the presence of a wet surgical field due to the diffusion of current by saline rich blood.

Teleologically then, the only selective indication for using the highly modulated 'coag' waveform during monopolar electrosurgery, is for the superficial coagulation of tissue along a large surface area. Exemplary needs for fulguration during laparoscopic surgery include the myometrial bed after myomectomy, the base of the ovarian cortex after cystectomy, and for oozing veins enwrapping Cooper's ligament during colposuspension. Since thermal effects are kept quite superficial by the rapid surface desiccation, fulgurative current is the best choice to superficially electrocoagulate areas of endometriosis over vital structures such as the bladder and ureter.

The Argon Beam Coagulator (ABC) is a true fulgurating electrosurgical device that utilizes the flow of argon gas through an electrode device to form a comparatively longer bridge of electric arcs to the tissue. This gas is easier to ionize than air allowing the electric arcs to create a more uniform surface coagulation effect. The high flow of gas (4 L/min) displaces oxygen and nitrogen as well as pooled blood, which focuses the effective surface area, and reduces the formation of smoke, carbonization, and tissue build-up on the tip of the electrode.

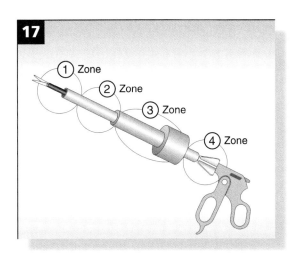

PROBLEMS OF MONOPOLAR ELECTROSURGERY DURING LAPAROSCOPIC SURGERY

Contrary to the open surgical environment during laparotomy, the bulk of most instruments and nearly all surrounding intraabdominal structures are not visualized during any laparoscopic procedure. Furthermore, nearly all of the potential conductors during laparoscopic electrosurgery are also out of the surgeon's field of view. Intended and unintended couriers of direct or induced currents include the abdominal wall, metallic trocar sheaths and instruments, the operating laparoscope, contiguous visceral tissues, and the active electrode (which is the only part of the circuit under view!) (Figure 17). It comes as no surprise that most accidental electrosurgical burns during laparoscopic surgery are undetected at the time of injury.

INSULATION FAILURE

Insulation failure occurs secondary to breaks or holes in the insulation caused by physical abruption during use (such as during passage through an incompletely engaged trumpet cannula) or during normal reprocessing procedures. Completely intact insulation (especially on disposable instrumentation) can be breached by very high voltage (e.g., during open circuit activation or using a modulated 'coag' waveform). Any break or breach in insulation may provide an alternate pathway for the flow of current. If the defective portion of insulation contacts tissue during electrode activation, an electric arc will bridge directly from the electrode through the defect to this tissue (Figures 18 and 19). Thermal damage will occur if the current density is high enough to significantly heat the tissue. Since these defects are usually out of the field of view, this type of injury usually occurs undetected at the time of insult.

Insulation failure can be minimized by periodically inspecting the insulation covering of all laparoscopic electrodes (especially at the shoulder) for small cracks and defects. Disposable monopolar electrodes should not be reused. The risk of high voltage can be eliminated by using the unmodulated

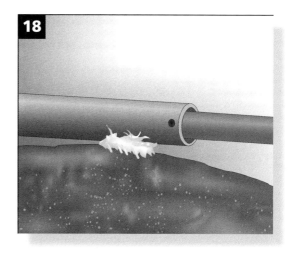

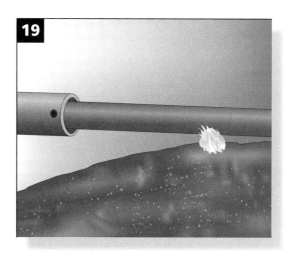

'cut' waveform, and avoiding open circuit activation.

DIRECT COUPLING

Direct coupling of current occurs when an activated electrode makes unintended contact with another metal object in the area of the surgical field. Accidental electrode contact with

Chapter 6

86 | USING ELECTROSURGERY AND ULTRASONIC ENERGY DURING OPERATIVE LAPAROSCOPY . . . .

a suction–irrigator probe, the operating laparoscope, or a metal cannula creates an alternate pathway that is normally conducted up through a metal trocar to the abdominal wall and back to the dispersive electrode. However, if any of these devices are isolated from direct contact with the abdominal wall by an insulator (e.g., plastic cannula or self-retaining device), the current may take an alternate pathway through a point of contact with adjacent tissue (Figure 20). Again, if the current density is high, thermal damage may occur.

Direct coupling can be avoided by never activating the generator when the electrode is touching or in near proximity to another metal object in the surgical field.

CAPACITIVE COUPLING

Capacitance is the property of an electrical circuit to store energy. Any device that creates capacitance is called a capacitor. A capacitor exists whenever two conductors that have different potentials are separated by an insulator. A difference of potential or voltage will exist between two conductors that have differing numbers of free electrons (an overall negative charge on the conductor with excess, and a positive charge on the electron-deficient conductor). Although separation by an

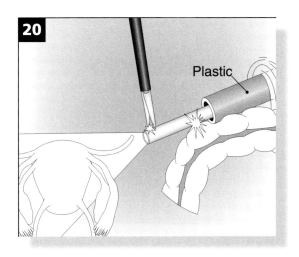

insulator prevents the flow of electrons between these conductors, the potential difference nevertheless creates an attraction or electrostatic force between them. This force results in an electric field and creates a reservoir of stored energy. When an alternating current flows through a circuit, the applied voltage and flow of current periodically changes direction. This means that a capacitor with alternating current is continuously 'charged' in alternating directions. With each reversal of current flow, the energy of the stored electric field is discharged. Although no actual current flows through the capacitor, the charged current from capacitance completes the circuit and in essence conducts the alternating current. Since the amount of capacitance is directly proportional to the voltage, capacitance is greatest during open circuit activation and with highly modulated current such as the 'coag' waveform.

Capacitive coupling is the induction of stray current to a surrounding conductor through the intact insulation of an active electrode. In fact, all of the necessary ingredients for the localized genesis of capacitance are provided by an activated monopolar electrode that is passed through a conductive sheath.

Two conductors of differing potentials, the active electrode and the metal sheath (e.g., trocar sheath, working channel of an operating laparoscope, irrigator–aspirator probe), are separated by the insulation of the electrode (Figures 21 and 22). On activation, up to 80% of the generator current is induced on the metal sheath by capacitance. Normally this stray current is safely returned to the dispersive electrode by conduction through the large area of contact between the metal trocar sheath and the abdominal wall. The magnitude of capacitance is greater with higher voltage, smaller cannulas, and longer electrodes. Furthermore, the induced current will persist until the electrode is deactivated or it is conducted via an alternate pathway.

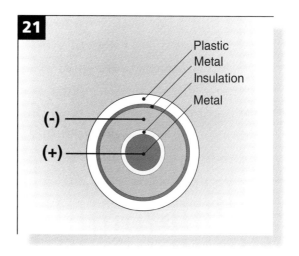

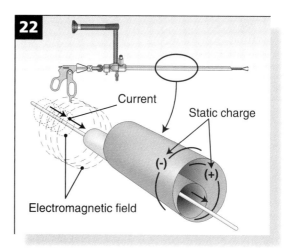

If the metal trocar sheath is attached to the abdominal wall by a nonconductive plastic device (e.g., hybrid trocar (metal/plastic) or plastic self-retaining screw device), the induced current becomes electrically isolated from the abdominal wall. Contact between the cannula and a visceral structure provides an alternate pathway for the stray current to discharge (Figure 23). Significant thermal damage will occur if the current density is sufficiently concentrated by a small area of contact. A similar phenomenon of capacitive coupling and isolation of current may occur during activation of an electrode placed through the working port of an operating laparoscope that is isolated from the abdominal wall by an all plastic cannula. In either case, the thermal injury is usually out of the surgeon's field of view.

Capacitance is minimized by using an unmodulated 'cut' waveform and avoiding open circuit activation (i.e., minimizing voltage). An all-metal system will suffice for the safe conduction of capacitively coupled current back to the dispersive electrode. Hybrid cannula systems (mixtures of plastic and metal) should not be used to house monopolar electrosurgical devices.

BIPOLAR ELECTROSURGERY

During monopolar electrosurgery, a high density of electrons leave the active electrode and are ultimately dispersed over the broad surface of a return electrode pad. The current returns to the generator after the electrons pass through the patient via a myriad of variably conductive pathways.

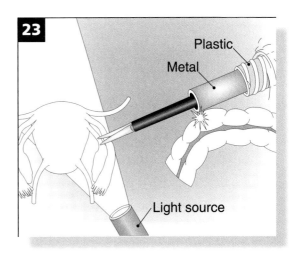

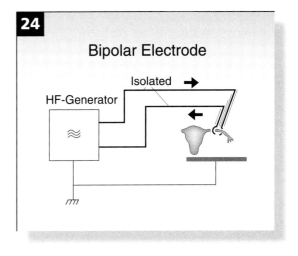

Bipolar technology consolidates an active electrode and a return electrode into an electrosurgical instrument with two small poles (e.g., tines of forceps or blades of scissors) (Figure 24). Rather than coursing through the patient, the flow of alternating current is symmetrically distributed through the tissue between the poles, reversing direction every 1/2 cycle. This eliminates the risk of capacitive coupling and alternate current pathways. Power requirements are significantly less than with monopolar surgery due to the current concentration between the poles. Therefore, an unmodulated 'cut'waveform with low peak-to-peak voltage is the generator output during bipolar electrosurgery (Figure 25). These factors intrinsically limit the thermal effects to desiccation and coagulation of tissue.

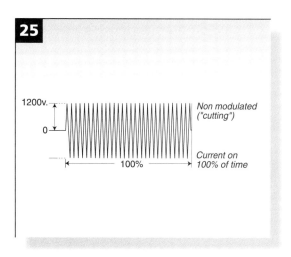

Bipolar electrosurgery is used for laparoscopic tubal sterilization by sequentially grasping and desiccating the midportion of the Fallopian tube and adjacent mesosalpinx with the Kleppinger forceps. Failure of this method usually results from incomplete destruction of the tubal lumen with persistent viability of the endosalpinx. Complete desiccation is best ensured by including the vascular portion of the tube in the forceps, coagulating at least 3 cm of contiguous areas along the ampullary portion of the tube, using relatively low power (25 W) and an inline ammeter to ensure that the tissue is completely desiccated (Figure 26).

The localization of current between the poles of the instrument during bipolar electrosurgery offers several distinct advantages. Thermal damage is generally limited to a discrete

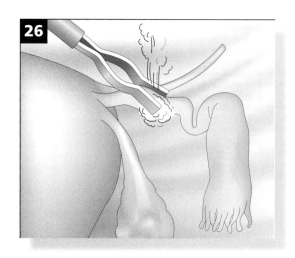

volume of tissue. The bipolar forceps can be used to coapt and thermally weld blood vessels. The concentrated current and small distance between the poles makes it possible to desiccate tissue that is immersed in fluid. The apparent disadvantages of this modality arise when open blood vessels are retracted or tissue pedicles are very thick.

Although the flow of current and primary thermal effects are restricted to the tissue between the poles, this does not remove the risk of thermal effects to tissue that is distant from the operative site. In fact, the net thermal effects are also governed by the physical parameters described during monopolar electrosurgery. The application of bipolar current leads to the gradual desiccation of the intervening tissue. The rate of tissue coagulation at any given power is moderated by the applied surface area of the poles, the thickness of the pedicle, the formation of a vapor layer between the poles and tissue, and the evanescing degree of tissue hydration. Impedance is maximal when the vapor phase is abolished as the tissue is completely desiccated. If the current is further applied and maintained more than several seconds, a secondary thermal bloom occurs to surrounding tissues from a correspondingly rapid rise in tissue temperature. Thus, tissues at some distance from the operative site may undergo subtle but irreversible thermal damage (e.g., the pelvic ureter during overzealous bipolar desiccation of the uterine artery).

During laparoscopic surgery, other than tubal sterilization, the spread of thermal damage during bipolar desic-

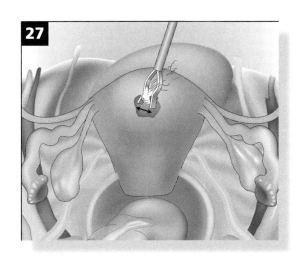

cation should be minimized by terminating the flow of current at the end of the vapor phase, cooling the surrounding tissues with irrigating solution, applying current in a pulsatile rather than continuous fashion, avoiding the use of an inline ammeter to determine the endpoint of desiccation, and securing vascular pedicles by using a stepwise process that alternates between partial desiccation and incremental cutting. The smallest depth of coagulative necrosis will occur when the sides or tips of a slightly open forceps are used to lightly 'paint' the tissue surface for directed hemostasis (Figure 27).

HARMONIC SCALPEL

The harmonic scalpel is an ultrasonically activated laparoscopic device that provides mechanical energy to cut and coagulate tissue. A piezoelectric crystal housed in the handpiece vibrates the tip of a titanium blade at 55,500 times/second over a variable excursion of 50-100 μm. Energy is transmitted through tissue primarily in a linear fashion, parallel to lines of force (Figure 28). Hydrogen bonds that maintain the configuration of tissue proteins are ruptured, gradually leading to a denatured protein coagulum up to 2 mm without significant desiccation or charring. Mechanical vibration and cavitational fragmentation of tissue parenchyma produce tissue cutting. Steam bubbles that form as the vaporization threshold is reduced by local changes in atmospheric pressure concurrently separate tissue planes in front of the tip.

Available 5-mm blades include a hook and curved electrodes for cutting and coagulating (Figures 29 and 30). The LCS-B5 is a 5-mm harmonic scalpel shear with a straight cylindrical active blade. Its shape is continuous circumferentially. The LCS-C5 is a 5-mm harmonic scalpel shear with a curved active blade. The curved blade has an increased amplitude compared to the straight blade, giving it an increased longitudinal motion, leading to increased cutting speed. The straight blade provides better hemostasis.

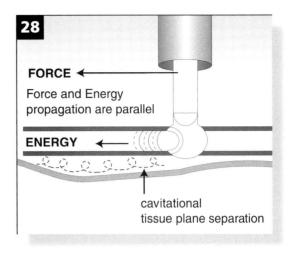

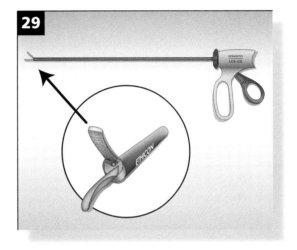

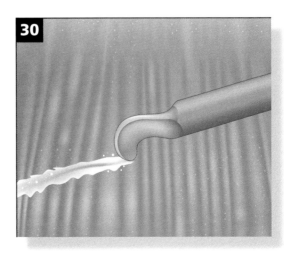

A 10-mm laparoscopic coagulating shears (LCS) provides coaptive coagulation and cutting by securing tissue between a grooved plastic pad and a 15-mm multipurpose rotational blade with sharp, blunt, and flat surfaces. By employing various combinations of blade configurations, blade excursion, and tissue tension, specific tissue effects are created with this device. Operationally, cutting should be considered the obverse of coagulation. Cutting velocity is proportional to blade excursion, tissue traction, and blade sharpness, and inversely related to density and elasticity of tissue. Coagulation is inversely related to tissue tension, blade sharpness, blade excursion, and cutting speed. Thus, the fastest cutting occurs when tissue is placed on tension and firmly squeezed, lifted, or rotated with the sharp side of the blade set at maximum excursion. Effective coagulation is best accomplished by relaxing tissue tension, minimizing blade excursion, and using a blunt edge or flattened surface. Although a zone of coagulation of less than 1 mm is typically created by coaptive incision with the LCS, it remains proportional to blade excursion, application time, and applied pressure.

Suggested Reading:

Ewing J. A Treatise on Tumors. 2nd ed. Philadelphia. WB Saunders. 1922:17

D'Arsonval MA. Action physiologique des courants alternaifs. Soc Biol 1891;43:283-286

Luciano A, Soderstrom R, Martin D. Essential principles of electrosurgery in operative laparoscopy. J Am Assoc Gynecol Laparosc 1994;1:189-195

Friedman J. The technical aspects of electrosurgery. Oral Surg 1973;36:177-187

Tucker RD, Benda JA, Sievert CE, et al. The effect of bipolar electrosurgical coagulation waveform on a rat uterine model of fallopian tube sterilization. J Gynecol Surg 1992;8:235-241

Erbe Elcktromedzin. Operating Instructions Manual. Erbotom ACC 450. Tubingen, Germany, 1990

Honig WM. The mechanism of cutting in electrosurgery. IEEE Trans Biomed Eng BME 1975;22:58-55

Sigel B, Dunn MR. The mechanism of bleed vessel closure by high frequency electrocoagulation. Surg Gynecol Obstet 1965;121:823-831

Nduka C, Super P, Monson J, et al. Cause and prevention of electrosurgical injuries in laparoscopy. J Am Coll Surg 1994;179:161

Wattiez A, Khandwala S, Bruhat MA. Electrosurgery in Operative Endoscopy. Oxford, Blackwell Science, 1995:81-92

Kelly HA, Ward GE. Electrosurgery. Philadelphia, WB Saunders, 1932

Vaincaillie TG. Electrosurgery at laparoscopy: Guidelines to avoid complication. Gynaecol Endosc 1994;3:143-150

Phipps JH. Thermometry studies with bipolar diathermy during hysterectomy. Gynaecol Laparosc 1994;3:5-7

Ryder RM, Hulka JF. Bladder and bowel injury after electrodesiccation with Kleppinger bipolar forceps: A clinicopathologic study. J Reprod Med 1993;3:595-598

Nezhat C, Crowgey Sr, Garrison CP. Surgical treatment of endometriosis via laser laparoscopy. Fertil Steril 1986;45:778-783

Reich J, MacGregor T III, Vancaillie T. CO_2 laser used through the operating channel of laser laparoscopes: In vitro study of power and power density losses. Obstet Gynecol 1991;77:40-47

Corson SL, Unger M, Kwa D, et al. Laparoscopic laser treatment of endometriosis with the Nd:YAG sapphire probe. Am J Obstet Gynecol 1989;160:718-723

Semm K. Endocoagulation: A new field of endoscopic surgery. J Reprod Med 1976;16:195-203

McCarus SD. Physiologic mechanism of the ultrasonically activated scalpel. J Am Assoc Gynecol Laparosc 1996;3:601-608

Hambley R, Hebda PA, Abell E. Wound healing of skin incisions produced by ultrasonically vibrating knife, scalpel, electrosurgery, and carbon dioxide laser. J Dermatol Surg Oncol 1988;14:1213-1217

Amaral JF, Chrostek C. Depth of thermal injury: Ultrasonically activated scalpel vs electro-surgery. Surg Endosc 1995;9:226

Luciano M, Whitman G, Maier DB, et al. A comparison of thermal injury, healing patterns, and postoperative adhesion formation following CO_2 laser and electromicrosurgery. Fertil Steril 1987;48:1025-1029

Tulandi T, Chan KL, Arseneau J. Histopathological and adhesion formation after incision using ultrasonic vibrating scalpel and regular scalpel in the rat. Fertil Steril 1994;61:548–560

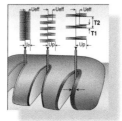

ALL YOU NEED TO KNOW ABOUT LAPAROSCOPIC SUTURING

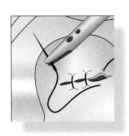

Resad Pasic, M.D., Ph.D.

Why do laparoscopic surgeons avoid suturing?

The perception is that it is cumbersome to learn and perform.

Surgeons are unfamiliar with:

- principles of needle introduction,

- principles of needle positioning and suturing, and knot tying techniques.

As laparoscopic hysterectomies, bladder suspensions, pelvic wall reconstructions and other advanced endoscopic procedures are becoming the accepted method of treatment, there is an increasing need for laparoscopic suturing techniques. Laparoscopic ligation and suturing is used for approximation of tissue planes and effectively provides hemostasis and prevents bleeding in laparoscopic surgery.

Laparoscopic suturing requires significant hand to eye coordination, since laparoscopic procedures are performed while monitoring a bidimensional TV screen with up to six times magnification; this eliminates depth perception and the direct tactile feeling of the tissue. Suturing represents the third level of laparoscopic skills.

The important steps in endoscopic suturing are:

1. Introduction of the needle and suture into the abdominal cavity;

2. Placement of the suture ligature;

3. Knot tying, either extracorporeal or intracorporeal.

The following equipment is required for laparoscopic suturing:

- laparoscopic needle holders;

- laparoscopic graspers;

- knot pusher;

- laparoscopic scissors;

- ligatures and sutures.

Two-handed manipulation is required to perform laparoscopic suturing and knot tying. This necessitates an assistant to hold the camera and laparoscope and to stabilize the laparoscopic ports. A zero-degree laparoscope should be used to permit a direct view. Proper placement of ancil-

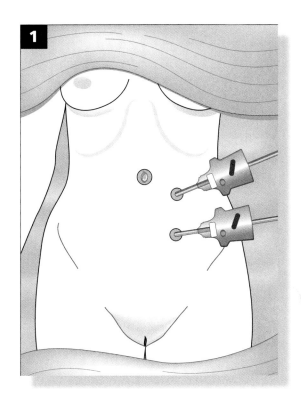

lary trocars is imperative for optimal suturing and knot tying. The tips of the instruments must be in front of the laparoscope, and should enter the field of view tangentially rather than in coaxial orientation, to prevent obscuring of the operative field. For laparoscopic surgery, the same principles of suture choice and suturing materials are applied as for conventional surgery.

For surgeons who are right handed, two ports above the pubic hairline, lateral to the deep epigastric vessels, on the patients left side are recommended for placement of laparoscopic needle-holder, and grasper (Figure 1). We recommend using another needle holder with articulating jaws, instead of the grasper, giving better needle handling during suturing, as well as the ability of placing a stitch with both hands.

Laparoscopic surgeries can be performed using 5-mm trocar sleeves, but a 10/11 disposable trocar for the introduction of the needle can also be used.

INSTRUMENTS

The needle holders have two designs: those with standard articulating jaws and self righting ones with fixed locking jaw mechanisms as in the Cook needle holder (Cook OB/GYN, Spencer, IN) which will not allow instrument tying.

Graspers can be used for tissue stabilization, needle holding or internal knot tying. Graspers with flat narrow tips are optimal, although some surgeons use two needle holders.

The laparoscopic knot pusher was first introduced by Dr. Courtenay Clarke in 1972. Clarke's horseshoe knot pusher (Marlow Surgical Technologies Inc., Willoughby, OH) is probably the most widely used.

For extracorporeal knot tying, a long ligature thread of at least 70 cm should be used. If an intracorporeal technique

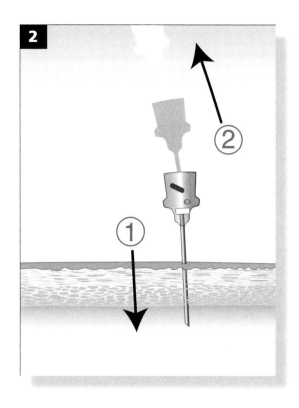

is utilized, the preferable ligature length is 10–12 cm.

Curved needles are increasingly utilized for hemostatic ligature placement, closure of tissue defects and suspension of organs. A majority of surgeons use CT-1, CT-2, or HS needles since they can be introduced into the peritoneal cavity through the disposable 10/11 trocar sleeves by grasping the suture near the needle hub with a 5-mm grasper and introducing it into the peritoneal cavity. Pop-off sutures should not be used in laparoscopic suturing. Techniques have also been described regarding the intraperitoneal introduction of any size needle for laparoscopic suturing without the use of large trocars.

INTRODUCTION OF A SUTURE IN THE PERITONEAL CAVITY

Dr. Harry Reich's technique allows the placement of any size curved needle into the abdominal cavity by using a 5-mm lower quadrant incision. This technique is shown in Figures 2–5.

The ancillary trocar is withdrawn from the abdominal wall. The trocar hole is plugged with the assistant's finger to prevent escape of gas from the peritoneal cavity (Figure 2).

The needle holder or grasper is inserted through the trocar sleeve, and the suture tail is grasped and pulled back through the trocar. The grasper is then reintroduced through the trocar along the suture and the suture is grasped about 3-4 cm above the needle hub (Figures 3 and 4).

The needle holder is then introduced into the peritoneal cavity through the same incision pulling the needle with it. When the needle is pulled into the abdominal cavity, the trocar sleeve is then pushed over the grasper using it as a guide to seal the incision in the abdominal wall (Figure 5).

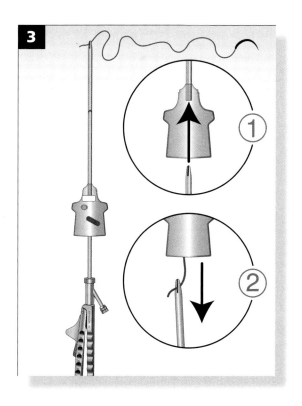

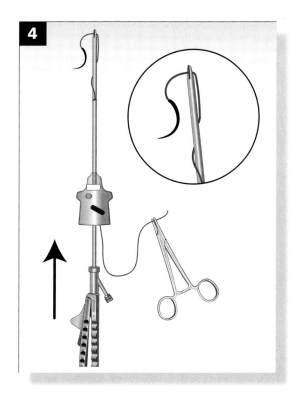

After introducing the needle into the abdominal cavity, the suture is fed into the abdominal cavity using a laparoscopic grasper. It is important to feed the suture into the abdominal cavity particularly if a helical, or figure of eight stitch is made. A small clamp is placed at the suture tail to prevent the tail of the suture from being pulled into the trocar.

HOW TO PLACE LIGATURES

In order to grasp the needle properly with the needle holder, the suture is held 1-2 cm above the needle hub and the needle is positioned so that the needle tip is facing toward the patient's left side. The laparoscopic needle holder is pushed forward to grasp the needle at a 90° angle 1/3 from the needle hub. A laparoscopic camera should be zoomed on the needle while the needle holder is grasping it and kept in the middle of the screen at all times (Figure 6).

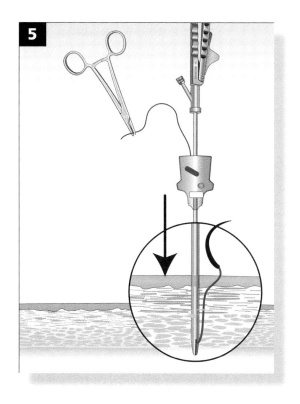

If the needle cannot be placed in a position to face toward the left side, it should be lowered down until it touches the bowel or pelvic structures, and then slowly turned and manipulated toward the patient's left.

When the needle is grasped with the needle holder, its position can be corrected by pulling the suture with the

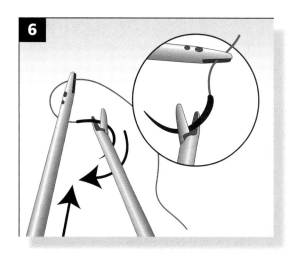

grasper, or by grasping the needle tip with the grasper and correcting its position while slightly loosening the needle holders grasp on the needle.

The grasper is used to hold the tissue being sutured, or it is pushed against the tissue to create a counter force while the needle is driven from the other side.

Due to the restricted instrument mobility in laparoscopic surgery, passing the needle through a tissue is limited by the trocar placement to a single rotating movement around the axis of the needle holder. Because of these limitations, it is crucial that the needle holder is secured with a firm grip onto the needle to avoid needle displacement and rotation in the needle holder's jaws. With practice, a good level of hand–eye coordination can be achieved.

When the needle is correctly grasped, suturing is performed by a gentle initial push followed by rotation of the wrist. When the needle tip is driven through the tissue it can be held by the grasper and pulled through by continuing the rotation of the needle and releasing the needle holder (Figure 7).

Some laparoscopic surgeons use straight needles for suturing. The straight needles can be easily introduced into the peritoneal cavity through 5-mm cannulas, and they are easily manipulated with laparoscopic instruments. The main disadvantage of

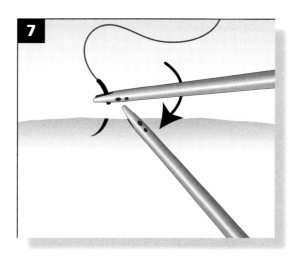

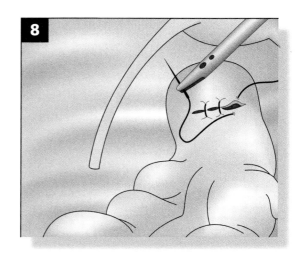

straight needles is that it is difficult to suture pedicles (Figure 8).

KNOT TYING

Secure knot formation is essential to laparoscopic suturing procedures. Knot tying can be divided into two general categories; extracorporeal knots formed outside of the body and pushed into the peritoneal cavity through the trocar sleeve by a knot pusher, and intracorporeal knots that are tied inside the abdominal cavity using laparoscopic instruments. Both techniques are safe and reliable and can be used in different clinical situations. The endoscopic surgeon should be familiar with both techniques in order to successfully perform advanced laparoscopic surgical procedures.

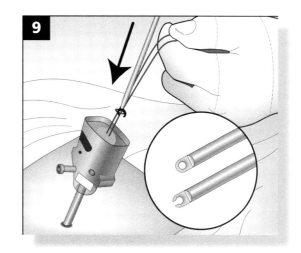

EXTRACORPOREAL KNOT TYING

After the suturing is completed, if the needle is introduced through a 5-mm port, the needle has to be cut off and temporarily parked in the anterior abdominal wall. If the needle was introduced through 10/11 trocar, it can be pulled out and cut off. If the needle is cut inside the peritoneal cavity, the suture end is grasped with the needle holder and pulled out through the same trocar sleeve where it was originally introduced. While the suture is drawn out of the abdomen, the rest of the ligature should be simultaneously fed into the peritoneal cavity to prevent pulling or sawing on the tissue.

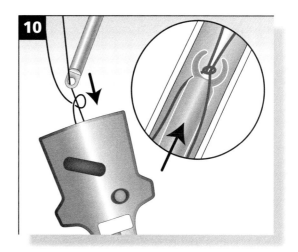

Holding both ends of the suture, a single simple knot is tied and pushed down with the knot pusher. Steady pressure should be maintained on the knot pusher and suture ends (Figures 9–11). Several knots should be placed on

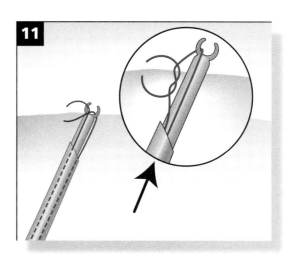

top of each other. The knot pusher sometimes may become dislodged during knot pushing because some polyfilament materials such as silk or catgut do not slide easily. If the knot pusher is dislodged the suture should be pulled with the grasper inside the peritoneal cavity until the knot can be located. The knot pusher is then placed on the knot under direct vision. If the knot cannot be seen, the whole suture should be pulled inside the abdomen, untangled, and both strings should be taken out through the trocar and a new knot placed.

Many surgeons prefer using the closed knot pusher for laparoscopic suturing (Figures 9 and 10). The closed knot pusher does not allow the knot to slip. One suture end is passed through the hole at the distal end of the knot pusher and a one-hand granny knot is tied with the other end of the suture and pushed into the abdomen with the knot pusher. After placing three knots, the other end of the suture is passed through the hole on the knot pusher, and the next three knots are placed. This maneuver locks the knots in place and prevents sliding.

After knot tying is completed and the suture has been cut, the needle is removed from the peritoneal cavity by grasping the suture about 2 cm away from the needle and extracting it

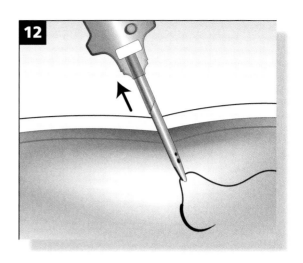

through a 10/11 trocar, or pulling it together with the 5-mm trocar sleeve, from the abdominal cavity. Careful observation of the needle is recommended to complete withdrawal (Figure 12).

INTRACORPOREAL KNOT TYING

The laparoscopic surgeon may choose to tie knots intraperitoneally. This technique involves instrument tying and requires certain skill. Intracorporeal knots are most often used for tissue fixation that does not require a lot of tension and less often for hemostasis since they cannot be tied with the same strength as extracorporeal knots. They are also used for anchoring a running suture, like those used for peritoneal closure, repair of bladder lacerations, or laparoscopic tubal reanastomosis. For intracorporeal knot tying, a short ligature of about 10–14 cm is used unless a running suture is placed, in which case a longer ligature is required. If the suture is too long, it can be very difficult to control the knot formation. The suture is passed into the peritoneal cavity as previously described, and following the suture placement, an instrument tie is performed within the peritoneal cavity. There are several types of intracorporeal knot tying, but only one is necessary. The surgeon must practice and learn the technique well.

SQUARE KNOT

This knot is tied utilizing the classic microsurgical technique of instrument tying. After the needle is passed through the tissue, the suture is pulled almost all the way, leaving only 1-2 cm of the suture tail at the site of the needle insertion. This knot is much easier to tie if the needle is attached to the suture. If the needle is still attached, it should be grasped with the left hand as shown in Figure 13. The grasper is held in the right hand and placed on top of the suture. The tip of the grasper is then moved in the rotating pathway describing a full circle down and back, and again forward through the needle. This motion of the grasper tip wraps

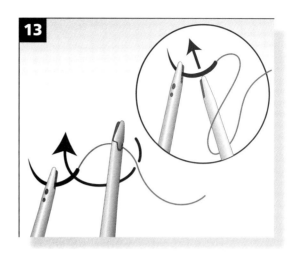

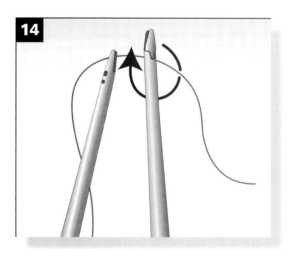

the suture around the grasper and forms the loop required for completion of the knot.

If the needle is not attached, the long tail of the suture is grasped with the needle holder, held in the left hand and rotated counterclockwise forming a mild upward curve of the suture. The grasper is introduced with the right hand parallel to the needle holder and placed forward on top of the suture (Figure 14). It is then moved in the rotating pathway, describing a full circle down and back, and again left and forward. This movement of the grasper forms the loop that wraps the suture around the grasper (Figures 15 and 16). Holding the jaws of the grasper open during this circular movement may help prevent the formed loop from slipping off its tip. After the loop is formed around the grasper, a short tail of the suture is grasped and pulled through the loop, while the needle holder provides countertraction on the opposite end of the suture. With this movement, the first flat knot is created (Figure 17).

The same procedure is repeated in the opposite direction, and a second locking knot is formed. A third optional opposing flat knot can be added in the same manner as the first knot.

LOOP LIGATURE

The loop ligature was originally demonstrated by Dr. Kurt Semm and was based on the Roeder Loop. The loop is closed when the distal portion is pulled while pushing the knot into place with the plastic slide. Ligation with the preformed loop has certain limitations, since it is restricted to open ended pedicles and utilizes a slip knot

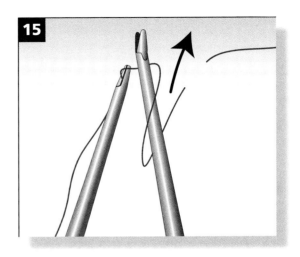

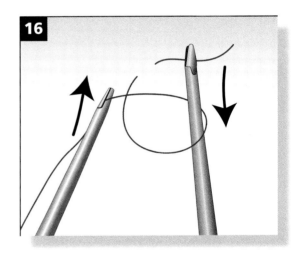

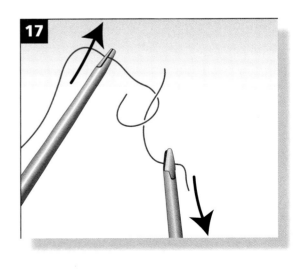

which may be prone to slipping, and requires a special introducer.

The loop ligature is back loaded into a hollow 3-mm tube called an applicator. The tube is then placed through a 5-mm trocar sheath. Loop ligature also can be directly placed through disposable 5 mm cannulas. The edges of the tissue to be adapted are then grasped through the loop with an appropriate instrument, and the loop is tightened. The tip of the loop applicator is placed on the exact spot where we want the knot to be and the loop is tightened (Figures 18 and 19). Scissors are introduced through a separate port and the loop ligature is cut.

This is the simplest way to close open pedicles; however, it may be more likely to produce adhesions. If prepackaged loop ligature is not available, a loop can be improvized by tying a Roeder knot extracorporeally, and using a suture applicator to push the knot into the abdominal cavity.

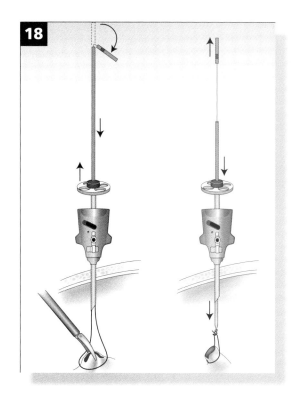

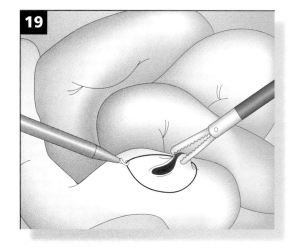

Suggested Reading:

Reich H, McGlynn F. Laparoscopic repair of bladder injury. Obstet Gyn 1990; 76: 909-10

Reich H. Laparoscopic hysterectomy. Surg Laparosc Endosc 1992; 2: 85-8

Liu CY, Paek W. Laparoscopic retropubic colposuspension (Burch procedure). J Am Assoc Gynecol Laparosc 1993; 1: 31-35

Soper NJ, Hunter JG. Suturing and knot tying in laparoscopy. Surg Clin N Am 1992; 72:1139-52

Clarke HC. Laparoscopy-new instruments for suturing and ligation. Fertil Steril 1972; 23: 274-77

Semm K. New method of pelviscopy for myomectomy, ovariectomy, tubectomy, and appendectomy. Endoscopy 1979; 11: 85-93

Reich H, Clarke HC, Sekel L. A simple method for ligating with straight and curved needles in operative laparoscopy. Obstet Gynec 1992; 79: 143-7

Semm K. Tissue-puncher and loop-ligation, new ideas for surgical therapeutic pelviscopy (laparoscopy) endoscopic intra-abdominal surgery. Endoscopy 1978; 10: 119-24

Hay LD, Levine RL, Von Frauenhopher AJ, Masterson JB. Chromic gut pelviscopic loop ligature effect of the number of pulls on the tensile strength. J Reprod Med 1990; 35: 260-2

Topel H. The video encyclopedia of endoscopic surgery for the gynecologist. Ed. Gerald S. Shirk. Tape 1, Medical Video Productions, 1994

Pasic R, Levine RL. Laparoscopic suturing and ligation techniques. J Am Assoc Gynecol Laparosc 1995; 3: 67-79

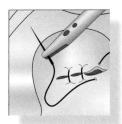

LAPAROSCOPIC TUBAL STERILIZATION

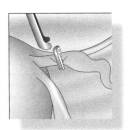

Ronald L. Levine, M.D.

Laparoscopic sterilization is the most common type of female sterilization surgery performed in the United States. There are essentially three major methods, however, occasionally a surgeon may still use thermal coagulation.

1. Electrosurgical:
   a. Monopolar
   b. Bipolar
2. Clips:
   a. Hulka
   b. Filshie
3. Bands (Fallope ring)
4. Thermal coagulation

All of the methods that will be described may be performed through either a single puncture technique using an operating laparoscope (Figure 1), or through a double puncture technique, using a 5-mm second puncture trocar that may be placed in the midline suprapubic area. The double puncture technique uses a 5 or 10-mm laparoscope that is inserted through the umbilical port (Figure 2). Our preference in recent years has been to use the single puncture technique unless there is difficulty in mobilizing the Fallopian tube. If the single puncture technique is the method of choice, it is very important that a well functioning uterine manipulator be employed. By moving the manipulator it is possible to stretch the tube laterally. The surgeon can control the operative field by moving the laparoscope in and out, to obtain close up or panoramic view, and by moving the instrument inserted through the operative channel.

One of the greatest causes of sterilization failure is the misidentification of either the round ligament or the uteroovarian ligament for the Fallopian tube. Therefore, it is vital to identify all three structures and to trace the tube to the fimbriae if at all possible, prior to performing the sterilization.

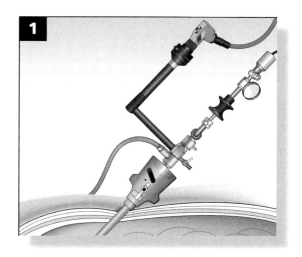

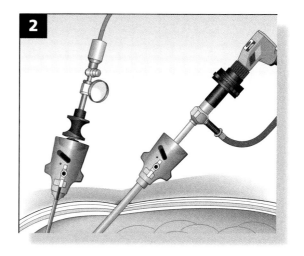

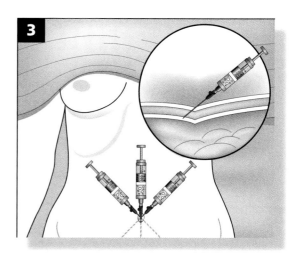

Although many of our sterilization procedures are performed under general anesthesia, a large number are accomplished under local. When local is the method, the skin and deeper tissues are blocked using lidocaine (Figure 3). The art, however, is to instill a mixture of 10 cc carbocaine and lidocaine transcervically via the uterine manipulator. The tubes can almost be seen to blanche (Figure 4). Prior to using the desired technique, we then drip another 10 cc of lidocaine along the length of the tube (Figure 5).

ELECTROSURGICAL

Monopolar electrosurgery is still used by some gynecologists, however, it has lost favor because of its risks of thermal bowel burns. The technique of bipolar coagulation, as originally described by Dr. Richard Kleppinger, is still the most popular form of laparoscopic sterilization and is our suggested form of electrosurgical management.

BIPOLAR

The bipolar Kleppinger type forceps have been described in Chapter 1. The tips of the forceps are where the energy is distributed from one tong to the other. It is therefore important that the tips enclose the tube as much as possible (Figure 6).

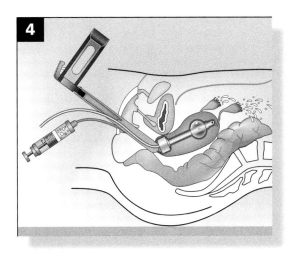

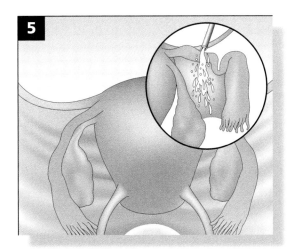

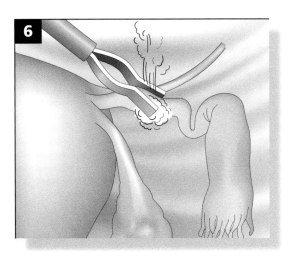

Bipolar coagulation provides a more localized area of tubal burn thus requiring at least 3 cm of tube to be coagulated. The tube is grasped in the isthmic portion of the tube at least 2 cm from the cornua (Figure 6). If too close to the uterus there is a risk of creating a uteroperitoneal fistula. The tips of the tongs should be minimally in the mesosalpinx to avoid too much damage to the blood supply of the tube and its anastamotic branches to the ovary. The electrosurgical generator should be set to deliver a power of 25 W in a non-modulated or cutting mode to desiccate the tissue sufficiently. If too much energy is used, the tube tends to be rapidly coagulated on the periphery, rather than through slow coagulation. This may lead to a sterilization failure. The tube should be coagulated with 2 to 3 contiguous burns to provide an area of about 3 cm of coagulation. The endpoint of coagulation is the cessation of current flow. This will supply a relatively accurate indication of complete

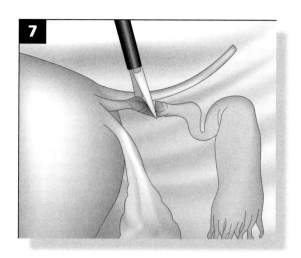

coagulation. Most electrosurgical generators have either a visual ammeter or an audio signal of this endpoint. After completing the coagulation, it has been our technique to sever the tube in the middle of the burn area with a laparoscopic scissors (Figure 7). However, there is some controversy regarding this and many surgeons do not cut the tube believing that it leads to a higher failure rate due to possible fistula formation.

CLIPS

Mechanical occlusion of the tube is most commonly performed using one of two types of clips. The most popular has been the Hulka-Clemens spring-loaded clip available since 1976. The clip itself is a plastic, hinged device that is closed by advancing a metal spring over the plastic jaws. The inner parts of the jaws have several small teeth that

---

IMPORTANT NUMBERS

2 CM FROM FUNDUS

3 CM OF TUBE

2-3 CONTINUOUS BURNS

25 W POWER

keep the clip in place (Figure 8). The clip requires a special laparoscopic applicator that may be passed through the single puncture operating laparoscope. This instrument is 7 mm and is inserted through the operating channel.

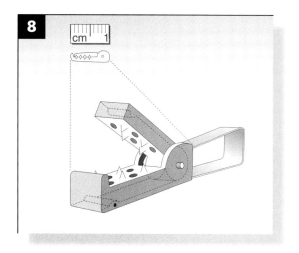

The clip applicator has four positions (Figure 9).

1. Safe open – In this position the clip is held on the end of the applicator and can be opened and closed without locking. This position is used when the applicator and clip are passed through the operating scope channel.

2. Safe closed – The tube is grasped with the clip and closed to this position. The clip may be removed by opening the clip applicator jaws.

3. Full closed – The thumb manipulator of the applicator drives the metal spring over the plastic jaws of the clip and locks it in place.

4. Full open – The ring on the handle is pulled back and the clip is thus removed from the applicator and left in place on the tube.

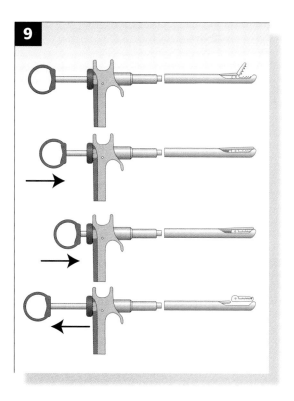

The applicator jaws are then closed and the instrument is removed. The clip should be applied on the isthmus at least 2 cm from the uterus and should be placed completely across the tube. This can be assured by observing that the tube rests completely against the hinge of the clip (Figure 10). With correct application, the mesosalpinx is pulled up to resemble the shape of an envelope flap. This is referred to as the 'Kleppinger envelope sign' (Figure 11). As noted above, because of a misapplication, it is sometimes necessary to apply more than one clip.

Although classically described, if the clip is in a bad position another clip should be placed because it was thought that the clip could not be removed. However, Dr. Walter Wolfe described a technique for removal of a clip that is simple and works well. A Kleppinger forcep may be passed using the tongs to grasp the sides of the clip (Figure 12). The Kleppinger holds the sides firmly and the clip easily is pulled off and is removed.

A secondary advantage of the clip is the fact that the area of damage to the tube is small. As such, a short segment of tube is destroyed and increases the ability for surgical reversibility.

Another style clip is the Filshie clip (Avalon Medical Corp., Williston, VT). Although first described in 1976 and used in the United Kingdom for many years, it was not approved in the United States until 1996. This clip is made of titanium with a silicone rubber lining that expands to keep the tube compressed as it flattens. This clip also requires a special applicator. It may

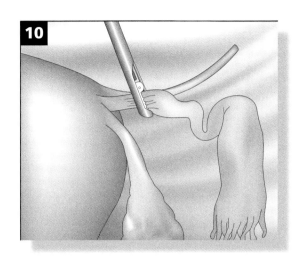

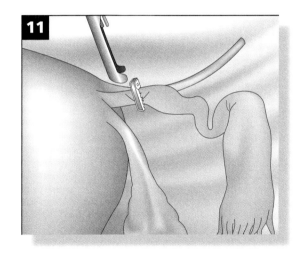

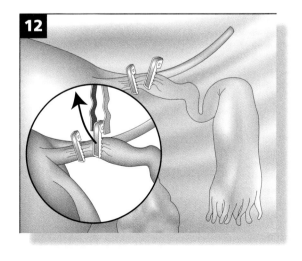

also be advanced into the abdomen through the operating channel of the single puncture operating laparoscope by half closing the upper jaw. When the finger bar is released the clip opens and is then placed (Figure 13). The Filshie clip is applied in a similar manner to the Hulka clip, on the isthmic portion of the tube. The bar is then squeezed to its limit thus closing the clip and releasing it from the applicator. The clip locks around the tube and cannot be removed. If misapplied another clip may be placed. A small area of the tube is crushed, so that similar to the Hulka clip, this method may yield a high success rate for surgical reversal. It has been stated by the CREST study that the Filshie clip has a relatively low failure rate.

BANDS

Yoon and associates introduced the silastic band in 1974. This small silastic band is applied to the tube by use of a special 8-mm applicator that may be used through the single puncture 12 mm operating laparoscope. The bands are preloaded onto the instrument using a special plastic loading device. The applicator is then passed down the channel and grasping hooks are deployed from the end of the applicator (Figure 14). The tube is grasped

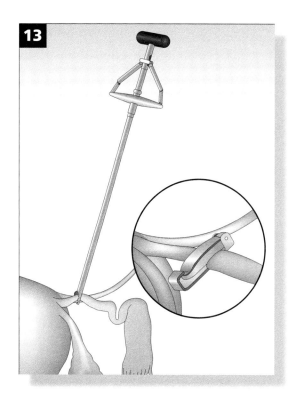

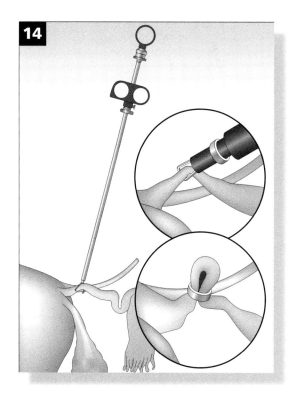

in the isthmic area about 3 cm from the cornua of the uterus. The tube is then drawn up into the inner cylinder of the applicator by the grasping hooks and the silastic band is applied by moving the outer cylinder forward. It is important that a sufficient knuckle of tube is brought back into the applicator to assure that two complete lumens have been occluded. After application of the band, the grasping tongs are moved forward out of the inner cylinder to release the occluded tube.

Several problems have been described with the bands. There have been a significant number of complications secondary to tears in the mesosalpinx. Bleeding from this problem can usually be controlled by bipolar coagulation. Postoperative pain is more frequent than with clips or bipolar coagulation. A large number of these patients require an oral analgesic for several days postoperatively.

THERMAL COAGULATION

Thermal coagulation is also known as tubal cautery. This technique has been

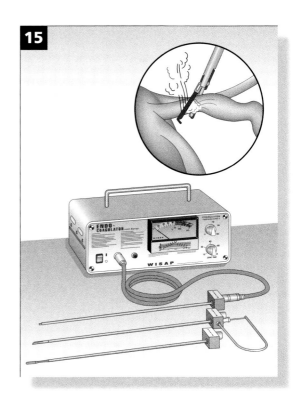

described primarily by Dr. Kurt Semm. He invented an instrument called the Semm Endotherm (Wisap, Lenexa, KS) (Figure 15). This instrument is best described as producing a soldering iron effect. The tips of the forcep are directly heated by an electric current to 120°C to 160°C. The tube is then grasped in a similar manner to the Kleppinger technique and the tube is held for 60 to 90 seconds to effect coagulation of the tissue.

SUGGESTED READING:

ACOG Technical Bulletin. Number 222. April 1996

Peterson, XIA and Hughes: The risk of pregnancy after tubal sterilization: Findings from the US Collaborative Review of Sterilization. Am J Obstet Gynecol 1996;174:1161-1170

The Contraception Report.Update on Female Sterilization. Editor: David Grimes.Vol VII, No. 3, Sept 1996

Christman GM,Vechi H. Female Sterilization 2000;25:48-58

ENDOMETRIOSIS

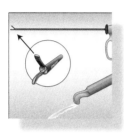

Dan Martin, M.D.

INTRODUCTION

Endometriosis presents in many fashions. Some of these are readily treated at laparoscopy while others may be better approached at laparotomy. The purpose of this chapter is to describe the recognition and treatment of those lesions which are most readily found at laparoscopy.

GOALS OF SURGERY

The type of surgery planned depends on the goals of treatment. For infertility, limited dissection and/or coagulation may help decrease adhesions. This may be better for fertility as it can cause fewer adhesions than extensive dissection. For pain, extensive dissection and complete removal of endometriosis appears to be a better approach for deep infiltration.

This may require deep dissection at laparotomy. If the purpose is tissue diagnosis, then excisional biopsy with tissue sent to pathology is necessary.

PURPOSE OF CONFIRMATION

Purposes of histologic confirmation can be clinical, audit or research. A primary clinical purpose of biopsy is to rule out cancer and/or other non-endometriotic pathology. Carbon, ectopic pregnancy, splenosis, hemangiomas, chlamydia and other diseases can look like endometriosis.

At an audit level, biopsy confirmation gives quality assurance. Although it appears that physicians interested in endometriosis can maintain greater than 70% confirmation and recognition, Walter suggests that this number may be less in usual care. This is discussed further in the last paragraph of recognition.

Confirmation of disease would appear to be essential for research studies.

RECOGNITION

Subtle appearing lesions may be more prevalent than dark lesions. Dark lesions are the easiest to see and to document (Figure 1). Subtle forms are more common. The limits of

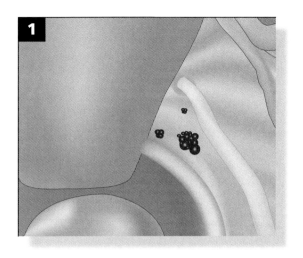

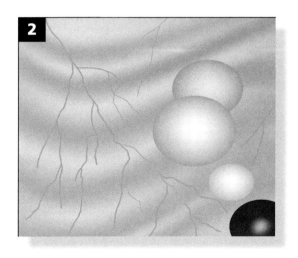

resolution for visualizing these lesions appears to be between 120 μm and 400 μm. These subtle lesions have many descriptions and appear to preceed darker lesions. Colorless, amenorrheic lesions were seen by Fallon in 1950. Karnaky published an age-dependent appearance of endometriosis starting with an initial water blister presentation in 1969

(Figure 2). Red glandular lesions are very active and can appear like native endometrium on histology.

The term 'typical' and 'atypical' are generally avoided in this chapter for two reasons. First, the most common appearances in my studies have been subtle. Second, the use of the term atypical is better reserved for histologic atypicality in premalignant or malignant processes.

Recognition of lesions appears to be related to the surgeon's experience and attention to this possibility. Physicians have failed to diagnose 59% of the endometriosis that was sent to the lab and to have as little as 53% confirmed by the pathologists. At the other extreme, 86% of the endometriosis sent to the lab was recognized by surgeons and 99% has been confirmed.

Physicians may desire to test their own sensitivity and predictivity. The sensitivity is the least expensive measure to produce. This requires that a physician ask for his or her pathology reports that are positive for endometriosis. These can be compared to the operative notes to determine what was seen and what was not. More time consuming is to keep track of every case for endometriosis that was diagnosed either by the surgeon or

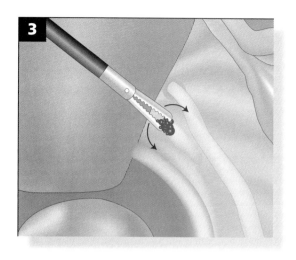

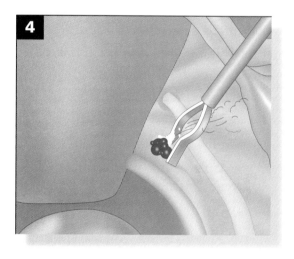

by pathology and compare this with the reports by Scott and Martin.

TREATMENT

PERITONEAL LESIONS

Peritoneal lesions can be diagnosed by grasping them and moving the peritoneum. If these move freely across loose connective tissue, then there is no evidence of deep infiltration (Figure

3). These type lesions are readily treated with any energy source when they are small (2 mm to 5 mm). This includes coagulation, excision and vaporization. Coagulation with bipolar electrosurgery is the technique available to all physicians trained to do bipolar tubal coagulations (Figure 4).

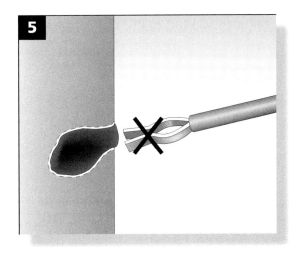

DEEP LESIONS

Deep endometriosis can be difficult to treat, as the depth can be frequently difficult to determine. Coagulation has limited usefulness with these lesions, as the risk of both adequate treatment and lateral damage is present. When the lesions are deeper than 5 mm, attempting to coagulate these can produce deep burns, which can include damage to organs such as the bowel or ureter (Figure 5). If inadequate coagulation is used, residual endometriosis can be found beneath the foreign body reaction from coagulation.

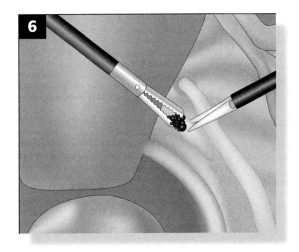

Vaporization has been used by authors who will vaporize to the level of healthy fat. Many surgeons find this depth to be very confusing and potentially dangerous. Personally, I took almost 3 years to learn what vaporizing fat looked like. I have ceased to do that as the margins are not sufficiently clear.

Excision appears to be the most useful technique. Sharp dissection

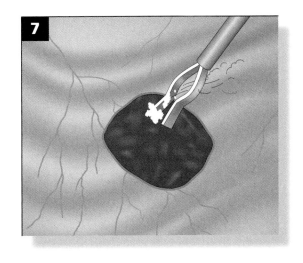

with scissors, incisions with monopolar electrosurgery or incision with lasers have been useful. Sharp scissors followed by bipolar electrosurgery are available in most operating rooms (Figure 6). Bipolar scissors are useful when the expense of disposable instruments can be justified. Lasers are useful but difficult to learn and expensive to maintain. The bleeding from the excised peritoneum usually stops spontaneously. If the excised area continues to bleed, superficial coagulation with bipolar forceps can be performed by touching the base of the lesion with a bipolar coagulator while keeping the blades slightly apart (Figure 7). Simultaneous irrigation and coagulation of small blood vessels with mini-bipolar forceps is effective (Figure 8).

Dissection at laparoscopy can be performed when visualization is adequate to differentiate loose connective tissue and fat from the appearance of endometriosis. Histologic presence of adequate healthy tissue at the margins confirms the ability to make this distinction. It has been useful in the past to look at slides after excision to confirm this.

On the other hand, manual palpation at laparotomy increases recognition of deep lesions, subperitoneal nodules, epiploic fat nodules, endometriosis in

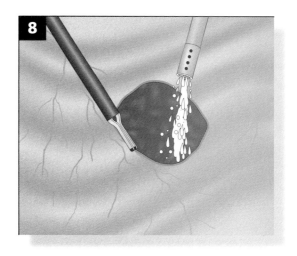

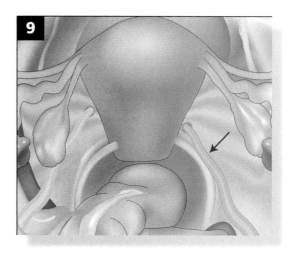

the mesentery appendix and infiltrating bowel lesions. Almost half of my appendiceal lesions have been found by palpation and not visualization. I have missed as many as 20 nodules in the bowel at laparoscopy.

MEDIAL DEVIATION

Of specific note, medial deviation of the ureter has been found in up to 25%

of patients with endometriosis (Figure 9). This may be as high as 100% of those with broad ligament pockets. Be careful to identify the ureter in the presence of a broad ligament pocket. Ureter is often the medial margin of the pocket and may be confused with the uterosacral ligament. After a round structure in this area is identified, follow it into the upper pelvis. The ureter could go over the pelvic brim and uterosacral ligament and go deep into the pelvis.

RETROCERVICAL ENDOMETRIOSIS

Retrocervical endometriosis may be easier to palpate in the office than to find at surgery. Careful mapping and intraoperative palpation may help better identify these lesions (Figure 10). If the cul-de-sac appears to be of normal depth, a rectal probe can be placed in the rectum, and a sponge stick in the vagina for better exposure of the lesion (Figure 11). Laparoscopic resection of the rectal lesion can be performed using sharp dissection with scissors. If the probe can be placed between the lesion and the rectum, a combined laparoscopic and vaginal approach may be useful. However, if these conditions are not met, then preparation for rectovaginal surgery and repair is needed.

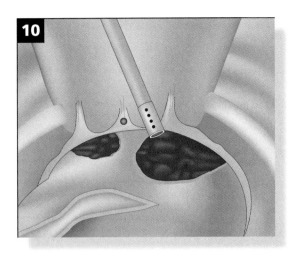

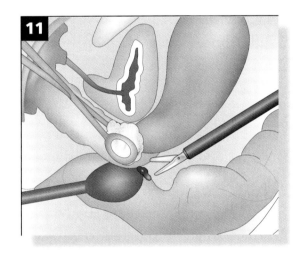

OVARIAN LESIONS

Ovarian lesions can infiltrate or invaginate into the ovary. While these are superficial, coagulation or vaporization may be useful. With deeper penetration, stripping or drainage of the chocolate cyst followed by coagulation of the inner lining may be useful.

Stripping of the pseudo-capsule of an endometrioma begins with opening of the endometrioma. This can be done in a linear or rounded fashion. The advantage of a round or oval opening is in finding the demarcation between healthy ovary and endometrioma (Figure 12). A linear incision directly across the endometrioma may have only abnormal tissue in the incisional area.

Once the demarcation between healthy and an endometriotic pseudo-capsule is recognized, slow tension is placed on both edges (Figure 13). If tension is inadequate, a third instrument is used to dissect in between the first two. This can be a pusher, spreader or scissors. If dissection is near the hilum, extra care is needed. If dissection is difficult in this area, the endometrioma is amputated so that the deep portion is left attached to the vessels to avoid excessive bleeding and damage to the ovary. This portion is coagulated.

When diagnosing chocolate cysts, the distinction between corpus luteum and endometrioma is clinically important. Corpus luteum can have a more clotted fluid and a more uniformly brown base. Endometriosis has a mottled base, which is generally brown and has red areas on a white pseudo-capsule. This occurs after washing the inner lining. Ongoing correlation with histology is needed in order to maintain quality control and to confirm recognition.

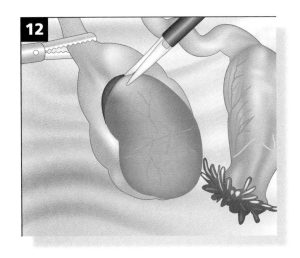

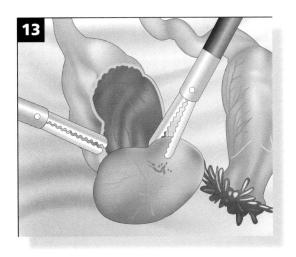

After stripping or coagulation of the base, sutures are avoided. Healing appears to be better without sutures than with them. Sutures appear to increase the chance of adhesions.

COMPLETION OF SURGERY

At the completion of surgery, considerations for flotation and adhesion prevention barriers may be important. In addition, Perry has shown that instillation of 1 to 2 L of fluid at the end of the laparoscopy significantly decreases the frequency of subdiaphragmatic and shoulder pain when sitting or standing. Flotation is used for this reason in all patients. There is also a chance that flotation may decrease adhesions between surfaces by letting them move easily across each other.

Surgical barriers such as Interceed™ (Johnson & Johnson Medical, Sommerville, NJ) may physically represent a barrier between tissue margins. There is potential for decreasing adhesions and Interceed™ has been used for this purpose in some studies. This does require complete hemostasis and is not generally used with flotation. I generally place a small amount of solution at the end of the procedure in order to float gas. I try to limit this so that it will not also float the Interceed™.

CONCLUSIONS

In summary, laparoscopy is excellent for superficial lesions and lesions which can be dissected. Deeper lesions and those involving the serosa or muscularis of the bowel may be better treated at laparotomy.

Suggested Reading:

Fallon J, Brosnan JT, Manning JJ, Moran WG, Meyers J, Fletcher ME. Endometriosis: a report of 400 cases. Rhode Island Med J 1950; 33:15-23

Fayez JA, Vogel MF. Comparison of different treatment methods of endometriomas by laparoscopy. Obstet Gynecol 1991; 78:660-665

Karnaky KJ. Theories and known observations about hormonal treatment of endometriosis-in-situ, and endometriosis at the enzyme level. Arizona Medicine 1969; 26:37-41

Martin DC, Hubert GD, Vander Zwaag R, El-Zeky FA. Laparoscopic appearances of peritoneal endometriosis. Fertil Steril 1989; 51:63-67

Martin DC, Ahmic R, El-Zeky FA, Vander Zwaag R, Pickens MT, Cherry K. Increased histologic confirmation of endometriosis. J Gynecol Surg 1990; 6:275-279

Perry CP, Tombrello R. Effect of fluid instillation on post laparoscopy pain. J Reprod Med 1993; 38:768-770

Redwine DB. Age-related evolution in color appearance of endometriosis. Fertil Steril 1987; 48:1062-1063

Scott RB, TeLinde RW. External endometriosis - the scourge of the private patient. Ann Surg 1950; 131:697–720

www.danmartinmd.com/endometriosis.htm

www.memfert.com/color_atlas.htm

LAPAROSCOPIC SURGERY FOR ADHESIONS

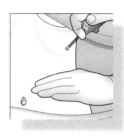

Harry Reich, M.D.

Lisa M. Roberts, M.D.

Jay Redan, M.D.

INTRODUCTION

Postoperative adhesions occur after almost every abdominal surgery and are the leading cause of intestinal obstruction. In one study, 93% of patients who had undergone at least one previous open abdominal operation had post surgical adhesions. This was not considered surprising, given the extreme delicacy of the peritoneum and the fact that apposition of two injured surfaces nearly always results in adhesion formation.

Adhesions are the most common cause of bowel obstruction and most likely result from gynecologic procedures, appendectomies, trauma and other intestinal operations. Adhesions have also been proposed to cause infertility and abdominal and pelvic pain. Although nerve fibers have been confirmed in pelvic adhesions, their presence is not increased in those patients with pelvic pain. In addition, there does not appear to be an association between the severity of adhesions and complaint of pain. It is generally accepted that adhesions may impair organ motility resulting in visceral pain transmitted by peritoneal innervation. Many patients experience resolution of their symptoms after adhesiolysis. This may be complicated by placebo effect as demonstrated by one study that showed no difference in pain scores between patients who were randomized to adhesiolysis versus expectant management.

In 1994, adhesiolysis procedures resulted in 303,836 hospitalizations, 846,415 days of inpatient care, and $1.3 billion in health care expenditures. Forty-seven per cent of these hospitalizations were for adhesiolysis of the female reproductive system, the primary site for these procedures. In comparison to similar data from 1988, the cost of adhesiolysis hospitalizations is down. One significant influence on this trend is the increased use of minimally invasive surgical techniques resulting in fewer days of inpatient care.

This chapter reviews the pathophysiology of adhesion formation, equipment and technique for adhesiolysis, and methods for adhesion prevention.

PATHOPHYSIOLOGY OF ADHESION FORMATION

Adhesion formation is initiated by peritoneal trauma. Its morphogenesis was described in detail by diZerega. Within hours at the site of injury, polymorphonuclear leukocytes appear in large numbers meshed in fibrin strands. At 24-36 hours, macrophages appear in large numbers and are responsible for regulating fibroblast and mesothelial cell activities. By day two, the wound surface is covered by macrophages, islands of primitive mesenchymal cells and mesothelial cells. By day four the islands of primitive mesenchymal cells have now come into contact with each other. Fibroblasts and collagen are now present and increasing. By day five, an organized fibrin interconnection is now seen composed of collagen, fibroblasts, mast cells, and vascular channels containing endothelial cells. The adhesion continues to mature as collagen fibrils organize into bands covered by mesothelium that contain blood vessels and connective tissue fiber.

EQUIPMENT

A review of standard equipment such as light sources and video systems is beyond the scope of this chapter. Equipment useful for advanced procedures and energy sources is included. However, the main technique for adhesiolysis with the least possibility for reformation can simply be described as 'cold scissors dissection with bipolar backup'.

LAPAROSCOPES

Four different laparoscopes should be available for adhesiolysis: a 10-mm 0° straight viewing laparoscope; a 10-mm operative laparoscope with 5-mm operating channel; a 5-mm straight viewing laparoscope for introduction through 5-mm trocar sleeves; and an oblique-angle laparoscope (30°–45°) for upper abdominal and pelvic procedures (Figure 1).

SCISSORS

Scissors are the preferred instrument to cut adhesions, especially avascular and/or congenital adhesions (Figure 2). Using the magnification afforded by the laparoscope, most anterior abdominal wall, pelvic, and bowel adhesions can be carefully inspected and divided with minimal bleeding, rarely requiring micro bipolar coagulation. Loose fibrous or areolar tissue is separated by inserting a closed scissors and withdrawing it in the open position (Figure 3), pushing tissue with the partially open blunt scissors tip is used to develop natural planes.

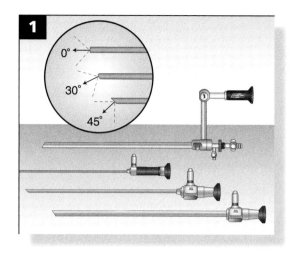

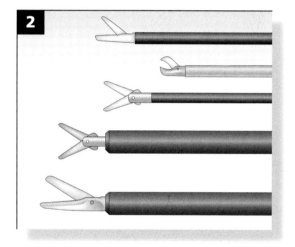

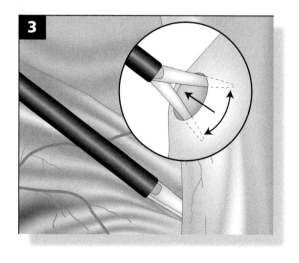

Reusable 5-mm blunt-tipped saw tooth scissors and curved scissors cut well without cautery. Blunt or rounded-tip 5-mm scissors with one stable blade and one moveable blade are used to divide thin and thick bowel adhesions sharply. Sharp dissection is the primary technique used for adhesiolysis to diminish the potential for adhesion formation; electrification and laser are usually reserved for hemostatic dissection of adhesions where anatomic planes are not evident or vascular adherences are anticipated. Thermal energy sources must be avoided as much as possible to reduce adhesion recurrence. Blunt-tipped, saw-tooth scissors, with or without a curve, cut well (Richard Wolf Medical Instruments, Vernon Hills, IL and Karl Storz Endoscopy, Culver City, CA). Many disposable scissors depend greatly on electrification for cutting. Hook-scissors are not very useful for adhesiolysis.

Surgeons should select scissors that feel comfortable. To facilitate direction changes, the scissors should not be too long or encumbered by an electrical cord. This author prefers to make rapid instrument exchanges between scissors and micro bipolar forceps through the same portal to control bleeding, instead of applying electrification via scissors.

ELECTROSURGERY

When discussing electrosurgery, the term 'cautery' should be abandoned. Cautery, thermocoagulation, or endo-coagulation refer to the passive transfer of heat from a hot instrument heated by electrical current to tissue. The temperature rises within the tissue until cell proteins begin to denature and coagulate with resultant cell death. Electrical current does not pass through the patient's body!

Monopolar cutting current can be used safely, as the voltage is too low to arc to organs even 1 mm away. Cutting current is used to both cut and/or coagulate (desiccate) depending on the portion of the electrode in contact with the

> MONOPOLAR ELECTROSURGERY SHOULD BE AVOIDED WHEN WORKING ON THE BOWEL UNLESS THE SURGEON IS WELL VERSED IN THIS MODALITY. THE EXPERT LAPAROSCOPIC SURGEON CAN USE MONOPOLAR ELECTROSURGERY SAFELY TO CUT OR FULGURATE TISSUE, BUT DESICCATION (COAGULATION) ON BOWEL SHOULD BE PERFORMED WITH BIPOLAR TECHNIQUES.

tissue. The tip cuts, while the wider body tamponades and coagulates.

Monopolar coagulation current which uses voltages over 10 times that of cutting current can arc 1 to 2 mm and is used in close proximity to tissue, but not in contact, to fulgurate diffuse venous and arteriolar bleeders. It takes 30% more power to spark or arc in CO_2 pneumoperitoneum than in room air; thus, at the same electrosurgical power setting, less arcing occurs at laparoscopy than at laparotomy.

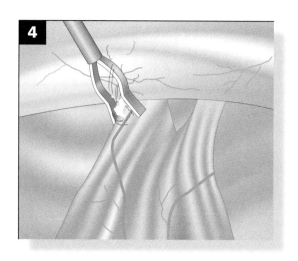

Electrosurgical injury to the bowel can occur beyond the surgeon's field of view during laparoscopic procedures from electrode insulation defects or capacitive coupling. While the surgeon views the tip of the electrode, electrical discharge may occur from its body (insulation failure) or from metal trocar cannulas surrounding the electrode if they are separated from the skin by plastic retention sleeves. These problems are eliminated by active electrode monitoring using the Electroshield EM-1 monitor system (Encision, Boulder, CO). This consists of a sheath surrounding the electrode and a sheath monitor (EM-1) to detect any insulation faults and shield against capacitive coupling.

Bipolar desiccation using cutting current between two closely opposed elec-

trodes is safe and efficient for large vessel hemostasis. Large blood vessels are compressed and bipolar cutting current passed until complete desiccation is achieved, i.e., the current depletes the tissue fluid and electrolytes and fuses the vessel wall (Figure 4). Coagulating current is not used as it may rapidly desiccate the outer layers of the tissue, producing superficial resistance thereby preventing deeper penetration.

Small vessel hemostasis necessary for adhesiolysis is best achieved by using micro bipolar forceps after precisely identifying the vessel with electrolyte solution irrigation. Micro bipolar forceps (Richard Wolf Medical Instruments, Vernon Hills, IL) with an irrigation channel work best for precise tissue desiccation with minimal thermal spread (Figure 5).

Harmonic Scalpel

The use of harmonic scalpel (Ethicon Endosurgery, Cincinnati, Ohio) for laparoscopic adhesiolysis is gaining popularity (Figure 6). Although it has its limitations, the benefit of this multifunctional instrument far outweighs any disadvantage. Many factors can be attributed to its progressive acceptance. The lack of electrical energy used to coagulate vessels and the smaller (2 mm) lateral energy spread make it more attractive than conventional electrosurgical instruments by potentially reducing the percentage of delayed postoperative bowel injuries (caused by electrical burns.) This is not to say however, that injury cannot occur. As with standard electrosurgical instruments, the harmonic scalpel, specifically the jaws, can become hot and cause tissue injury if not used in a prudent manner. Although harmonic scalpel has the ability to grasp, cut, and cauterize simultaneously, making it a useful instrument for a judicious operator (requiring fewer instrument changes in and out of port sites), the inability to cut without applying energy assures the need for a sharp pair of conventional scissors in laparoscopic adhesiolysis.

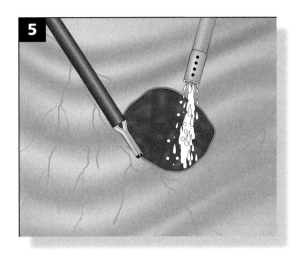

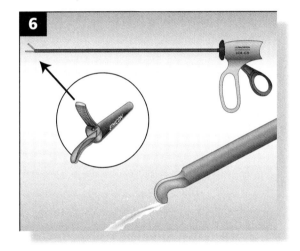

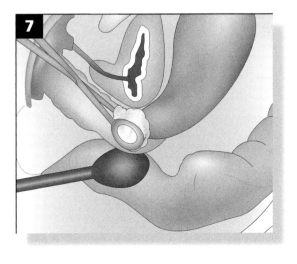

RECTAL AND VAGINAL PROBES

A sponge on a ring forceps is inserted into the vagina or the posterior vaginal fornix, and an 81-French probe is placed in the rectum to define the rectum and posterior vagina for lysis of pelvic adhesions and/or excision of endometriosis when there is a significant degree of cul-de-sac obliteration. Whenever rectal location is in doubt, it is identified by insertion of the rectal probe (Figure 7).

CO$_2$ LASER

The CO$_2$ laser, with its 0.1 mm depth of penetration and inability to traverse through water, allows the surgeon some security when lysing adhesions especially in the pelvis. The Coherent 5000L laser (Palo Alto, CA), by using a 11.1 μm wavelength beam, maintains a 1.5-mm spot size at all power settings allowing for more precision than most standard 10.6 μm wavelength CO$_2$ lasers.

AQUA DISSECTION

Aqua dissection is the use of hydraulic energy from pressurized fluid to aid in the performance of surgical procedures. The force vector is multidirectional within the volume of expansion of the uncompressible fluid;

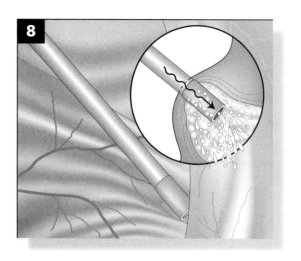

the force applied with a blunt probe is unidirectional. Instillation of fluid under pressure displaces tissue, creating cleavage planes in the least resistant spaces (Figure 8). Aqua dissection into closed spaces behind peritoneum or adhesions produces edematous, distended tissue on tension with loss of elasticity, making further division easy and safe using blunt dissection, scissors dissection, laser, or electrosurgery.

Suction-irrigators with the ability to dissect using pressurized fluid should have a single channel to maximize suctioning and irrigating capacity. This allows the surgeon to perform atraumatic suction-traction-retraction, irrigate directly, and develop surgical planes (aqua dissection). The distal tip should not have side holes as they impede these actions, spray the surgical field without purpose, and cause unnecessary tissue trauma when omentum, epiploic appendices, and adhesions become caught. The shaft should have a dull finish to prevent CO_2 laser beam reflection, allowing it to be used as a backstop. The market is crowded with many aqua dissection devices.

PLUME ELIMINATOR

Smoke evacuation during electro-surgery or CO_2 laser laparoscopy is expedited using most of the suction irrigation cannula.

LAPAROSCOPIC PERITONEAL CAVITY ADHESIOLYSIS

Adhesiolysis by laparoscopy and laparotomy can be very time-consuming and technically difficult and is best performed by an expert surgeon. However, despite lengthy laparoscopic procedures (two to four hours), most patients are discharged on the day of the procedure, avoid large abdominal incisions, experience minimal complications, and return to full activity within one week of surgery.

In this section, general adhesiolysis, pelvic adhesiolysis, ovariolysis, salpingo-ovariolysis, and salpingostomy are described. The laparoscopic treatment of acute adhesions has not been included. However, the best treatment

for sexually transmitted disease adhesive sequelae may be prevention through early laparoscopic diagnosis and treatment of acute pelvic infection, including abscesses. Acute adhesiolysis will often prevent chronic adhesion formation.

CLASSIFICATIONS

Extensive peritoneal cavity adhesion procedures need a classification system that relates to their degree of severity and the surgical expertise necessary for adhesiolysis. The single best indicator of the degree of severity and expertise necessary for adhesiolysis is the number of previous laparotomies. The frequency of small bowel obstruction symptoms indicates the need for surgery.

Peritoneal adhesiolysis is classified into enterolysis including omentolysis and female reproductive reconstruction (salpingo-ovariolysis and cul-de-sac dissection with excision of deep fibrotic endometriosis). Bowel adhesions are divided into upper abdominal, lower abdominal, pelvic, and combinations. Adhesions surrounding the umbilicus are upper abdominal as they require an upper abdominal laparoscopic view for division. The extent, thickness, and vascularity of adhesions vary widely. Intricate adhesive patterns exist with fusion to parietal peritoneum or various meshes.

Extensive small bowel adhesions are not a frequent finding at laparoscopy for pelvic pain or infertility. In these cases, the Fallopian tube is adhered to the ovary, the ovary is adhered to the pelvic sidewall, and the rectosigmoid may cover both. Rarely, the omentum and small bowel are involved. Adhesions may be the result of an episode of pelvic inflammatory disease or endometriosis, but most commonly are caused by previous surgery. Adhesions cause pain by entrapment of the organs they surround. The surgical management of extensive pelvic adhesions is one of the most difficult problems facing surgeons today.

SURGICAL PLAN FOR EXTENSIVE ENTEROLYSIS

A well-defined strategy is important for small bowel enterolysis. For simplification, this is divided into three parts:

Time frequently dictates that all adhesions cannot be lysed. From the history, the surgeon should conceptualize the adhesions most likely to be causing the pain, i.e., upper or lower abdomen, left or right, and clear these areas of adhesions.

PREOPERATIVE PREPARATION

Patients are informed preoperatively of the high risk for bowel injury during laparoscopic procedures when extensive cul-de-sac involvement with endometriosis or adhesions is suspected. They are encouraged to hydrate and eat lightly for 24 hours before admission. A mechanical bowel preparation is administered orally the afternoon before surgery to induce brisk, self-limiting diarrhea to cleanse the bowel. The patient is usually

1. DIVISION OF ALL ADHESIONS TO THE ANTERIOR ABDOMINAL WALL PARIETAL PERITONEUM. SMALL BOWEL LOOPS ENCOUNTERED DURING THIS PROCESS ARE SEPARATED USING THEIR ANTERIOR ATTACHMENT FOR COUNTERTRACTION INSTEAD OF WAITING UNTIL THE LAST PORTION OF THE PROCEDURE (RUNNING OF THE BOWEL).

2. DIVISION OF ALL SMALL BOWEL AND OMENTAL ADHESIONS IN THE PELVIS. RECTOSIGMOID, CECUM, AND APPENDIX OFTEN REQUIRE SOME SEPARATION DURING THIS PART OF THE PROCEDURE.

3. RUNNING OF THE BOWEL. USING ATRAUMATIC GRASPING FORCEPS AND USUALLY A SUCTION-IRRIGATOR FOR SUCTION TRACTION, THE BOWEL IS RUN. STARTING AT THE CECUM AND TERMINAL ILEUM, LOOPS AND SIGNIFICANT KINKS ARE FREED INTO THE HIGH UPPER ABDOMEN TO THE LIGAMENT OF TREITZ.

4. (OPTIONAL) FINALLY TUBOOVARIAN PATHOLOGY IS TREATED IF INDICATED.

admitted on the day of surgery. Lower abdominal, pubic, and perineal hair is not shaved. Patients are encouraged to void on call to the OR, and a Foley catheter is inserted only if the bladder is distended or a long operation anticipated. A catheter is inserted during the operation and removed in the recovery room when the patient is aware of its presence, to prevent bladder distension. Antibiotics (usually cefoxitin) are administered in all cases.

PATIENT POSITIONING

All laparoscopic surgical procedures are done under general anesthesia with endotracheal intubation. An orogastric tube is placed routinely to diminish the possibility of a trocar injury to the stomach and to reduce small bowel distention. The patient's arms should be tucked on both sides so that the surgeon's position is comfortable and not limited. The patient's position is flat (0°) (Figure 9) during umbilical trocar sleeve insertion and anterior abdominal wall adhesiolysis but a steep Trendelenburg position (30°), reverse Trendelenburg position, and side-to-side rotation are used when necessary. Lithotomy position, with the hip extended (thigh parallel to abdomen) is obtained with Allen stirrups (Edgewater Medical Systems, Mayfield Heights, OH) or knee braces, which are adjusted individually to each

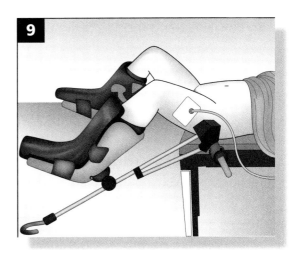

patient before she is anesthetized. Anesthesia examination is performed prior to prepping the patient.

INCISIONS

In the absence of suspected periumbilical adhesions, an intraumbilical vertical incision is made through the skin of the inferior umbilical fossa extending to and just beyond its lowest point. A Veress needle is placed through this low point while pulling the umbilicus towards the pubic symphysis and insufflation with CO_2 is continued until an intraabdominal pressure of 25–30 mmHg is obtained.

Special alternate entry sites and techniques are used when there is a high suspicion for periumbilical adhesions in patients who have undergone multiple laparotomies, have lower abdominal incisions traversing the umbilicus, or who have extensive adhesions either clinically or from a previous operative record. Open laparoscopy at the umbilicus carries the same risk for bowel laceration if the bowel is fused to the umbilical undersurface.

One alternate site is in the left ninth intercostal space, anterior axillary line (Figure 10). Adhesions are rare in this area, and the peritoneum is tethered to the undersurface of the ribs, making peritoneal tenting away from the needle unusual. A 5-mm skin incision is made over the lowest intercostal space (the 9th) in the anterior axillary line. The Veress needle is grasped near its tip, like a dart, between thumb and forefinger, while the other index finger spreads this intercostal space. The needle tip is inserted at a right angle to the skin (a 45° angle to the horizontal) between the ninth and tenth ribs. A single pop is felt on penetration of the peritoneum. Pneumoperitoneum to a pressure of 30 mmHg is obtained. A 5-mm trocar is then inserted through this same incision that has migrated downward below the left costal margin because of the pneumoperitoneum. (Figure 11)

Another alternate entry site is Palmer's point located 3 cm inferior to the subcostal arch in the left medioclavicular line (Figure 12). Also, if the uterus is present and thought to be free of adhesions, the surgeon may consider

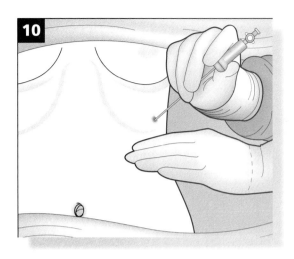
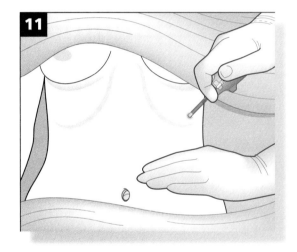
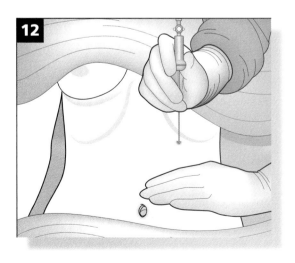

inserting a long Veress needle transvaginally through the uterus (Figure 13).

When unexpected extensive adhesions are encountered initially surrounding the umbilical puncture, the surgeon should immediately seek a higher site. Thereafter, the adhesions can be freed down to and just beneath the umbilicus, and the surrounding bowel inspected for perforations. The umbilical portal can then be reestablished safely for further work.

Other laparoscopic puncture sites are placed as needed, usually lateral to the rectus abdominis muscles and always under direct laparoscopic vision.

If an umbilical insertion is possible and extensive adhesions are present close to but below the umbilicus, the operating laparoscope with scissors in the operating channel is the first instrument used. If a left upper quadrant 5-mm incision is necessary, there is usually room for another puncture site to perform initial adhesiolysis with scissors.

ABDOMINAL ADHESIOLYSIS

Anterior abdominal wall adhesions involve the parietal peritoneum stuck to the omentum, transverse colon, and small bowel with varying degrees of fibrosis and vascularity. Adhesions may be filmy and avascular, filmy and vas-

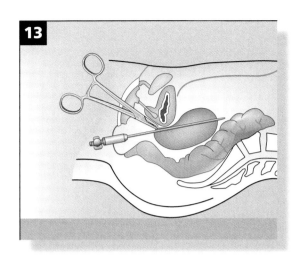

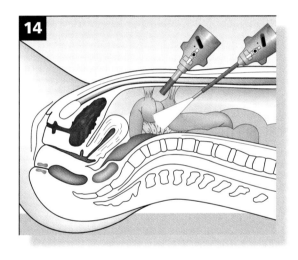

cular, or dense, fibrous and vascular. All of these adhesions to the anterior abdominal wall are released. If adhesions extend from above the level of the laparoscope in the umbilicus, another trocar is inserted above the level of the highest adhesion and the laparoscope is inserted there (Figure 14). Adhesions are easier to divide when working above them, instead of within them, as gravity helps to delineate the plane for separation after which the CO_2 pneumoperitoneum can disperse into the dissection plane.

Adhesiolysis is done using scissors alone if possible. Electrosurgery, CO_2 laser, and the harmonic scalpel are used. In most cases, the initial adhesiolysis is performed with scissors. CO_2 laser through the laparoscope on adhesions close to the trocar insertion often results in reflection with loss of precision. Electrosurgery (cutting current) is used only when there is little chance that small bowel is involved in the adhesion.

Initially, blunt-tipped scissors in the operating channel of an operating laparoscope are inserted into the interface between the anterior abdominal wall parietal peritoneum and the omentum (Figure 15). Rotating the laparoscope so that the scissors exit at 12 o'clock instead of 3 o'clock facilitates early adhesiolysis. Blunt dissection is performed by inserting the scissors at the interface, opening, and withdrawing them. This maneuver is repeated many times to delineate the thin avascular adhesions from thicker vascular fibrotic attachments that are individually coagulated and divided. Frequently, adhesions can be bluntly divided by grasping the adhesion in the partially closed scissors, and gently pushing the tissue. If the plane of adhesions cannot be reached with the tip of

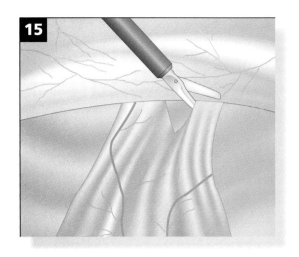

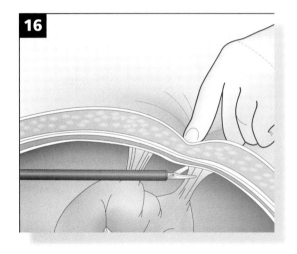

the scissors, abdominal wall can be pressed from above with the finger to make it accessible to the scissors (Figure 16).

After initial adhesiolysis, visualization is improved allowing better access and exposure for further adhesiolysis. Secondary trocar sites can now be placed safely. After their insertion, the remainder of the adhesions can now be lysed using scissors with micro bipolar backup for rare arteriolar bleeders. Small venule bleeders are left alone. On occasion, in operations in which symptomatic bowel adhesions are not the main problem, an electrosurgical spoon or knife is used to divide the remaining omental adhesions if bowel is not involved. If bowel is involved, dissection proceeds with scissors, without electrosurgery, through the second puncture site, aided by traction on the bowel from an opposite placed puncture site (Figure 17). Rarely, the CO_2 laser may be used through the operating channel of the operating laparoscope. When using the CO_2 laser for adhesiolysis, aqua dissection is performed to distend the adhesive surface with fluid before vaporizing the individual adhesive layers. The suction-irrigator can also be used for suction traction, instead of a laparoscopic Babcock, and as a backstop to prevent thermal damage to other structures. The suction irrigator is also used to clean the laparoscopic optic, which is then wiped on the bowel serosa before continuing. Denuded areas of bowel muscularis are repaired transversely using a 3-0 or 4-0 Vicryl seromuscular stitch. Denuded peritoneum is left alone. Minimal oozing should be observed and not desiccated unless this bleeding hinders the next adhesiolysis step or persists towards the end of the

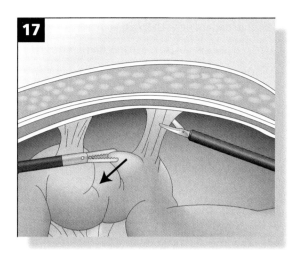

operation. With perseverance, all anterior abdominal wall parietal peritoneum adhesions can be released.

The harmonic scalpel is also useful for adhesiolysis. It bears repeating, the harmonic scalpel is not a scissor. This instrument works by coagulating tissue in between the blades and allowing it to be 'pressed apart' after full coagulation of the tissue between the active blade and the compressing surface. Tissue is first grasped between the blades of the harmonic scalpel, steadily compressed, and the blade is activated allowing the tissue to separate once it is fully coagulated (Figure 18). Any tissue between the blades of the harmonic scalpel will be heated and then be allowed to fall apart. This includes all blood vessels up to 3 mm in diameter incorporated in the tissue between the blades. As stated before, the harmonic scalpel can be used to grasp tissue in a general manner when the blades are not active. However, prior to grasping any tissue, the operator must allow the active blade to cool sufficiently so it will not burn any tissue it may come in contact with. The operator must remember that a harmonic scalpel does not replace the scissor, especially when dealing with bowel in the same proximity to an adhesion plane. Harmonic scalpel comes in 5- and 10-mm size instrumentation with active jaws as well as adaptable adjuncts to the instrument such as a spatula type dissector, 'ball' type dissector and hook dissector. All of these type instruments can be used in the same location as you would normally use a monopolar electrode; bear in mind once again that the lateral energy spread is only 2 mm with the harmonic scalpel.

PELVIC ADHESIOLYSIS

The next step is to free all bowel loops in the pelvis. Small bowel attached to the vesicouterine peritoneal fold, uterus or vaginal cuff, and the rectum is liberated. There are three key points when performing bowel adhesiolysis within the pelvis: scissors dissection without electrosurgery, countertraction and blunt dissection. The bowel is gently held with an atraumatic grasper and lifted away from the structure to which it is adhered,

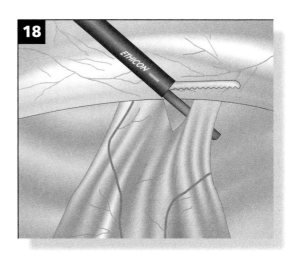

exposing the plane of dissection. When adhesive interfaces are obvious, scissors are used. The blunt-tipped scissors are used to sharply dissect the adhesions in small, successive cuts taking care not to damage the bowel serosa. Countertraction will further expose the plane of dissection and ultimately free the attachment. Electrosurgery and laser are generally not used for adhesiolysis involving the bowel due to the risk of thermal damage and recurrent adhesion formation. However, when adhesive aggregates blend into each other, initial incision is made very superficially with laser, and aqua dissection distends the layers of the adhesions, facilitating identification of the involved structures. Division of adhesions continues with laser at 10-20 W in pulsed mode. The aqua dissector and injected fluid from it are used as a backstop behind adhesive bands that are divided with the CO_2 laser.

The rectosigmoid can be adhered to the left pelvic sidewall obscuring visualization of the left adnexa. Dissection starts well out of the pelvis in the left iliac fossa. Scissors are used to develop the space between the sigmoid colon and the psoas muscle to the iliac vessels, and the rectosigmoid reflected toward the midline. Thereafter, with the rectosigmoid placed on traction, rectosigmoid and rectal adhesions to the left pelvic sidewall are divided starting cephalad and continuing caudad (Figure 19).

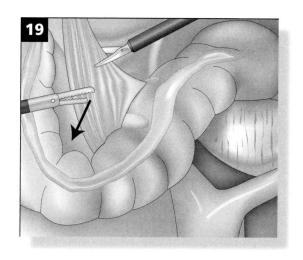

Cul-de-sac adhesions can cause partial or complete cul-de-sac obliteration from fibrosis between the anterior rectum, posterior vagina, cervix, and the uterosacral ligaments. The technique of freeing the anterior rectum to the loose areolar tissue of the rectovaginal septum before excising and/or vaporizing visible and palpable deep fibrotic endometriosis is used (Figure 20).

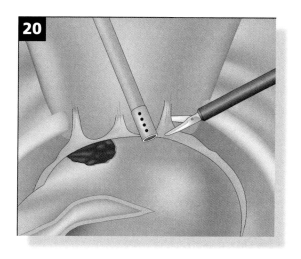

Attention is first directed to complete dissection of the anterior rectum throughout its area of involvement until the loose areolar tissue of the rectovaginal space is reached. Using the rectal probe as a guide, the rectal serosa is opened at its junction with the cul-de-sac lesion. Careful dissection ensues using aqua dissection, suction-traction, laser, and scissors until the rectum is completely freed and identifiable below the lesion. Excision of the fibrotic endometriosis is done only after rectal dissection is completed.

Deep fibrotic, often nodular, endometriotic lesions are excised from the uterosacral ligaments, the upper posterior vagina, (the location of which is confirmed by the Valtchev retractor or a sponge in the posterior fornix), and the posterior cervix (Figure 21). The dissection on the outside of the vaginal wall proceeds using laser or scissors until soft pliable upper posterior vaginal wall is uncovered. It is frequently difficult to distinguish fibrotic endometriosis from cervix at the cervicovaginal junction and above. Frequent palpation using rectovaginal examinations helps identify occult lesions. When the lesion infiltrates through the vaginal wall, an 'en bloc' laparoscopic resection from cul-de-sac to posterior vaginal wall is done, and the vagina is repaired laparoscopically with the pneumoperitoneum maintained with a 30-cc Foley balloon in the vagina. Or, more recently, the vaginal lesion is mobilized vaginally, the vagina closed over the mobilized portion, and the en bloc lesion excision completed laparoscopically. Sometimes the fibrotic cul-de-sac lesion encompassing both uterosacral ligament insertions and the intervening posterior cervix–vagina and anterior rectal lesion can be excised as one en bloc specimen.

Endometriotic nodules infiltrating the anterior rectal muscularis are excised, usually with the surgeon's or his assistant's finger in the rectum just beneath the lesion (Figure 22). In some cases, the anterior rectum is reperitonealized by plicating the uterosacral ligaments and

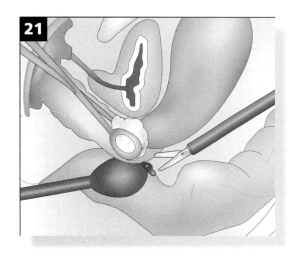

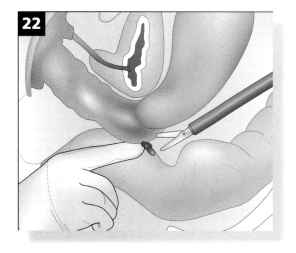

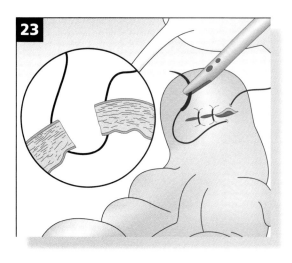

lateral rectal peritoneum across the midline. Deep rectal muscularis defects are always closed with suture. Full thickness rectal lesion excisions are suture repaired laparoscopically (Figure 23).

When a ureter is close to the lesion, its course in the deep pelvis is traced by opening its overlying peritoneum with scissors or laser (Figure 24). On the left, this often requires scissors reflection of the rectosigmoid, as previously described, starting at the pelvic brim. Bipolar forceps are used to control arterial and venous bleeding.

ADNEXAL ADHESIOLYSIS (SALPINGO-OVARIOLYSIS)

Ovarian adhesions to the pelvic sidewall can be filmy or fused. Initially, adhesions between the ovary and Fallopian tubes and other peritoneal surfaces are identified. It is imperative that the surgeon knows the surrounding anatomy prior to cutting any tissue to avoid damage to vital structures. The plane of dissection is identified and followed to avoid damage to other structures. The uteroovarian ligament may be held with an atraumatic grasper to facilitate countertraction and expose the line of cleavage. During ovariolysis, it is important to preserve as much peritoneum as possible while freeing the ovary. Dissection starts either high in the pelvis just beneath the infundibu-

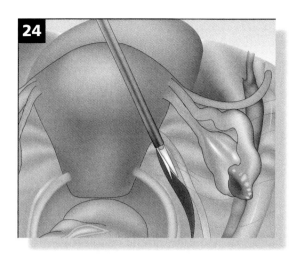

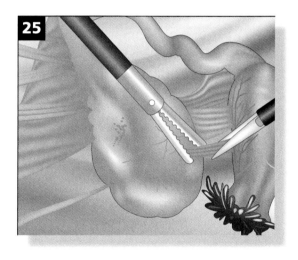

lopelvic ligament or deep on the pelvic sidewall beneath the ureter in the pararectal space. In each case, scissors are used both bluntly and sharply to mobilize the ovary from the sidewall (Figure 25). Alternatively, aqua dissection may be used to facilitate identification of adhesion layers and to provide a safe backstop for the CO_2 laser. Once an adhesion layer is identified, the aqua dissector can also be placed behind this ridge and used as a backstop during CO_2 laser adhesiolysis. Adhesiolysis is performed sharply and bluntly in a methodical manner working caudad until the cul-de-sac is reached.

If fimbrioplasty is to be performed, then hydro distension is achieved by transcervical injection of dilute indigo carmine through a uterine manipulator (Figure 26). This distends the distal portion of the tube, which is stabilized, and the adhesive bands are freed using scissors, laser or micropoint electrosurgery. If necessary, the fimbriated end can be progressively dilated using 3 mm alligator-type forceps. The closed forceps are placed through the aperture, opened, and removed (Figure 27). This is repeated one or more times. If the opening does not remain everted on its own, the intussusception salpingostomy method of McComb is used to avoid thermal damage to the ciliated tubal epithelium from CO_2 laser or electrosurgery. The tip of the aqua dissector is inserted approximately 2 cm into the newly opened tube, suction applied, and the tube fimbrial edges pulled around the instrument to turn the tube end inside-out. The borders of the incision act as a restrictive collar to maintain the mucosa in this newly everted configuration (Figure 28). In some cases, the ostial margin is sutured to the ampullary serosa with 6-0 suture (Figure 29).

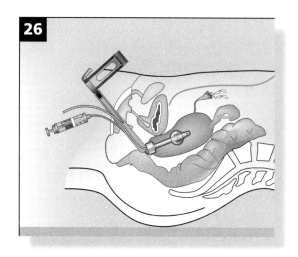

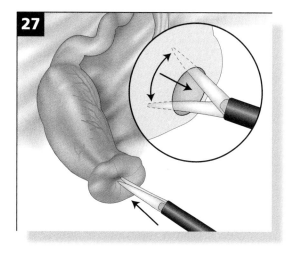

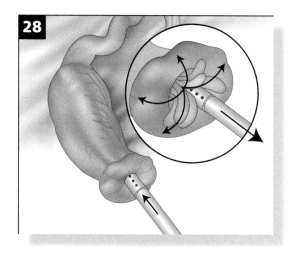

UNDERWATER SURGERY AT THE END OF EACH PROCEDURE

At the close of each operation, an underwater examination is used to document complete intraperitoneal hemostasis in stages; this detects bleeding from vessels and viscera tamponaded during the procedure by the increased intraperitoneal pressure of the CO_2 pneumoperitoneum. The integrity of the rectum and rectosigmoid is often checked at this time by instillation of dilute indigo carmine solution or air transanally through a 30 cc Foley catheter (Figure 30).

The CO_2 pneumoperitoneum is displaced with 2 to 5 L of Ringer's lactate solution, and the peritoneal cavity is vigorously irrigated and suctioned until the effluent is clear of blood products, usually after 10-20 L. Underwater inspection of the pelvis is performed to detect any further bleeding which is controlled using microbipolar-irrigating forceps to coagulate through the electrolyte solution. First, hemostasis is established with the patient in Trendelenburg position, then per underwater examination with the patient supine and in reverse Trendelenburg, and, finally, with all instruments removed, including the uterine manipulator.

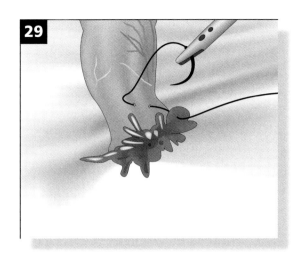

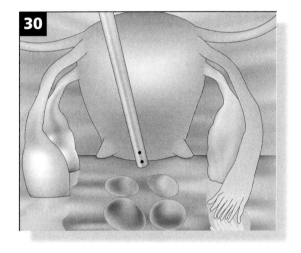

To visualize the pelvis with the patient supine, the 10-mm straight laparoscope and the actively irrigating aqua dissector tip are manipulated together into the deep cul-de-sac beneath floating bowel and omentum. During this copious irrigation procedure, clear fluid is deposited into the pelvis and circulates into the upper abdomen, displacing upper abdominal bloody fluid, which is suctioned after flowing back into the pelvis. An 'underwater' examination is then performed to observe the completely separated tubes and ovaries and to confirm complete hemostasis (Figure 31).

A final copious lavage with Ringer's lactate solution is undertaken and all clots directly aspirated; at least 2 L of lactated Ringer's solution are left in the peritoneal cavity to displace CO_2 and to prevent fibrin adherences from forming by separating raw operated-upon surfaces during the initial stages of reperitonealization. Displacement of the CO_2 with Ringer's lactate diminishes the frequency and severity of shoulder pain from CO_2 insufflation. No other anti–adhesive agents are employed. No drains, antibiotic solutions, or heparin are used.

HANDOSCOPY

Hand assisted laparoscopy or 'handoscopy' has become popular over the last 5 years, mainly in the field of solid organ surgery and bowel surgery. The main advantage of handoscopy is that it allows the surgeon to regain the tactile feel of surrounding tissues previously lost to 'laser' laparoscopists and permits a more purposeful manipulation of larger organs. Often, it is the use of handoscopy for tissue palpation, that enables a successful laparoscopic adhesiolysis. At times, during laparoscopic procedures, visualization can be

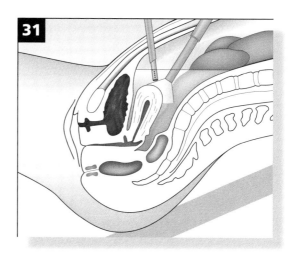

poor due to dense adhesions and the inability to determine tissue planes. With the placement of the operator's hand inside the peritoneal cavity, the surgeon is usually able to palpate surrounding organs and allow for a better tissue dissection plane that otherwise may not have been possible through direct visualization only. Not only can the use of a hand port facilitate an otherwise tedious procedure, it effects a safer operation for the patient with less chance of bowel injury. If bowel resection should become necessary, the use of the hand port allows for exteriorization of the segment that requires resection once again making the procedure easier and less time consuming. A handoscopy incision is usually only 7-8 cm and is either placed in the left or right lower portion of the abdomen with insertion of the operator's non-dominant hand (Figures 32 and 33). The muscle splitting technique is used in a similar method as in performing an open appendectomy. The entire peritoneal cavity can be examined through either one of these incisions with the operator's hand and it can be used for organ extraction as well. Several different types of handoscopy ports are available and all provide equal access to the peritoneal cavity (Figure 34).

When placing a handoscopy port for adhesiolysis, the operator must first choose a location on the abdominal wall that will allow optimal access to the point where adhesions are greatest. After the hand port location is chosen, a marking pen should be used to outline the area of the abdominal wall where the hand port is to be placed. The area for the incision should be anesthetized with bupivicaine for postoperative pain control and an incision should then be made into the skin. The size of the incision should be the same size as the operator's glove size. After this is completed, a muscle splitting technique should be used to enter the peritoneal cavity just as the operator would in performing an open appendectomy. Once the peritoneal cavity is entered, the hand port can then be placed. All of the hand port apparatus require that any adhesions on the peritoneal side of the incision be lysed prior to inserting the handoscopy device. Additionally, these devices

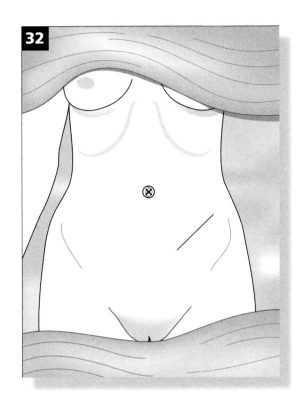

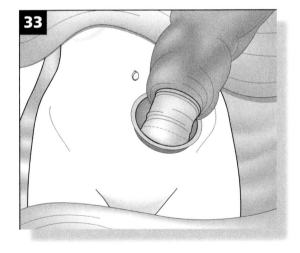

should not be placed over any bony prominences, i.e., iliac crest or encompassing any bowel in the peritoneal ring surface as to injure any bowel in the abdomen. If the handoscopy port is placed in the upper abdomen, the falciform ligament may require division prior to inserting the ring. Once the handoscopy device is in place the lysis of adhesions can proceed in an orderly fashion by identifying the tissue planes by feel with the operator's fingers and additionally being able to provide appropriate traction and countertraction to allow for a safe adhesiolysis. Incidental enterotomies can be sutured with conventional suture and then tied using one hand knot-tying technique with the intraabdominal hand. Should any bowel resections be required the hand port can be used as a mini laparotomy site for extraction of any specimens and for exteriorizing any bowel that may require resection and or repair. Additionally all handoscopy devices that are placed through the abdominal wall act as a wound protector and may minimize postoperative wound infections as well as protect from any potential tumor seeding if the operation is for malignancy. The opening of the Ethicon Lap-Disc™ is like a camera shutter that can be reduced to seal the pneumoperitoneum around any size trocar (Figure 35).

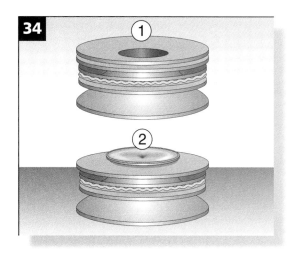

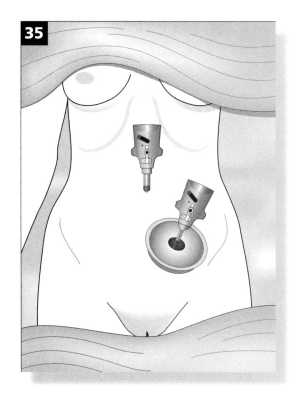

Once the procedure is completed the hand port device is removed, anterior and posterior rectus sheath muscle fascia are closed with either 0 or 2-0 absorbable suture and the skin is then closed in a subcuticular manner. Additionally, a variety of 'pain buster' catheters are now available for insertion into the supra fascia layer of the wound which allow for excellent postoperative analgesia. These help to minimize postoperative narcotic requirements thereby facilitating an earlier return of bowel function and more expedient discharge from the hospital. It has been the author's personal experience that patients undergoing a handoscopy type of operation parallel their recovery in the same manner as a conventional laparoscopic

> ANY MESENTERY DEFECT CAUSED BY A SMALL BOWEL RESECTION SHOULD BE CLOSED WITH A RUNNING LOCKING 0 OR 2-0 ABSORBABLE SUTURE. MESENTERIC DEFECTS NEED NOT BE CLOSED AFTER LARGE BOWEL RESECTIONS

case with a delay of only one day in recovery. If a bowel resection should be required, the patient usually only requires to be NPO overnight and clear liquids may be started on the first postoperative day. The patient is maintained on clear liquids until passing flatus and moving bowels. Most patients are discharged home on the second postoperative day if a bowel resection has been required.

In the event that a bowel resection is required, stapling instruments are used routinely for division of the bowel and anastomosis. The mesentery of the bowel can be divided with the use of surgical ties, harmonic scalpel, or vascular cartridge stapling devices. Bowel resection is preceded by first identifying the lines of resection, the use of stapling devices to transect the bowel proximally and distally, division of the mesentery, followed by re-anastomosis once again using stapling devices and closing the enterotomy required by the tines of the stapling device with an additional stapling device.

OPEN ADHESIOLYSIS

In certain situations an open adhesiolysis is best for the patients. It is usually performed after an attempted laparoscopic approach has been abandoned. If a pelvic adhesiolysis is needed, a Pfannenstiel incision usually is adequate. However, if the entire peritoneal cavity is encased in dense fibrotic adhesions a midline incision is usually required. Open adhesiolysis should be reserved for the worst possible cases where laparoscopic adhesiolysis has failed, where there have been several incidental enterotomies made, or adhesiolysis cannot be performed secondary to encasement of the bowel. Open adhesiolysis should also be considered in a patient unable to tolerate CO_2 insufflation.

An open adhesiolysis is performed in the exact same way as a laparoscopic adhesiolysis. First, all adhesions are taken down from the abdominal wall usually with the Metzenbaum scissors. Second, all loops of bowel are extracted out of the pelvis. Finally, all interloop adhesions are lysed from the ligament of Treitz to ileo-cecal valve. Any incidental enterotomies should be repaired at the time of discovery to avoid intraperitoneal contamination and development of an infection. Hemostasis must be meticulous during the entire dissection as in a laparoscopic procedure. An abundant use of warm irrigation fluid should be made as well. It is extremely important to keep the tissues moist to prevent desiccation from atmospheric air as this can stimulate adhesion reformation. It has been a personal experience that the use of adhesion barriers has been ineffective in open procedures on the bowel and is not indicated.

ADHESION PREVENTION

Intraoperatively, the surgeon can minimize adhesion formation through careful tissue handling, complete hemostasis, abundant irrigation, limited thermal injury, infection prophylaxis, and minimizing foreign body reaction. A recent Cochrane Database Systematic Review investigated whether pharmacological and liquid agents used as adjuvants during pelvic surgery in infertility patients lead to a reduction in the incidence or severity of postoperative adhesion (re-)formation, and/or an improvement in subsequent pregnancy rates. The results of this review are as follows: there is some evidence that intraperitoneal steroid administration decreases the incidence and severity of postoperative adhesion formation; intraperitoneal administration of dextran did not decrease postoperative adhesion formation at second look laparoscopy; there is no evidence that intraabdominal crystalloid instillation, calcium channel blocking agents, non-steroidal antiinflammatory drugs and proteolytics decrease postoperative adhesion formation.

Barrier agents for prevention of adhesion formation are commercially available. The Cochrane Menstrual Disorders and Subfertility Group investigated the effects these agents have on postoperative adhesion formation. The 15 randomized controlled trials comprised laparoscopic and laparotomy surgical techniques. Results of the investigation were as follows: oxidized regenerated cellulose Interceed™ (Johnson & Johnson Medical, Somerville, NJ) reduces the incidence of adhesion formation and re-formation at laparoscopy and laparotomy in the pelvis; polytetrafluoroethylene Gore-Tex™ (W.L. Gore & Associates, Flagstaff, AZ) appears to be superior to Interceed™ in preventing adhesion formation in the pelvis but is limited by the need for suturing and later removal; Seprafilm™ (Genzyme, Cambridge, MA) does not appear to be effective in preventing adhesion formation.

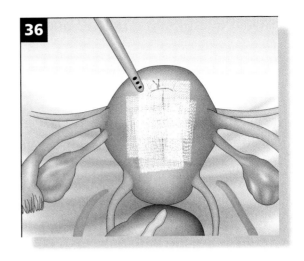

If Interceed™ is to be used for prevention of adhesion formation, the intrapelvic fluid should be completely aspirated. A piece of Interceed large enough to cover the at-risk area is placed and moistened with a small volume of irrigant (Figure 36). Complete hemostasis must be achieved prior to placing the material. If hemostasis has not been achieved, the Interceed will turn brown or black and must be replaced as this may actually increase adhesion formation. Animal studies and clinical trials of a gel form of modified hyaluronic acid, a naturally occurring glycosaminoglycan, show evidence for reducing de novo adhesion formation. Intergel™ (Gynecare – Johnson and Johnson Inc., Somerville, NJ) is commercially available for open surgery use (Figure 37).

The ideal barrier material should be easy to apply, both in open and laparoscopic surgeries. Additionally, it should be nonreactive, persist during the critical wound reepithelization period, stay in

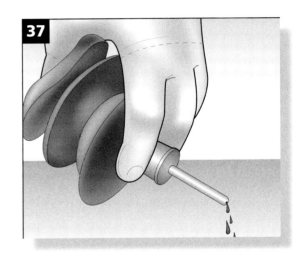

place on the target tissue for several days, and eventually be resorbed following peritoneal healing.

A new product, currently undergoing clinical trials, SprayGel™ (Confluent Surgical, Waltham, MA), also meets these criteria. The gel remains intact for the next 5 to 7 days before breaking down by hydrolysis, and eventual clearance through the kidneys. Preclinical safety studies of SprayGel™ adhesion barrier demonstrate that it is a remarkably inert, biocompatible material, resulting in no signs of toxicity at multiple time points, even when tested at 25 times the anticipated normal dose. Clinical studies in Europe and the US further support the safety profile of this material as an implant. Preliminary prospective randomized clinical trials have evaluated SprayGel™ adhesion barrier in open and laparoscopic myomectomy surgery, as well as in laparoscopic ovarian surgery. In the European myomectomy study, a significant improvement was demonstrated in the tenacity of adhesions between the treated and control populations, when comparing the initial procedures and second-look laparoscopies, as evaluated by the surgeon. The product is currently under review in a multicenter pivotal clinical trial in the US.

CONCLUSION

Adhesion formation after gynecologic surgery is common. When compared to laparotomy, laparoscopy has been shown to result in less de novo adhesion formation, but adhesion reformation continues to be a problem. Sequelae of intraabdominal adhesion formation can be fatal, result in infertility and may be a source of chronic pelvic pain. Minimally invasive surgical management of adhesion formation affords the patient all of the known benefits of laparoscopic surgery including less postoperative analgesics, shorter hospital stays, and more rapid convalescence and return to normal activities. Unfortunately, recurrence rates after adhesiolysis for intestinal obstruction are reported to range from 8% to 32%. Thus, for some patients, adhesiolysis may become a repeat surgical procedure.

No longer can the surgeon ignore the benefits of minimally invasive surgery for adhesiolysis. While these techniques and procedures are not without risk, patients should not be denied their inherent advantages. Astute clinicians must work together to discern the most appropriate uses for this therapy.

Suggested Reading:

Ellis H. The clinical significance of adhesions: Focus on intestinal obstruction. Eur J Surg 1997; Suppl 577:5-9

Bryant T. Clinical lectures on intestinal obstruction. Med Tim Gaz 1872;1:363-5

Welch JP. Adhesions. In: Welch JP, ed. Bowel obstruction. Philadelphia: WB Saunders, 1990:154-65

Kligman I, Drachenberg C, Papdimitriou J, et al. Immunohistochemical demonstration of nerve fibers in pelvic adhesions. Obstet Gynecol 1993;82:566-568

Kresch AJ, Seifer DB, Sachs LB, et al. Laparoscopy in 100 women with chronic pelvic pain. Obstet Gynecol 1984; 64:672-674

Steege JF, Stout AL. Resolution of chronic pelvic pain after laparoscopic lysis of adhesions. Am J Obstet Gynecol 1991;165:278-81

Chan CL, Wood C. Pelvic adhesiolysis: The assessment of symptom relief by 100 patients. Aust NZ Obstet Gynaecol 1985;25:295-298

Daniell JF. Laparoscopic enterolysis for chronic abdominal pain. J Gynecol Surg 1990;5:61-66

Sutton C, MacDonald R. Laser laparoscopic adhesiolysis. J Gynecol Surg 1990;6:155-159

Peters A, Trimbos-Kemper G, Admiraal C, et al. A randomized clinical trial on the benefit of adhesiolysis in patients with intraperitoneal adhesions and pelvic pain. Br J Obstet Gynaecol 1992;99:59-62

Fox Ray N, Denton WG, Thamer M, Henderson SC, Perry S. Abdominal adhesiolysis: Inpatient care and expenditures in the United States in 1994. J Am Coll Surg 1998;186(1):1-9

DiZerega GS. Contemporary adhesion prevention. Fertil Steril 1994;61(2):219-235

Reich H. Laparoscopic treatment of extensive pelvic adhesions including hydrosalpinx. J Reprod Med 1987;32:736

Odell R. Principles of Electrosurgery. In Sivak M, ed. Gastroenterologic Endoscopy. New York: W.B. Saunders Company, 1987:128

Reich H, Vancaillie T, Soderstrom R. Electrical Techniques. Operative Laparoscopy. In Martin DC, Holtz GL, Levinson CJ, Soderstrom RM, eds. Manual of Endoscopy. Santa Fe Springs: American Association of Gynecologic Laparoscopists, 1990:105

Reich H, McGlynn F. Laparoscopic oophorectomy and salpingo-oophorectomy in the treatment of benign tuboovarian disease. J Reprod Med 1986;31:609

Reich H. Laparoscopic oophorectomy and salpingo-oophorectomy in the treatment of benign tubo-ovarian disease. Int J Fertil 1987;32:233

Reich H, McGlynn F. Laparoscopic treatment of tubo-ovarian and pelvic abscess. J Reprod Med 1987;32:747

Henry-Suchet J, Soler A, Lofferdo V. Laparoscopic treatment of tubo-ovarian abscesses. J Reprod Med 1984;29:579

Reich H. Endoscopic management of tuboovarian abscess and pelvic inflammatory disease. In Sanfilippo JS and Levine RL, eds. Operative Gynecologic Endoscopy. New York: Springer-Verlag, 1989:118

Reich H. Laparoscopic bowel injury. Surg Laparosc Endosc 1992;2:74

Palmer R. Safety in laparoscopy. J Reprod Med 1974;13:1-5

Fu-Hsing Chang, Hung-Hsueh Chou, Chyi-Long Lee, et al. Extraumbilical insertion of the operative laparoscope in patients with extensive intraabdominal adhesions. J Amer Assoc Gynecol Laparosc 1995;2(3):335-337

Pasic R, Wolfe WM. Transuterine insertion of Veress needle. N Z Med J 1994;107(987):411

Reich H, McGlynn F, Salvat J. Laparoscopic treatment of cul-de-sac obliteration secondary to retrocervical deep fibrotic endometriosis. J Reprod Med 1991;36:516

Peacock LM, Rock JA. Distal Tubal Reconstructive Surgery. In Sanfilippo J ed. Operative Gynecologic Endoscopy. New York: Springer, 1996:182-191

McComb PF, Paleologou A. The intussusception salpingostomy technique for the therapy of distal oviductal occlusion at laparoscopy. Obstet Gynecol 1991;78:443

Reich H. New techniques in advanced laparoscopic surgery. In Sutton C, ed. Laparoscopic Surgery. Bailliere's Clinical Obstetrics and Gynaecology. London: WB Saunders, 1989:6551

Singhal V, Li T, Cooke I. An analysis of the factors influencing the outcome of 232 consecutive tubal microsurgery cases. Br J Obstet Gynaecol 1991;98:628-36

Winston R, Margara R. Microsurgical salpingostomy is not an obsolete procedure. Br J Obstet Gynaecol 1991; 98:637-42

Watson A, Vandekerckhove P, Lilford R. Liquid and fluid agents for preventing adhesions after surgery for subfertility. Cochrane Database of Systematic Reviews. Issue 4, 2000

Farquhar C, Vandekerckhove P, Watson A, Vail A, Wiseman D. Barrier agents for preventing adhesions after surgery for subfertility. Cochrane Database of Systematic Reviews. Issue 4, 2000

Diamond MP, Linsky CB, Cunningham TC, et al. Synergistic effects of Interceed (TC7) and heparin in reducing adhesion formation in the rabbit uterine horn model. Fertil Steril 1991;55:389-94

Burns JW, Skinner K, Yu LP, et al. An injectable biodegradable gel for the prevention of postsurgical adhesions: Evaluation in two animal models. In Proceedings of the 50th Annual Meeting of the American Fertility Society, San Antonio, Texas, November 5-10, 1994

Johns DB, Keyport GM, Hoehler F. diZerega GS. Reduction of post surgical adhesions with Intergel® adhesion prevention Solution: a multicenter study of safety and efficacy after conservative gynecologic surgery. Fertil Steril 2001; 76: 595-604

Operative Laparoscopy Study Group. Postoperative adhesion development after operative laparoscopy: evaluation at early second look procedures. Fertil Steril 1991;55:700-4

Close MB, Chistensen NM. Transmesenteric small bowel plication or intraluminal tube stenting. Am J Surg 1979;138:89-91

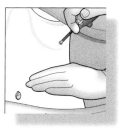

ECTOPIC PREGNANCY

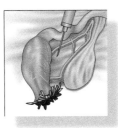

Gerard Roy, M.D.

Anthony Luciano, M.D.

INTRODUCTION

Pregnancy outside the confines of the uterine cavity has been described for hundreds of years. In the 1800s, the mortality associated with ectopic pregnancy was >60%. Today it accounts for 9% of pregnancy related mortality and less than 1% of overall mortality in women. Figure 1 depicts this data from 1970-92. Here we see a greater than 90% reduction in mortality despite more than a 5-fold increase in the overall incidence.

Although ectopic pregnancy has been recognized for over 400 years, it continues to be an ever-increasing affliction affecting greater than 2% of all pregnancies. The rising incidence of ectopic pregnancies in the past 25 years has been attributed to a number of different risk factors, listed in Table 1. Theoretically, anything that impedes migration of the conceptus to the uterine cavity may predispose a woman to

Table 1

MAJOR CONTRIBUTING FACTORS AND ASSOCIATED RELATIVE RISK FOR ECTOPIC PREGNANCY.*

RISK FACTOR	RELATIVE RISK
Current use of IUD	11.9
Use of clomiphene citrate	10.0
Prior tubal surgery	5.6
Pelvic inflammatory disease	4.0
Infertility	2.9
Induced abortion	2.5
Adhesions	2.4
Abdominal surgery	2.3
T-shaped uterus	2.0
Myomata	1.7
Progestin only oral contraceptives	1.6

*Adapted from Marchbanks PA et al: Risk factors for ectopic pregnancy: A population based study. JAMA 1988; 259:1823–7.

Table 2

SIGNS AND SYMPTONS SUGGESTIVE OF ECTOPIC PREGNANCY

- Nausea, breast fullness, fatigue, amenorrhea
- Lower abdominal pain, heavy cramping, shoulder pain
- Uterine bleeding/spotting
- Pelvic tenderness, enlarged, soft uterus
- Adnexal mass, tenderness
- Positive pregnancy test
- Serum levels of hCG <6000 mIU/mL at 6 weeks
- Less than 66% increase in hCG titers in 48 hours.
- Serum progesterone <25 ng/mL
- Aspiration of non-clotting blood on culdocentesis
- Absence of gestational sac in the uterus by U/S when the hCG titer exceeds 2500 mIU/mL
- Gestational sac outside the uterus by U/S

develop an ectopic gestation. These may be intrinsic anatomic defects in the tubal epithelium, hormonal factors that interfere with normal transport of the conceptus, or pathologic conditions that affect normal tubal functioning. Besides the symptoms commonly associated with early pregnancy, women with ectopic pregnancy commonly experience pelvic pain and bleeding. The bleeding is variable and may only be a sign of a complication. Up to 20% of women with first trimester bleeding will go on to have a

Table 3

DIFFERENTIAL DIAGNOSIS IN CASES OF SUSPECTED ECTOPIC PREGNANCY

- Spontaneous abortion
- Ruptured ovarian cyst
- Corpus luteum hemorragicum
- Adnexal torsion
- Pelvic inflammatory disease
- Endometriosis
- Urolithiasis
- Urinary tract infection
- Appendicitis
- Other lower gastrointestinal tract Disease

healthy pregnancy. Table 2 lists some of the more common signs and symptoms that need to be differentiated from other gynecologic and non-gynecologic causes. The differential diagnosis for cases of suspected ectopic pregnancies are listed in Table 3.

Until 1970, more than 80% of ectopic pregnancies were diagnosed after rupture, resulting in significant morbidity and mortality. With excellent resolution obtained from pelvic ultrasound, highly sensitive radioimmunoassays for human chorionic gonadotropin (hCG) and increased vigilance by clinicians, greater than 80% of ectopic pregnancies are now diagnosed intact which allows more conservative management.

Awareness of the possibility of an ectopic pregnancy is most critical for early detection. Measurement of hCG with a doubling time of 2-3 days should occur if it is a normal gestation. A note of caution is that approximately 10% of normal pregnancies do not follow this doubling time.

When hCG levels are >1000 mIU/mL, transvaginal ultrasound is reliable in diagnosing the location of the gestation approximately 98% of the time. If using an abdominal ultrasound, then the hCG needs to be above 6000

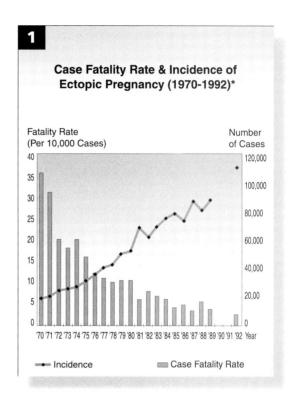

Case Fatality Rate & Incidence of Ectopic Pregnancy (1970-1992)*

mIU/mL to make an accurate diagnosis. Progesterone can also be used to help differentiate a viable from nonviable gestation. A progesterone level of greater than 25 ng/mL is indicative of a healthy gestation and a level lower than 15 ng/mL may signal an abnormal pregnancy. Values between those are more ambiguous.

The incidence of ectopic pregnancy based on location has been relatively unchanged for many years. Figure 2 shows the location of various ectopic pregnancies and their incidence in each location. The ampullary portion of the Fallopian tube is the site of the majority of ectopic pregnancies. This may be due to the fact that it is where the tube begins to narrow, where fertilization begins, or that it may be the most distal point of the majority of ascending infections that will still allow fertilization. Infectious damage to the fimbria typically causes phymosis and infertility. The ampullary portion of the tube lends itself extraordinarily well to minimally invasive surgical correction.

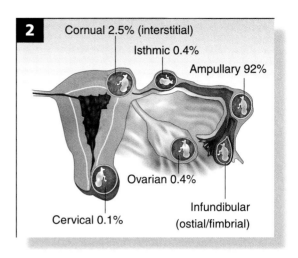

ANATOMY OF THE FALLOPIAN TUBE

The oviduct or tube is approximately 10-12 cm long. The tube itself can be functionally and anatomically divided into four parts (Figure 3). The intramural or interstitial portion of the tube is approximately 1 cm long and traverses through the myometrium and opens in the endometrial cavity. This is the 'valve' where the sperm line up to start their journey up the oviduct. It is also a highly vascular area and makes conservative surgical management more difficult.

The isthmus of the tube is approximately 4-6 cm in length. It is composed of a double layer of muscle and inner lumen. The outer muscle layer runs longitudinal to the axis of the tube and is thicker than the inner muscle layer, which is oriented in a circular fashion.

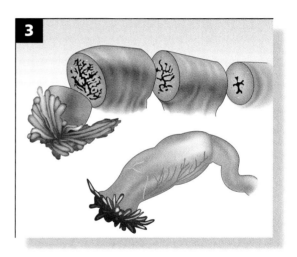

The lumen of the isthmus is approximately 1-2 mm until it gets to the ampulla where it enlarges.

The ampulla is the longest segment of the tube and makes up approximately 2/3 of the total length. Beneath the mucosa of the ampullary portion of the tube there is a series of large blood vessels – mostly veins originating from the uterine/ovarian supply to the tube. These become engorged at the time of ovulation to bring the fimbrae closer to the ovary. They can also be problematic during surgical treatment for an ectopic pregnancy. These vessels travel in a thick longitudinal muscle layer. The lumen of the tube is wider here and the mucosa has more rugae, which are covered with ciliated and secretory cells. These cells may be damaged with infection, previous ectopic or surgery predisposing patients to a greater risk of tubal pregnancy.

The final portion of the tube is the infundibulum of the oviduct. It is funnel shaped and its most distal end is called the fimbriae. There are greater concentrations of ciliary cells here that facilitate transport of the ovum into the ampulla.

The blood supply to the tube arises from a cascade of vessels originating from an arcuate formed by a branch of the ovarian artery and a tubal branch of the uterine artery (Figure 4). This arcuate is located in the mesosalpinx, between the Fallopian tube and ovary. Vessels then perforate the medial side of the tube and travel in the intimal layer.

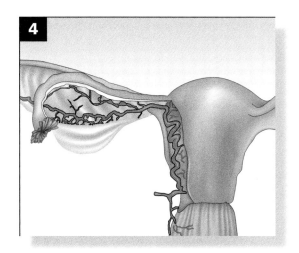

TREATMENT OPTIONS

Treatment options for ectopic pregnancy have broadened substantially in the past 10-15 years. Prior to this, laparotomy with salpingectomy was the standard of care. Now in an attempt to preserve tubal function, a more conservative approach has been taken. This is due to better resolution ultrasound and earlier diagnosis, improved microsurgical laparoscopic techniques and chemotherapeutics. Laparoscopic treatment of this condition is growing in popularity and is currently considered the standard of care. Even hemodyamic instability is not an absolute contraindication to laparoscopy. The availability of optimal anesthesia, advanced cardiovascular monitoring, ability to convert quickly to laparotomy, and superior magnification given by laparoscopy make it a viable option and possibly the best choice.

Some studies have shown that laparoscopy achieves superior pregnancy rates to laparotomy. It also carries decreased morbidity, length of hospital stays and costs as well as less need for analgesia.

Since the 1970s, a conservative approach to unruptured ectopic pregnancy has been advocated by many of the leading authorities in our field. There are several different types of conservative surgery that can be performed. These include linear salpingostomy, partial salpingectomy with anastomosis, and 'milking' the pregnancy from the distal ampulla.

SURGICAL MANAGEMENT BASED ON LOCATION

The location, size, and extent of the tubal pregnancy are observed laparoscopically. The management of each ectopic pregnancy is based upon these factors. Whatever the surgical approach chosen, adequate hemostasis with minimal trauma is optimal and should be obtained with as little cauterization as possible. All surgical approaches start by identification and mobilization of the involved Fallopian tube and inspection of the uninvolved side.

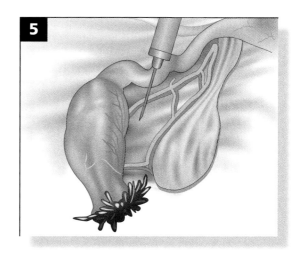

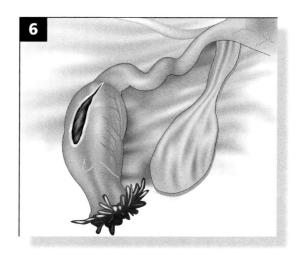

Ampullary ectopic: Once diagnosed, if the pregnancy is in the mid-ampullary segment as in the majority of cases, a 5-7 mL dilute solution of vasopressin (20 U/100mL of NS) is used. This is injected with a laparoscopic needle into the mesosalpinx just below the pregnancy and over the anti-mesenteric surface of the segment containing the gestation (Figure 5). It is extremely important to make sure that the vasopressin is not injected directly into a blood vessel as it can cause arterial hypertension, brady-cardia and death. Using a laser, micro-electrode, scissors, or harmonic scalpel a linear incision is made over the pregnancy approximately 1–2 cm in length (Figure 6). As one makes this incision the contents of the pregnancy usually begins to extrude. This can be completed by hydro dissection or using gentle traction with laparoscopic forceps (Figure 7). In some cases, more forceful irrigation in the salpingostomy incision may be required to dislodge the pregnancy from its implantation site. Occasionally, coagulation is used to secure hemostasis and is best accomplished with bipolar micro-forceps. Oozing from the tubal bed is common and usually ceases spontaneously. Copious irrigation is used to dislodge trophoblastic tissue and remove blood from the peritoneal cavity. The tubal opening is left to heal by secondary intention, unless the defect is wide and the edges do not come together spontaneously. For such cases, the edges may be approximated with a single 4–0 absorbable suture.

If the pregnancy is located in the distal ampullary segment of the tube, then, occasionally, the tubal segment

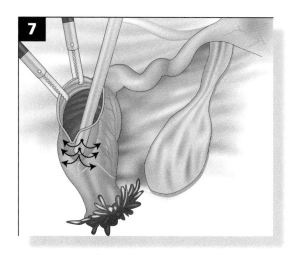

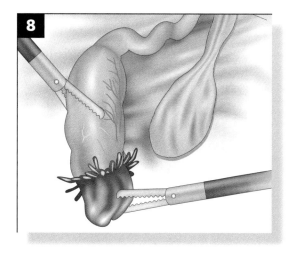

can be grasped and the pregnancy 'milked' out the fimbriae of the tube (Figure 8). This can also be done for partially extruded tubal pregnancies and infundibular pregnancies.

Isthmic ectopic: When the ectopic pregnancy implants in the isthmic portion of the tube, linear salpingostomy is not as successful because typically these pregnancies grow through the lumen of the tube and erode the muscularis.

Isthmic ectopic pregnancies have a higher rate of persistence and tubal patency is seldom preserved. With isthmic tubal pregnancy, segmental tubal resection is preferred. This can be accomplished by various means (i.e. bipolar, laser, sutures, or stapling devices). Bloodless resection is optimal and may be accomplished by using bipolar forceps, grasping both proximal and distal to the gestation and coagulating from the anti-mesenteric surface to the mesosalpinx (Figure 9). This is then cut and the mesosalpinx cauterized and cut in a similar fashion (Figure 10). The tube may be reanastomosed at a later date if desired.

Salpingectomy: This technique is chosen in the presence of uncontrolled bleeding, tubal destruction, recurrent ectopic in that tube, patient desire, or severe adhesion or hydrosalpinx. The tube is removed from its anatomical attachments. This can be accomplished by numerous methods including laser, stapling devices, harmonic energy, endoloops, or progressive bipolar coagulation. Progressive coagulation and cutting the mesosalpinx begins at the proximal isthmus of the tube and progresses to the fimbriated end (Figures 11 and 12). The products of conception can

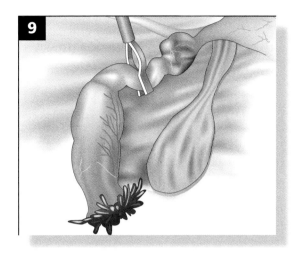

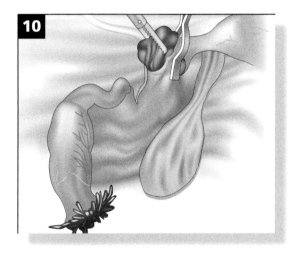

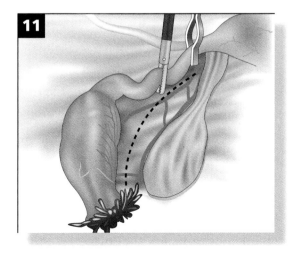

be removed through a 10-mm trocar sleeve with or without the use of a plastic bag (Endo-pouch, Ethicon, Inc.,Cincinnati, OH or Cook Sac).

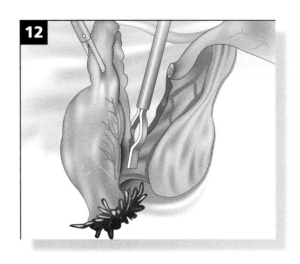

Interstitial/cornual ectopic: Fortunately, these types of ectopic pregnancies are rare with a prevalence of 1 in 5000 live births. Late diagnosis of this type of ectopic pregnancy, and the vascular nature of the cornua account for a mortality rate of 2-2.5%. Two to 4% of all ectopic gestations are interstitial/cornual. The traditional management of this type of ectopic gestation is laparotomy with salpingectomy and/or cornual resection. This surgery occasionally culminates in hysterectomy. It is important, however, to make a distinction between the interstitial ectopic and a true cornual ectopic pregnancy. The interstitial portion of the Fallopian tube is approximately 1 cm long, has a narrow lumen and follows a tortuous course through a thick layer of myometrium. The cornual pregnancy implants in this section of tube but opens to the uterine cavity. This allows hysteroscopy to be a potential method of surgical correction. However, the interstitial pregnancy implants deeper in this segment of the Fallopian tube and is not accessible from the uterine cavity, thus, it is not amenable to hysteroscopic resec-

tion. If the diagnosis is made early and the patient is stable, more conservative approaches should be considered. These options include methotrexate locally or systemically, potassium chloride injections locally and prostaglandin administration. Once the diagnosis is confirmed and medical management is not possible, surgical treatment options are explored and consist of immediate laparotomy or a combined laparoscopic, and hysteroscopic approach.

If the overlying myometrium is thin, a laparoscopic resection may be possible. Figure 13-1 demonstrates the appearance of an interstitial pregnancy laparoscopically. This pregnancy was managed using bipolar coagulation on the thinnest portion of the interstitium, and scissors were then used to enter the gestational sac. The fetus and gestation were then removed from this incision and bleeding was controlled with bipolar coagulation. The uterus was then closed with two intracorporeal figure of eight sutures (Figure 13-2). Early detection may afford one the option of a combined treatment using laparoscopy/hysteroscopy and methotrexate. If the gestation is truly cornual and accessible by hysteroscopy, it is resected using electrosurgery and removed.

For larger gestations that are accessible through the uterus, it may be safer and faster to do a gentle curettage under laparoscopic guidance. Remember that the cornua are extremely vascular and profuse bleeding can occur rapidly. Therefore, it is always prudent to have these patients typed and crossed for several units of packed red blood cells as well as consented for laparotomy.

Ovarian pregnancy: Pregnancy located in the ovary itself is a rare occurrence. The incidence is 1 in 6970 deliveries and 0.7 per 100 ectopic gestations. Table 4 delineates Speigelberg's criteria for the diagnosis of ovarian pregnancy established in 1878 and still used today. Management of ovarian pregnancy can be either medical or surgical. Typically, they are diagnosed in

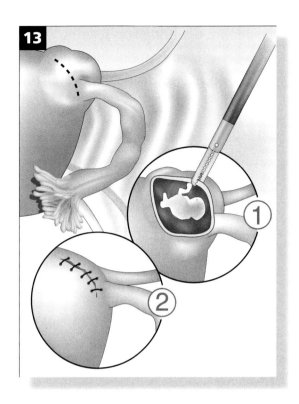

the first trimester and can be definitively treated by oophorectomy.

The ovarian ligament is grasped with bipolar forceps, cauterized and cut (Figure 14). The mesoovarium is then

Table 4

SPIEGELBERG'S CRITERIA FOR OVARIAN ECTOPIC PREGNANCY

1. Fallopian tube on the affected side must be intact

2. Fetal sac must occupy the position of the ovary

3. Ovary must be connected to the uterus by the ovarian ligament

4. Definite ovarian tissue must be found in the sac wall

taken down in a progressive fashion. This can also be performed using an endoloop or with the harmonic scalpel.

Cervical pregnancy: This type of ectopic pregnancy is also very rare and in the past was treated by hysterectomy. Management now is by medical therapy with methotrexate when possible. This has been proven safe, effective and preserves the patient's fertility options for the future.

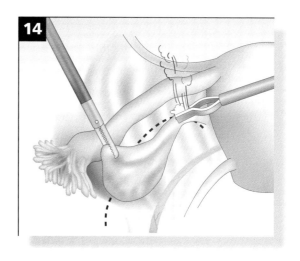

Abdominal pregnancy: This type of ectopic can either be primary or secondary based on the initial implantation site. Occasionally, a tubal pregnancy will rupture and implant abdominally and continue to evolve. This can also occur with tubal abortions. The management for abdominal ectopic is strictly by laparotomy as these pregnancies are usually not diagnosed until third trimester. Figure 15 shows a schematic of a possible implantation of an abdominal pregnancy. Realize that this implantation can occur on any organ in the abdominal cavity. The delivery is by laparotomy and there is controversy on removal of the placenta at that time or at a later date. It may be more prudent to leave the placenta in situ after delivery and use the interventional radiologist to embolize the placental bed prior to removal in an attempt to conserve

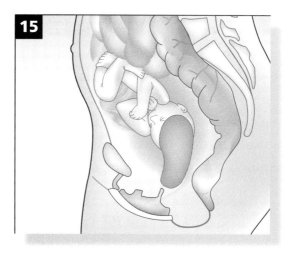

blood loss in this potentially catastrophic situation.

Management of ruptured ectopic pregnancy: Laparoscopy is considered to be presently the gold standard in treating patients with an unruptured ectopic pregnancy. Sometimes patients may present with ruptured ectopic pregnancy and surgical abdomen full of blood and blood clots.

Those patients may frequently be approached laparoscopically and there may be no need for laparotomy in patients with a ruptured ectopic pregnancy. There are several factors you need to keep in mind when performing laparoscopy in these patients.

Establishment of the pneumoperitoneum and placement of the trocar may be just as quick as performing laparotomy. When placing the Veress needle in the abdomen filled with blood, you may encounter higher initial insufflation pressures, since the tip of the needle may be immersed in blood. Only a sponge stick should be placed in the vagina for uterine manipulation, to avoid disruption of a possible intrauterine pregnancy.

After the placement of the umbilical trocar and insertion of the laparoscope, the patient should be placed in steep Trendelenburg position and a suprapubic port should be inserted and grasper introduced for quick localization of the ruptured tube, and to tamponade the bleeding site. After the bleeding area has been compressed, attention should be turned toward the removal of blood and blood clots. A cell saver is a great way to replace the patient's blood loss with her own blood and it may be utilized whenever a large blood loss is encountered.

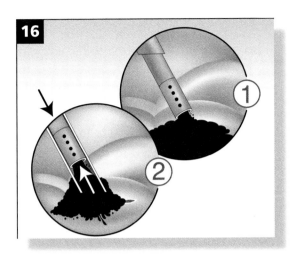

Blood clots should be removed with the help of the 5-mm laparoscopic suction device. The 10-mm suction does not offer any advantages since it is reduced to 5-mm in the instrument's handle. The best way to remove blood clots is to apply constant suction on the suction device, and to aspirate the clots and break them by pulling the suction tip into the 5 mm trocar. This maneuver breaks the clots and helps to evacuate them through the suction aspirator (Figure 16). Try to avoid excessive irrigation since the fluid in the abdomen lifts the bowel, which in turn decreases your area of vision.

After the blood has been removed from the abdominal cavity, proper assessment of the ectopic pregnancy can be made and an adequate treatment plan developed.

MEDICAL MANAGEMENT

The use of methotrexate has enabled the treatment of ectopic pregnancy to be even more conservative than laparoscopy. It can be used in all types of ectopic gestation and used either intramuscularly or directly into the gestation. Not all patients are candidates for medical management. Table 5 shows some of the criteria used to delineate the appropriate patients. If the criteria are met then 50 mg/m² are given in a single IM dose. Quantitative hCG is checked on day 4 and 7.

Table 5

INDICATIONS FOR THE USE OF METHOTREXATE IN ECTOPIC PREGNANCY

- Patient is reliable, compliant, healthy and hemodynamically stable
- Ultrasound notes definite ectopic gestation
- Pregnancy sac is less than 4 cm
- hCG titers <10,000 IU/mL
- Progesterone levels <10 ng/mL
- Absent fetal cardiac activity
- Normal liver function test, CBC
- Give Rhogam if Rh negative

Weekly titers are then obtained until the titer is negative. A drop in titers of 15% should be seen from the day 4 value to the day 7 value. Less than 10% of patients need a second injection of methotrexate. This method is 80-90% effective but runs the risk of emergent surgical correction for rupture. Therefore, the patient must be reliable and compliant and aware of this risk.

CONCLUSION

Ectopic pregnancy remains an increasing health problem. Its incidence continues to rise, paralleling the progressive increase in the incidence of its etiologic factors, especially, sexually transmitted diseases. With the advent of technology, improved ultrasonography and minimally invasive techniques, the surgical management of this worrisome condition can be less damaging. This may improve a patient's future fertility by enabling medical management as well as microscopic surgical techniques with similar success as more radical approaches to this life threatening condition.

SUGGESTED READING:

Nezhat,C., Seigler, Nezhat,F., et al. Operative Gynecologic Laparoscopy: Principles and Techniques, 2nd edn. McGraw-Hill Co. 2000:211-31

Speroff, Glass, Kase, Clinical Gynecologic Endocrinology and Infertility, 6th edn. Lippin-cott Williams&Wilkins, 1999:1149-67

Jain, Solima, Luciano, Ectopic Pregnancy, The J AAGL 1997;Vol4, No. 4:513-30

Marchblanks PA, JF Aneger, CB, Coulman,et al., Risk factors for ectopic pregnancy: A population based study. JAMA 1988;259: 1823-1827

Westrom L, Bengtsson LP, Mardh PA. Incidence, trends, and risks of ectopic pregnancy in a population of women. Br Med J (Clin Res Ed.) 1981; 282(6257): 15-8

Shepherd RW, Patton PE, Novy MJ, Burry KA. Serial data-hCG measurements in the early detection of ectopic pregnancy. Obstet Gynecol 1990; 75: 417-20

Kadar NG, Devore R, Romero. Discriminatory hCG zone: its use in the sonographic evaluation for ectopic pregnancy. Obstet Gynecol 1981; 58(2): 156-61

Decherney AH, Kase N. The conservative surgical management of unruptured ectopic pregnancy. Obstet Gynecol 1979; 54: 451-3

Tuomivaara LA, Kappila. Radical or conservative surgery for ectopic pregnancy? A follow up study of fertility of 323 patients. Fertil Steril 1988; 50: 580-583

Vermish M, Silva PD, Rosen GF, et al. Management of unruptured ectopic gestation by linear salpingostomy: A prospective randomized clinical trial of laparoscopy versus laparotomy. Obstet Gynecol 1989; 73: 400-3

Bruhat MA, H. Mahnes, G. Mage, et al. Treatment of ectopic pregnancy by means of laparoscopy. Fertil Steril 1980; 33: 411-14

Brumstead JC, Kessler C, Gibson,et al. A comparison of laparoscopy and laparotomy for the treatment of ectopic pregnancy. Obstet Gynecol 1988; 71: 889-92

Stenman UH, Tenhunen A, Ylikorkala O. Conservative treatment of ectopic pregnancy. Ann New York Academy Sciences 1991; 626: 516-23

Trio D, Strobelt N, Picciolo C, et al. Prognostic factors for successful expectant management of ectopic pregnancy. Fertil Steril 1995, Mar; 63(3): 469-72

Stovall TG, Ling FW, Gray LA. Single-dose methotrexate for treatment of ectopic pregnancy. Obstet Gynecol 1991, May; 77(5): 754-7

Lipscomb GH, McCord ML, Stovall TG, et al. Predictors of success of methotrexate treatment on women with tubal ectopic pregnancies. N Engl J Med 1999; 341: 1974-8

Graczykowski JW, Mishell DR. Methotrexate prophylaxis for persistent ectopic pregnancy after conservative treatment by salpingostomy, Obstet Gynecol 1997; 89: 118-22

Bremer T, Cela V, Luciano A. Surgical management of interstitial pregnancy. J AAGL 2000; 7, no.3:387-89

ENDOSCOPIC SURGERY FOR CHRONIC PELVIC PAIN

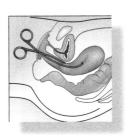

David L. Olive, M.D.

SUMMARY

Chronic pelvic pain should not be considered a primary surgical disease, but in some cases laparoscopic intervention may prove to be of value. Three procedures detailed here have some application to this problem; each can be helpful in specific instances where patients have been thoroughly evaluated and a number of diagnoses excluded. Thus, it is imprudent to think of these procedures as generalized approaches to the problem of chronic pelvic pain. Rather, these surgeries represent highly specialized techniques to combat specific pathologies.

A second aspect these three procedures share is a lack of proven efficacy. While all seem theoretically sound, only the laparoscopic uterosacral nerve ablation has undergone testing via randomized clinical trial, and even here the numbers are small and follow-up is brief. Before these procedures are adopted as routine, more rigorous testing and evaluation are clearly needed.

Chronic pelvic pain (CPP) is the bane of many gynecologists' existence: it is difficult to diagnose, and treatments are often of questionable efficacy. Medical therapy is generally the initial therapy; only when this has failed do gynecologists resort to surgical intervention. Even in this situation, directly viewing the pelvis can be problematic: in a review by Howard, 61% of patients with chronic pain had pathology at laparoscopy versus 28% in the control group. However, less than half these women experienced pain relief with surgical intervention. This raises several important issues regarding the role of endoscopic surgery for pelvic pain:

1. Can surgery help identify factors critical to the etiology of pelvic pain?

2. Can surgical targets be identified that will modify the pain experienced by those with CPP?

3. Does surgical intervention provide an advantage over medical therapy in the treatment of CPP?

Several chapters in this textbook consider procedures directed at pathology believed to contribute to pelvic pain (see Chapter 9 on Endometriosis, Chapter 10 Adhesiolysis, and Chapter 19 on Presacral Neurectomy). This chapter will review additional procedures used to combat pelvic pain. The first, laparoscopy under local anesthesia/con-scious sedation, is used to map the pain and attempt to determine the potential for surgical and medical intervention. The second, laparoscopic uterosacral nerve abla-tion/resection, is an attempt to alter the transmission pathway of pain from the central pelvis. Finally, uterine suspension is a procedure used to alter anatomic relationships in an attempt to reduce a specific type of pain: dyspare-unia. These procedures will be reviewed in detail in terms of their indications, methodology, and rates of success.

MICROLAPAROSCOPY UNDER LOCAL ANESTHESIA AND CONSCIOUS SEDATION

When patients present to the physician's office with CPP, the physician generally develops a differential diagnosis and investigates those etiologies thought to be of reasonable likelihood. Often that involves pathology that could be easily viewed at laparoscopy: examples include endometriosis and pelvic adhesions. However, an assumption is often made that pathology seen is causative of, or directly related to, the pelvic pain. In addition, patients with no visible pathology are often assumed to be disease free despite continual pain. When the patient is under general anesthesia, no feedback can be obtained that will add information beyond visual inspection of the pelvis.

Pain mapping during laparoscopy under local anesthesia/conscious sedation allows evaluation of the internal anatomy as a causative factor for chronic pain. The technique is as follows:

A uterine manipulator is placed within the cervical canal, with only local anesthesia (or none). Intrauterine balloons or heavy instruments with traction should be avoided, as they produce significant pain in a large number of patients (Figure 1).

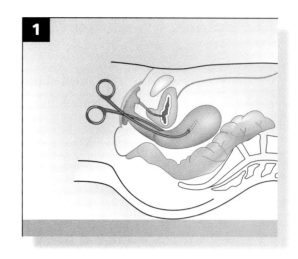

The patient, having been administered mild intravenous sedation (medazolam 1 mg, fentanyl 0.025 mg), is now given local anesthetic in the umbilicus (1% lidocaine and 0.25% bupivacaine in a 1:1 mixture). The local anesthesia is injected first superficially, then deep into the subcutaneous tissue and fascia (Figure 2).

After waiting approximately one minute, a small (2 mm) incision is made in the umbilicus. The lower abdomen is grasped and raised, and a Veress needle with microlaparoscopic sheath is inserted directly into the peritoneal cavity. No insufflation is performed initially; instead, the laparoscope is inserted to determine if placement is correct. If so, insufflation is carried out slowly under direct visualization (Figure 3).

Once the pelvis can be seen, the patient is placed in steep Trendelenburg position and the insufflation turned off (Figure 4).

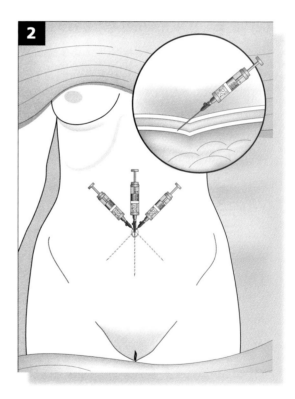

A second puncture site is chosen in the midline just above the pubic symphysis. Local anesthesia, incision, and Veress needle/trocar placement are performed as with the umbilical incision, but this time under direct visualization (Figure 5).

Complete, systematic inspection of the pelvis is now performed. Using a blunt probe in the second trocar site, pressure is applied to each area of normal anatomy and pathology. This can be done most consistently by developing a routine. Our technique is to begin in anterior cul-de-sac and move in a clockwise fashion, thus: (A) the anterior cul-de-sac, (B) right adnexa, (C) posterior cul-de-sac, (D) rectum, (E) utero-sacral ligaments, (F) left adnexa, and (G) uterus are all observed and prodded. The patient is asked to rate each area, when probed, on a scale of 0–10, as well as to state whether or not the pain is identical to that responsible for her symptoms (Figure 6).

If areas of pathology are noted, these too are examined for eliciting pain, utilizing the same technique as above (Figure 7). If a distinct area of pain is noted, local anesthesia can be applied directly to the area and pain relief is assessed (Figure 8).

If a uterosacral nerve ablation is contemplated in the future, injection of the uterosacral ligaments under direct visualization is performed in an attempt to predict efficacy (Figure 9). Similarly, if a presacral neurectomy is considered, injection of anesthetic into this area can help determine its likely value (Figure 10).

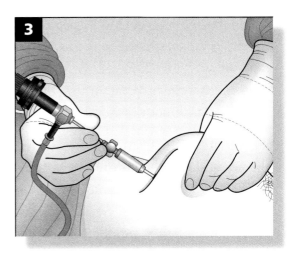

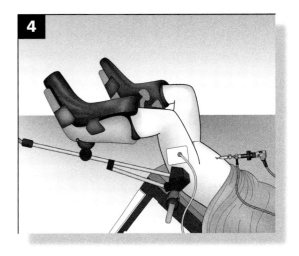

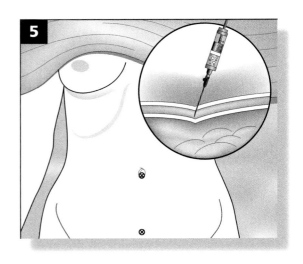

When the procedure is complete, all instruments are removed. Sutures are not needed to close incisions; small bandages are all that is required.

Results of pain mapping with micro-laparoscopy under conscious sedation reveal it to be an extremely well tolerated procedure (Table 1). However, patients with pelvic pain do respond more poorly than those undergoing the procedure for other indications.

Three overall patterns of response have been observed. In some patients, pain is either not elicited or is uniformly present at a low level. A second group of patients exhibit focally painful areas with a rating significantly greater than background. This finding of focal pain is often independent of identifiable pathology. While these patients may be regarded as surgical candidates, it must be realized that long-term follow-up studies have not been performed to test this hypothesis. A final subset of patients exhibits what we have called generalized visceral hypersensitivity (GVH): these women have pain in virtually all areas probed. It is our hypothesis that these patients will do poorly at surgery; however, this too is untested.

LAPAROSCOPIC UTEROSACRAL NERVE ABLATION (LUNA)

The central portion of the pelvis receives the bulk of its nerve supply from

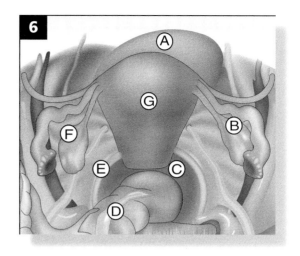

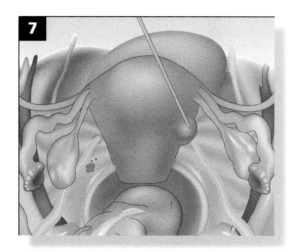

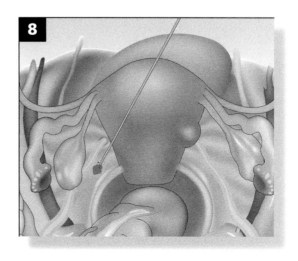

sympathetic nerve branches and parasympathetic fibers that pass through the uterosacral ligament. One approach to reducing central pelvic pain has been to surgically interrupt these fibers. Two approaches have been utilized: (1) presacral neurectomy (see Chapter 19) and (2) uterosacral nerve ablation. Both can be performed via the endoscope; the latter is described here.

The surgeon must begin by closely examining the pelvic anatomy of the posterior cul-de-sac. If adhesion formation is present, this must by lysed and structures identified prior to any tissue destruction for pain relief. In particular, the ureters must be clearly identified and distinguished from the uterosacral ligaments; these can be closely approximated or even confused with one another in the presence of substantial pathology.

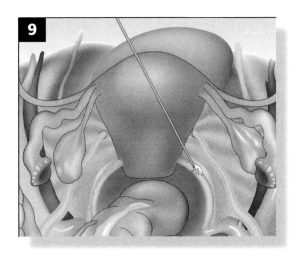

Table 1

RESULTS OF OFFICE MICROLAPAROSCOPY UNDER LOCAL ANESTHESIA

	All	CPP	INF	p Value
AGE (YEARS)	35.33	36.45	34.56	NS
GRAVIDY	0.96	1.55	0.56	<0.05
OPERATIVE TIME (MINS)	20.85	23.91	18.75	NS
RECOVERY TIME (MINS)	51.65	51.64	51.67	NS
FENTANYL (MG)	81.48	90.91	75.00	0.05
VERSED (MG)	3.20	4.00	2.66	<0.05
PAIN SCALE SCORE	5.87	7.00	5.04	<0.05
30 MIN POSTOP PAIN SCORE	1.48	3.17	0.53	<0.005
TIME TO NORMAL ACTIVITY (DAYS)	1.88	1.73	2.01	NS
TIME TO RETURN TO WORK (DAYS)	1.70	2.23	1.29	<0.05
TIME TO RESUME INTERCOURSE (DAYS)	4.61	5.42	4.21	NS
POSTOPMED USAGE (TABLETS IBUPROFEN)	4.88	9.45	1.53	<0.005

Once the uterosacral ligaments have been clearly isolated from surrounding structures, they are grasped. The ligament is mobilized medially by longitudinally incising the peritoneum lateral to the structure and medial to the ureter (Figure 11).

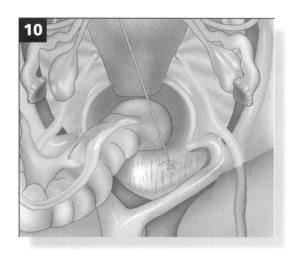

The uterosacral ligament is then incised at the cervico-utero-ligament junction. The uterosacral ligament is similarly incised approximately 2 cm distally (Figure 12).

The ligament is now dissected free of all underlying tissue, and the peritoneum medial to the structure is incised, resulting in complete excision of this portion of the uterosacral ligament (Figure 13). The entire procedure is carried out bilaterally.

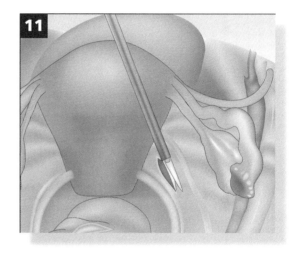

Results of uterosacral nerve ablations show the procedure to be highly efficacious initially in the treatment of dysmenorrhea. However, the amount of pain relief appears to decline substantially over time, and the procedure has produced results inferior to those of presacral neurectomy at 12 months.

Significant complications have been reported for the LUNA. Ablating or resecting the uterosacral ligaments may result in a loss of pelvic support and ultimately prolapse. Significant bladder voiding dysfunction has also occurred. Finally, ureteral damage due to incorrect

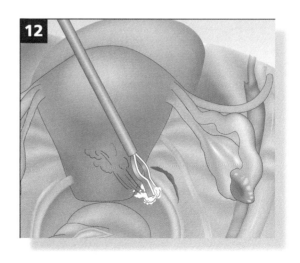

identification and isolation of structures is reported.

UTERINE SUSPENSION

Displacement of the uterus posteriorly was regarded for some time as a pathologic entity, but recent evidence suggests that few disorders are truly linked to such displacement. Contact dyspareunia has been noted in selected women with retropositioned uteri; correction of the uterus to a more anterior position has been used as an attempt to remedy the symptom. Additionally, it is often desirable following extensive surgery of the posterior cul-de-sac to prevent uterine retropositioning in the postoperative period, thereby minimizing adhesion formation in this compartment.

The uterine suspension is best performed laparoscopically with specialized instruments designed to grasp the round ligament and pass suture via small abdominal incisions. A permanent suture is also advised for long-term stability of the repair.

Initially, a small 2-mm incision is made in the skin just above the insertion of the round ligament into the abdominal wall (Figure 14). Using a grasping instrument, the round ligament is grasped and placed in tension to provide a straight course. A suture passer is

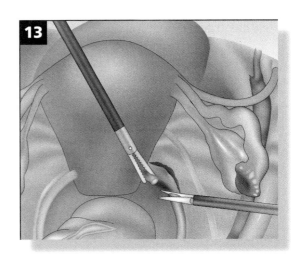

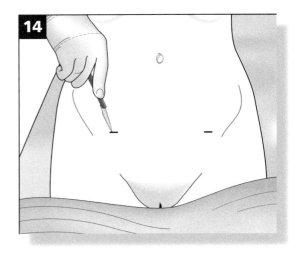

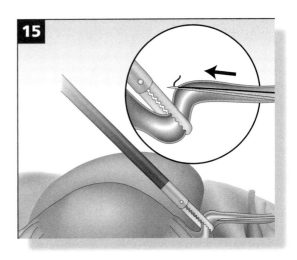

inserted through the abdominal wall and within the round ligament to within 1–2 cm of the uterus (Figure 15).

The passer then exits the round ligament, the suture is released, and the grasper is used to grasp the suture end (Figure 16). The passer is removed, then reinserted and pushed through a second exit point. The free suture end is then grasped by the passer (Figure 16 B).

The free end is withdrawn with the passer, and the suture is tied above the abdominal wall fascia, shortening and strengthening the round ligament (Figures 17 and 18). The procedure is then repeated on the opposite side.

Outcome measurement for this procedure is restricted to uncontrolled trials, all of which demonstrate significant pain relief in a carefully selected group of patients. A true randomized clinical trial of the procedure has not been performed; thus, further studies are necessary before a definitive conclusion about the value of uterine suspension can be made.

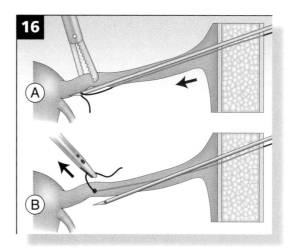

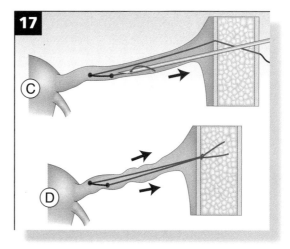

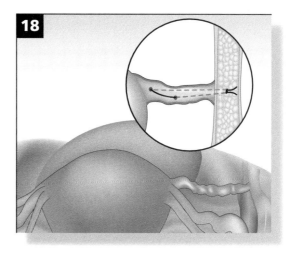

Suggested Reading:

Howard FM. The role of laparoscopy in chronic pelvic pain: promise and pitfalls. Obstet Gynecol Surg 1993;48:357-387.

Palter SF, Olive DL. Office laparoscopy under local anesthesia for chronic pelvic pain. J Am Assoc Gynecol Laparosc 1996;3:359-364.

Palter SF. Office-based surgery and its role in the management of pelvic pain. In Black-well RE, Olive DL, eds. Chronic pelvic pain: evaluation and management. New York, Springer-Verlag, 1998:167-182.

Lichten EM, Bombard J. Surgical treatment of primary dysmenorrhea with laparoscopic uterine nerve ablation. J Reprod Med 1987;32:37-41.

Chen FP, Chang SD, Chu KK, et al. Comparison of laparoscopic presacral neurectomy and laparoscopic uterine nerve ablation for primary dysmenorrhea. J Reprod Med 1996;41:463-466.

Davis GD. Uterine prolapse after laparoscopic uterosacral transection in nulliparous air-borne trainees: a report of three cases. J Reprod Med 1996;41:279-282.

Fitzpatrick CC, Flood H, Punch M, et al. Bladder dysfunction after repeat laparoscopic uterine nerve ablation (LUNA). Int Urogynecol J 1995;6:31-33.

Sharp HT. Surgical management of pelvic pain. In Blackwell RE, Olive DL, eds. Chronic pelvic pain: evaluation and management. New York, Springer-Verlag, 1998, pp 153-166.

Carter, JE. Carter-Thomason uterine suspension and positioning by ligament invest-ment, fixation, and truncation. J Reprod Med 1999;44:417-422.

Ivey J. Laparoscopic uterine suspension as an adjunctive procedure at the time of laser laparoscopy for the treatment of endometriosis. J Reprod Med 1992;37:759-765.

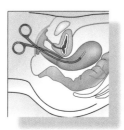

EVALUATION AND MANAGEMENT OF ADNEXAL MASSES

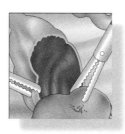

Resad Pasic, M.D., Ph.D.

It is estimated that 5-10% of women in the United States will undergo a surgical procedure for a suspected ovarian neoplasm during their lifetime, and 13-20% of these women will be diagnosed with an ovarian malignancy. The ultimate question when surgery is planned for an adnexal mass is whether the mass is benign or malignant? If the mass is benign, the laparoscopic approach is preferred. However, if there is suspicion of malignancy, other questions arise, such as:

1. What is the possibility that the entire mass can be removed laparoscopically without intraabdominal spillage?

2. If the spillage does occur, will it compromise the patient's survival?

3. If malignancy is discovered will it be possible to perform adequate surgical staging?

Therefore, a thorough preoperative evaluation is required before deciding on the surgical approach to an adnexal mass. A complete family history, physical examination, and ultrasonic imaging are vital in evaluating a suspected ovarian mass. The patient's age is an important factor in discriminating malignant from benign disease. In postmenopausal women, serum CA 125 determination further improves sensitivity and specificity. The majority of reproductive age women have benign adnexal masses. The risk of ovarian cancer in premenopausal women with an ovarian mass is 4/1000. The overall risk of malignancy in a persistent mass in a postmenopausal woman is much higher and is estimated to be between 20% and 30%. Therefore, it is impor-

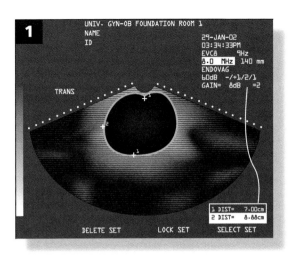

tant to divide patients into premenopausal versus postmenopausal when planning management.

Transvaginal sonography plays an important role in preoperative evaluation of patients with a pelvic mass. It provides useful information about the nature of the mass that can influence the clinical decision regarding selection of the operative approach via laparoscopy versus laparotomy, especially when malignancy is suspected. The accuracy of ultrasound in detecting the presence, size, location, and texture of a pelvic mass is in the range of 90% according to a number of studies and is definitely superior to manual examination. Ultrasonographic criteria for predicting a low risk of malignancy include size, unilaterality, a unilocular cyst with smooth borders, and no peritoneal fluid

MANAGEMENT OF ADNEXAL MASS DEPENDS UPON:

1. AGE AND MENOPAUSAL STATUS
2. SIZE OF THE MASS
3. ULTRASONOGRAPHIC FEATURES
4. LEVEL OF CA 125
5. PRESENCE OF SYMPTOMS
6. UNILATERAL VS. BILATERAL MASS

(Figure 1). A pelvic mass should be considered suspect for malignancy when it appears solid, fixed or with irregular borders (Figure 2).

SELECTION CRITERIA FOR MALIGNANT OVARIAN MASSES

SUSPICION FOR MALIGNANCY

Ultrasound cannot identify small endometriotic implants, and definitive diagnosis of endometriosis requires laparoscopic visualization and tissue confirmation. The sonographic appearance of larger endometriotic lesions can be cystic, solid or both and the images obtained by ultrasound can often be highly suggestive of the disease (Figure 3). Recurrences of endometriomas are often visible on ultrasound examination. In women with known pathology transvaginal scanning can be useful in monitoring disease activity. Endometriomas and hemorrhagic cysts present with regular borders, slightly thicker walls and sometimes with internal echoes.

The addition of color flow Doppler (CDS) to routine vaginal scanning can help in evaluation of ovarian torsion, diagnosis of pelvic congestion assessment of utero-ovarian perfusion and

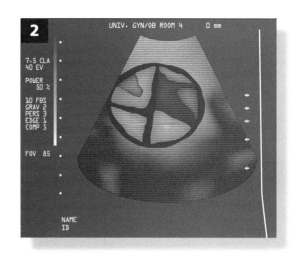

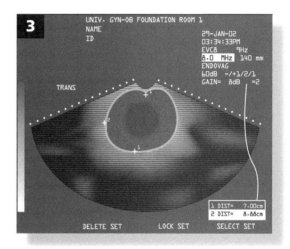

- PATIENT'S AGE (POSTMENOPAUSAL)
- SIZE OF THE MASS > 8 CM
- IRREGULAR BORDERS
- PRESENCE AND THICKNESS OF SEPTATIONS
- PAPILLARY EXCRESCENCES
- CA 125 > 35
- PULSATILITY INDEX < 0.7
- FIXED IMMOBILE MASS

differentiation of benign from malignant ovarian masses. The waveform shape obtained by CDS provides a rough indication of the type of blood flow within the vessel. Tumor vessels typically have continuous high diastolic flow with low pulsatility due to the lack of a muscular layer in the vessel wall. Normal arterioles have a muscular layer that helps regulate parenchymal perfusion. This is associated with lack of continuous diastolic flow, high pulsatility, a resistance index higher than 0.7 and presence of a diastolic notch (Figure 4).

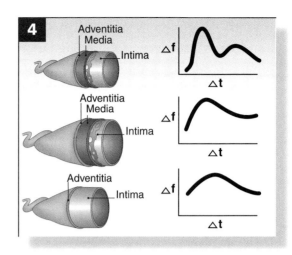

Areas of abnormal vascularity can be used as a means to distinguish benign from malignant masses. The absence of neovascularization and presence of a high pulsatility index can be used to exclude an invasive primary ovarian cancer. Therefore, indices of blood flow in adnexal masses differentiating benign and malignant lesions on the basis of their vascularity may improve the specificity of the ultrasound screening procedures for early detection of ovarian cancer. Using the color Doppler to exclude the presence of malignancy in an ovarian mass permits us to consider a less aggressive surgical approach, such as laparoscopy.

There are a variety of benign lesions that may demonstrate low impedance or high diastolic flow. These include hemorrhagic luteal cysts, dermoid cysts and inflammatory masses such as tubo-ovarian abscesses. Although differential diagnosis of pelvic masses by their morphology can achieve good accuracy, a secondary test such as CA 125 and a

TYPICAL TV-CDS PARAMETERS

BENIGN

- HIGH PULSATILITY INDEX
- HIGH RESISTANCE INDEX
- FLOW SEEN IN PERIPHERY
- PRESENT DIASTOLIC NOTCH

MALIGNANT

★ LOW RESISTANCE INDEX

★ FLOW IN CENTER

★ ABSENT DIASTOLIC NOTCH

color Doppler is occasionally necessary to establish the correct diagnosis.

The most clinically useful serum marker of epithelial ovarian cancer is glycoprotein CA 125. However, its low specificity and high false-positive rate make it unreliable as a screening test among premenopausal women. Elevated levels may result from many non-malignant conditions such as menstruation, pregnancy, pelvic inflammatory disease, endometriosis, adenomyosis, and peritonitis. Elevated levels of CA 125 also may result from carcinoma of the endometrium, endocervix, pancreas and breast or colorectal cancers. Normal CA 125 values are not highly predictive of the presence or absence of disease. In postmenopausal women using a threshold of 35 U/ml, the positive predictive value is 87% to 98% and the negative predictive value is 72% to 80%. Postmenopausal women tend to have lower CA 125 levels, which increases the sensitivity and specificity of this assay in this age group. Elevated levels are of value in predicting disease in postmenopausal patients and persistent disease during therapy. However, CA 125 has not proved to be effective in screening for ovarian cancer in asymptomatic women. Unfortunately, only 50% of Stage I ovarian cancer patients will have an elevated CA 125 value.

Development of new technologies for the detection of early stage ovarian cancer such as bioinformatics tools identifying proteomic patterns in serum show promising results for distinguishing neoplastic from non-neoplastic disease within the ovary.

OPERATIVE TECHNIQUE

When all of the selection criteria have been satisfied, an operative approach for a benign adnexal mass by laparoscopy may be considered. A 1990 survey conducted by the American Association of Gynecologic Laparoscopists suggests that operative laparoscopic management of benign adnexal masses can be appropriately accomplished in the majority of patients.

Functional cysts often regress spontaneously. If cysts found on an ultrasound appear to be functional, ultrasound reevaluation can be performed in three months to document regression. Placing patients on birth control pills may not influence the regression of the cyst. Simple cysts, however, may be good predictors of benign disease. According to standard sonographic criteria, cysts with distinct borders, less than 10 cm in diameter with no irregular or solid parts and no thick septa nor ascites, and a normal CA 125 level can be managed laparoscopically. All masses that meet strict ultrasonic selection criteria should be considered for the laparoscopic approach.

Hemorrhagic cysts, dermoids and endometriomas can be removed endoscopically. During laparoscopy, if there is suspicion of malignancy or excrescences are found they should be biopsied and sent for frozen section. If frozen sections are positive, or ascites or obvious malignancy is found a staging laparotomy through a midline incision should be performed without delay. Many investigators have lately questioned the standard approach of removing persistent cystic lesions in postmenopausal women. The majority of cystic adnexal masses in postmenopausal women are found to be histologically benign. Postmenopausal women with a subclinical simple cyst less than 5 cm in diameter detected on ultrasound with normal CA 125 values can be offered expectant management.

A patient scheduled for operative laparoscopy should also consent to possible laparotomy. The procedure is performed under general anesthesia in the lithotomy position. A Foley catheter is inserted in all patients to avoid bladder injury and a bowel prep is ordered if there is any suspicion of malignancy or if extensive adhesiolysis is anticipated. A 10-mm diagnostic laparoscope is uti-

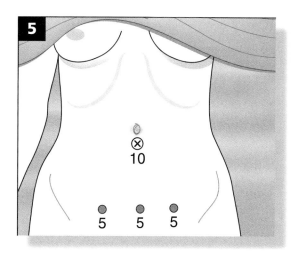

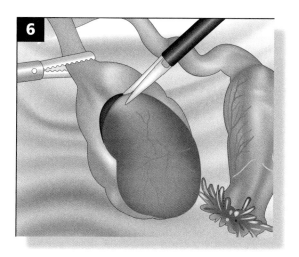

lized because it affords excellent field of vision and three 5-12 mm ancillary ports are utilized as needed (Figure 5).

CYSTECTOMY

Aspiration of a simple ovarian cyst is not recommended since the recurrence rate is high. Cytological analysis of aspirated cyst fluid has a high false negative rate and is not usually recommended.

Therefore, cystectomy or oophorectomy is the procedure of choice. The surgeon should focus his/her attention on removing the entire mass without rupturing it. It is preferable to identify the cyst wall by making the incision on the border of normal ovarian tissue and the cyst and to dissect the cyst without rupturing it (Figures 6 and 7). Since rupture of a malignant ovarian cystic mass at the time of surgery and its impact on survival is still controversial, the surgeon should focus his/her attention on removing the entire mass without rupture. However, this is not always possible.

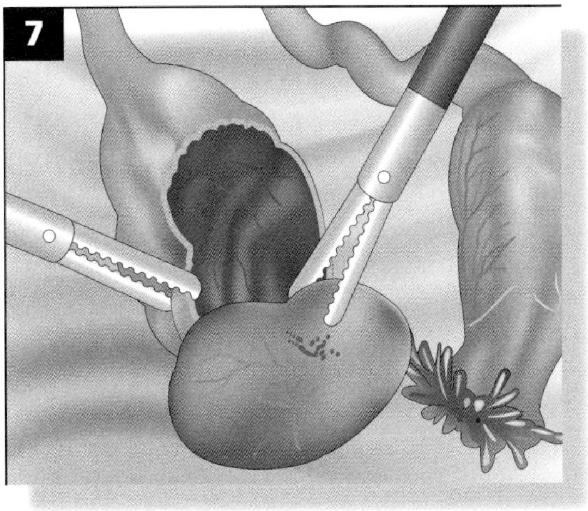

If the cyst appears benign and is too large to dissect, the cyst wall is punctured with the needle attached to suction tubing, minimizing spillage of the cystic fluid (Figure 8). After most of the fluid has been removed, the ovary is grasped with the grasper and a small incision is made with laparoscopic scissors (Figure 9). The cystic cavity is then irrigated with the suction cannula and inspection of the cavity is performed via the laparoscope (Figure 10). Any suspicious areas discovered during surgery should be biopsied and sent for frozen section. If the destruction of the ovarian tissue is substantial, resection of the cyst wall should be performed (Figure 11). The cyst wall is identified and peeled off the ovary with the help

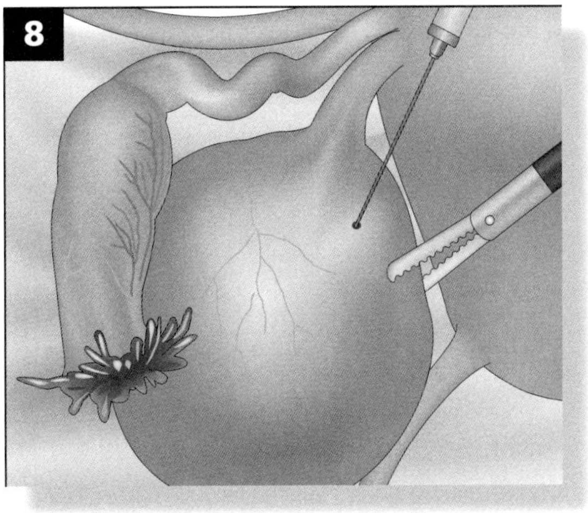

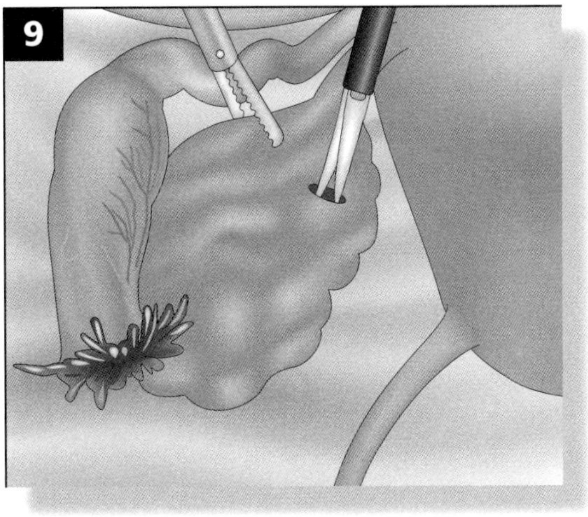

of a traumatic grasper by holding the capsule and rotating it around the grasper. Another grasper is used to provide counter traction by grasping the ovarian capsule (Figure 12). The resected tissue and the ovarian capsule are removed through a laparoscopic port by rotating the grasper and pulling it through the port. If the tissue is too big, it should be placed into a removal bag that is introduced through a 10-mm port. Bleeding from the ovary is usually self-limited or it can be controlled with a spot coagulator or bi-polar forceps.

ADNEXECTOMY

If the cyst has completely replaced normal ovarian tissue or if a large dermoid cyst is diagnosed, adnexectomy should be performed using a bipolar coagulator, harmonic scalpel™ (Ethicon Endosurgery, Cincinnati OH), Endocutter™ (Ethicon Endosurgery, Cincinnati OH) or the Roeder Endoloop™ (Ethicon Endosurgery, Cincinnati OH). The ovary or Fallopian tube should be grasped from a contralateral side and pulled medially to expose the IP ligament. The ureter should be identified, usually located about 2 cm below the IP ligament on the pelvic side wall. Removal of the ovary is usually started by coagulating and cutting the IP ligament with the bipolar forceps or harmonic scalpel introduced through the ipsilateral trocar

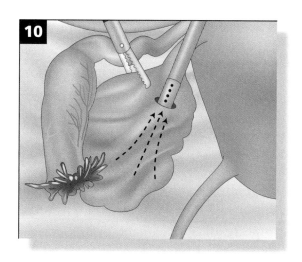

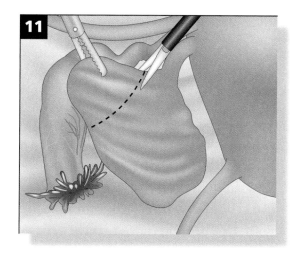

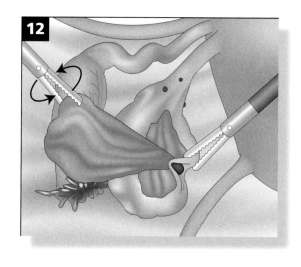

port and extending the line of coagulation dissection toward the utero-ovarian ligament (Figure 13).

If cystic fluid or the contents of a dermoid has been spilled, the peritoneal cavity should be thoroughly irrigated and aspirated. Dermoid cysts or any suspicious ovarian mass should be placed in a pouch before removing it from the peritoneal cavity (Figure 14). The bag should be introduced through an 11-mm port, which usually requires switching to a 5-mm laparoscope. The tissue should be held with a grasper and placed into the bag. The bags with a self-opening mechanism are easier to

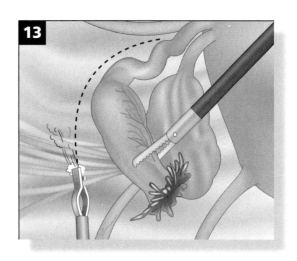

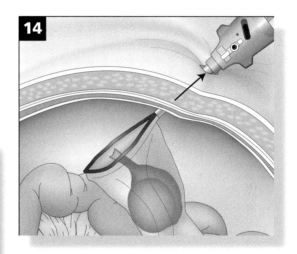

- GRASP THE OVARY OR TUBE FROM THE CONTRALATERAL SIDE

- PULL THE OVARY AND PLACE IP LIGAMENT ON STRETCH

- INTRODUCE THE BIPOLAR COAGULATOR FROM THE IPSILATERAL SIDE

- IDENTIFY THE URETER UNDERNEATH THE IP LIGAMENT

- INTRODUCE THE SCISSORS THROUGH THE MIDDLE PORT

- START THE COAGULATION/CUTTING FROM THE IP LIGAMENT

- KEEP THE OVARY ON STRETCH TOWARD MEDIAL

- PROGRESSIVE COAGULATION /CUTTING TOWARD THE UTERUS

manipulate. Two graspers are often required to facilitate the placement of the tissue into the bag. Once the tissue is placed, the bag should be slowly pulled through an 11-mm trocar cannula by pulling the cannula and the bag applicator together out of the abdomen. The bag should be pulled against the abdominal wall and its contents should be carefully morcellated using hemostat clamps and scissors then removed through the opening on the abdominal wall (Figure 15). Sometimes the abdominal incision has to be enlarged to facilitate removal of the mass within the bag.

SALPINGECTOMY

This technique is presented in Chapter 11. Numerous methods can be used, including bipolar coagulation and cutting, harmonic scalpel, laser, stapling devices or endoloops. The tube can be removed by coagulation of the mesosalpinx at the isthmus of the tube and progress to the fimbriated end. The preferred technique is to grasp the fimbrial end of the tube from the contralateral side and place it on stretch toward the midline. Start the coagulation of the mesosalpinx at the fimbrial end and work progressively toward the isthmic part of the tube (Figure 16). The whole tube can be removed by coagulation/cutting, or at some point the endoloop can be placed around the proximal part of the tube. It is not recommended to include a big pedicle of mesosalpinx into the endoloop. After the tube has been removed the proximal stump of the Fallopian tube should be coagulated to prevent ectopic pregnancy. The tube can be removed directly through a 10-mm trocar, or it can be placed into a bag for removal.

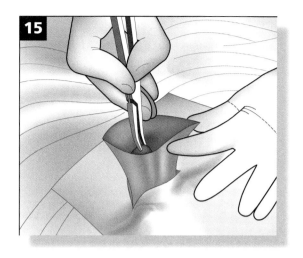

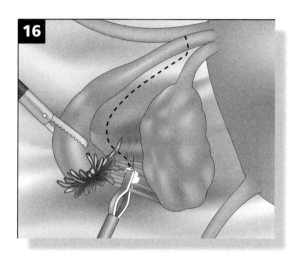

LAPAROSCOPY AND OVARIAN CANCER

Approximately 1 in 70 women will develop ovarian cancer in their lifetime making it the leading cause of death from gynecologic malignancy in the United States. Unfortunately there are no reliable means of early detection, and more than 65% of cases of ovarian cancer are not diagnosed until advanced stage III and IV.

Laparoscopy was first utilized as a 'second look' procedure in patients with ovarian malignancies and now is being considered for surgical staging and treatment of early ovarian cancer. The use of laparoscopy for staging early ovarian cancer appears to be a valuable alternative to traditional surgical staging and an increasing number of gynecologic oncologists are adopting the procedure as they become more experienced with laparoscopy.

RISK OF OVARIAN CANCER		
GENERAL POPULATION	1/70	
FIRST DEGREE RELATIVE	1/20	5%
TWO RELATIVES	1/14	7%
SYNDROMIC CANCER	1/2	40%

Laparoscopy offers excellent magnification, which is important for inspection of the peritoneal surfaces and the diaphragm, but is compromised by limited exposure of the lesser omental sac and diminished tactile feeling. Laparoscopy also offers absence of a midline incision and better patient tolerance as well as shorter hospitalization and recovery. Laparoscopy is much more reliant on equipment and trained operating room staff since minor equipment failure or staff unfamiliarity with laparoscopic surgery can make a very simple procedure impossible to perform. Advanced laparoscopic surgery training is essential when performing these procedures, and many gynecologic oncologists will initially find their experience with laparoscopy difficult.

A second look laparotomy or laparoscopy in many centers is no longer considered routine practice for patients who achieve complete remission after a course of chemotherapy. Second-look laparoscopy, when technically feasible, appears equally as effective as laparotomy in detecting persistent or recurrent malignancy and offers better patient comfort, less morbidity, shorter hospitalization and decreased cost.

Patients with advanced disease involving intraperitoneal metastasis are not candidates for laparoscopic surgery although laparoscopic debulking of advanced ovarian cancer in the setting of neoadjuvant chemotherapy has been performed. Those patients will benefit from comprehensive cytoreductive surgery by laparotomy and systemic chemotherapy.

SUGGESTED READING:

Nezhat F, Nezhat C, Welander CE, et al. Four ovarian cancers diagnosed during laparoscopic management of 1011 women with adnexal mass. Am J Obstet Gynecol 1992; 167: 790-6

El-Minawi MF, el-Halafawy AA, Abdel-Hadi M, et al Laparoscopic, gynecographic and ultrasonographic vs. clinical evaluation of pelvic mass. J Reprod Med 1984; 29: 197-9

Lande IM, Hill MC, Cosco FE, et al. Adnexal and cul-de-sac abnormalities: Transvaginal sonography. Radiology 1988; 166: 325-32

Frederic JL, Paulson RJ, Sauer MV. Routine use of vaginal ultrasound in the preoperative evaluation of gynecologic patients, an adjunct to resident education. J Reprod Med 1991; 36:779-82

Petricoin EF, Ardekani AM, Hitt BA, et al. Use of proteomic patterns in serum to identify ovarian cancer. Lancet 2002; 359: 572-7

Venezia R, Zangara C. Echohysterosalpingography: new diagnostic possibilities with S HU 450 Echovist. Acta Eur Fertil 1991; 22: 279-82

Reich H, McGlynn F. Treatment of ovarian endometriomas using laparoscopic surgical techniques. J Reprod Med 1987; 32: 747-52

Nezhat C, Winer W, Nezhat F. Laparoscopic removal of dermoid cysts. Obstet Gynecol 1989; 73: 278-81

Kurjak A, Zalud I, Alfirevic Z. Evaluation of adnexal masses with transvaginal color ultrasound. J Ultrasound Med 1991; 10: 295-7

Fleisher AC, Rogers WH, Ras BK, et al. Assessment of ovarian tumor vascularity with transvaginal color Doppler ultrasound. J Ultrasound Med 1991; 10: 563-8

Zalud I. Doppler evaluation of the ovary: clinical applications and challenges. Contemporary. Obstet Gynecol 2002;47:36-59

Vasilev S, Schlaerth J Campeau J, et al. Serum CA 125 levels in the preoperative evaluation of pelvic masses. Obstet Gynecol 1988;71:751-5

Parker WH. Management of adnexal masses by operative laparoscopy. J Reprod Med 1992; 37: 603-6

Jacobs I, Bast R. The CA 125 tumor associated antigen: A review of the literature. Human Reprod 1989; 4: 1-6

Rulin M, Preston A. Adnexal masses in postmenopausal women. Obstet Gynecol 1987; 70: 578-81

Parker WH, Berek JS. Management of the adnexal mass by operative laparoscopy. Clin Obstet Gynecol 1993; 36: 413-22

Wolf SI, Gosnik BB, Feldesman Mr, et al. The prevalence of simple adnexal cysts in post-menopausal women. Radiology 1991; 180: 65-71

Hulka J, Parker W, Surrey M, Phillips J. Management of ovarian masses: AAGL 1990 Survey. J Reprod Med 1992; 7: 599

Dembo AJ, Davy M, Stenwig A, et al. Prognostic factors in patients with stage I epithelial ovarian cancer. Obstet Gynecol 1990; 75: 263-7

Cutler SJ, Young JL, Eds. Third National Cancer Survey: Incidence Data, National Cancer Institute. Monogt 41, DHEW Pub (NIH) 75-77. Washington, DC : US Government Printing Office: 1975

Pasic R, Hilgers RD, Levine RL. The role of laparoscopy in management of gynecologic malignancies. J Surg Oncol 2000; 75: 60-71

Ozols RF, Fisher RI, Anderson C, et al. Peritoneoscopy in the management of ovarian cancer. Am J Obstet Gynecol 1981; 140:611-4

Berek JS, Griffiths CT, Leventhal JM. Laparoscopy for second look evaluation in ovarian cancer. Obstet Gynecol 1981; 58:192-5

Reich H., McGlynn F, Wilkie W. Laparoscopic management of stage I ovarian cancer: A case report. J Reprod Med 1990; 35:601-5

Nezhat C, Burrell M, Nezhat F, et al. Laparoscopic radical hysterectomy with periaortic and pelvic node dissection. Am J Obstet Gynecol 1992; 166: 864–73

Pomel C, Provencher D, Dauplat J, et al. Laparoscopic staging of early ovarian cancer. Gynecol Oncol 1995; 58: 301–6

Freidman JB, Weiss NS. Sounding board: Second thoughts about second look laparotomy in advanced ovarian cancer. N Engl J Med 1990; 322:1079–83

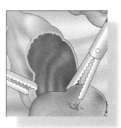

LAPAROSCOPIC HYSTERECTOMY

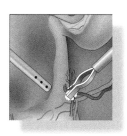

John Y. Phelps, M.D.

C. Y. Liu, M.D.

The advent of advanced laparoscopy has resulted in its frequent use to remove the uterus. The extent to which laparoscopy is used varies depending on the underlying pathology, uterine mobility, vaginal accessibility and the laparoscopic skills of the gynecologic surgeon. The laparoscopic approach is more commonly used to facilitate a vaginal hysterectomy. However, for the advanced laparoscopic surgeon, the uterus can be completely detached from its surrounding structures laparoscopically. In this chapter we will illustrate the various steps of hysterectomy using laparoscopy. We recommend the novice laparoscopic surgeon master the initial, more basic, steps of performing a hysterectomy laparoscopically prior to proceeding with the more advanced steps. Conversion to an abdominal hysterectomy should never be considered a complication; rather it is a prudent surgical decision when the surgeon becomes uncomfortable with the laparoscopic approach.

DEFINITIONS

To help delineate the extent to which the laparoscopy is used for removal of the uterus, the following descriptive system is proposed. This system incorporates, and is a modification of, a classification system previously published. However, the AAGL has published a recent abbreviated classification system (Table 1) that may also be utilized for reference.

Table 1

ABBREVIATED CLASSIFICATION SYSTEM FOR LAPAROSCOPIC HYSTERECTOMY

- TYPE O

  LAPAROSCOPIC-DIRECTED PREPARATION FOR VAGINAL HYSTERECTOMY

- TYPE I

  OCCLUSION AND DIVISION OF AT LEAST ONE OVARIAN PEDICLE, BUT NOT INCLUDING UTERINE ARTERIES

- TYPE II

  TYPE I PLUS OCCLUSION AND DIVISION OF THE UTERINE ARTERY, UNILATERAL OR BILATERAL

- TYPE III

  TYPE II PLUS A PORTION OF THE CARDINAL-UTEROSACRAL LIGAMENT COMPLEX, UNILATERAL OR BILATERAL

- TYPE IV

  COMPLETE DETACHMENT OF CARDINAL-UTEROSACRAL LIGAMENT COMPLEX, UNILATERAL OR BILATERAL, WITH OR WITHOUT ENTRY INTO THE VAGINA

Diagnostic laparoscopy with vaginal hysterectomy: The laparoscopic approach is used for diagnostic purposes only. Pelvic adhesions, uterine or ovarian pathology are excluded to assure the vaginal approach is safe. Laparoscopic visualization of the pelvis prior to a planned vaginal hysterectomy is justified in women with pelvic pain, history of endometriosis, previous abdominal or pelvic surgery and in women with questionable uterine or ovarian pathology.

Operative laparoscopy with vaginal hysterectomy: The laparoscopic approach is used to lyse adhesions to facilitate a planned vaginal hysterectomy. Laparoscopic oophorectomy, excision or ablation of endometriosis, in conjunction with a vaginal hysterectomy, would also be included in this term. No vascular or ligamentous supporting attachments to the uterus are ligated.

Laparoscopic assisted vaginal hysterectomy (LAVH): Part, or the majority, of the vascular and ligamentous attachments to the uterus, above the uterine artery, are ligated laparoscopically. The uterine arteries are subsequently ligated vaginally. It is the ligation of the uterine arteries vaginally that distinguishes this procedure from a laparoscopic hysterectomy in which the uterine arteries are ligated laparoscopically.

Laparoscopic supracervical hysterectomy: The laparoscopic approach is used to completely detach the uterus from the cervix. The cervix, cardinal ligaments and uterosacral ligaments are left intact.

Laparoscopic hysterectomy: The uterine arteries are secured laparoscopically while the remaining cardinal and uterosacral ligaments are secured vaginally.

Total laparoscopic hysterectomy: The laparoscopic approach is used to completely detach the uterus and cervix from their surrounding structures including the uterine arteries, cardinal ligaments, uterosacral ligaments and vagina. The vaginal cuff is closed laparoscopically or vaginally.

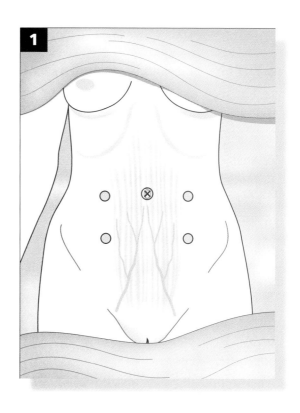

TROCAR PLACEMENT

Trocar placement varies depending on the preference of the surgeon. We routinely place a 12-mm trocar through a vertical intraumbilical incision for insertion of a 10-mm laparoscope. Four additional 5-mm trocars are then placed into the peritoneal cavity. The lower pair is placed lateral to the inferior epigastric vessels approximately two fingerbreadths above the pubis. The upper pair is placed lateral to the abdominal rectus muscles at a level slightly inferior to the umbilicus (Figure 1).

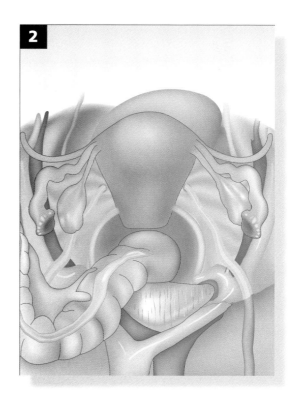

IDENTIFICATION OF THE URETERS

The ureters should be identified prior to ligating any supporting structures to the uterus. Knowledge of pelvic anatomy and the course of the ureter are crucial (Figure 2). In most cases the ureters are visible through the peritoneum. As long as the ureters are clearly identified through the peritoneum, it is reasonable not to dissect them when performing procedures such as a laparoscopic assisted vaginal hysterectomy or supracervical hysterectomy. However, when performing more advanced steps of the hysterectomy laparoscopically, we recommend dissecting the ureters to the level of the ureteric canal prior to ligating the uterine arteries laparoscopically.

To identify the ureters, incise the peritoneum just above the ureters. In Figure 3, laparoscopic scissors are used to incise the peritoneum just above the right ureter. Alternatively, a laser could be used. Graspers are used to separate the peritoneum from the ureter (Figure 4). With the peritoneum separated from the ureter, incise the peritoneum along the course of the ureter towards the cardinal ligament. Figure 5 shows the course of the right ureter in relation to the right uterosacral ligament. With meticulous dissection the ureter can be seen passing beneath the uterine artery at the level of the ureteric canal.

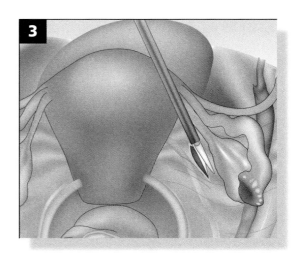

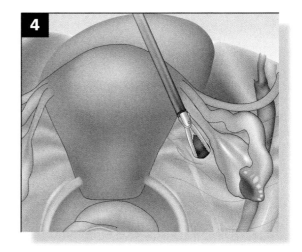

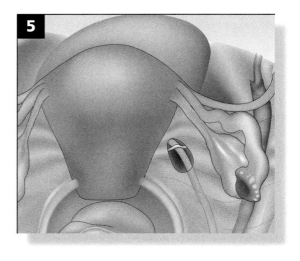

LIGATION OF THE INFUNDIBULOPELVIC LIGAMENTS

For women desiring removal of the ovaries, the infundibulopelvic ligaments are ligated bilaterally incorporating the ovaries and Fallopian tubes. Figures 6 and 7 show ligation of the right infundibulopelvic ligament with 1-0 Vicyrl suture on a CT-1 needle. To avoid back bleeding, two separate sutures are placed around the infundibulopelvic ligament which is divided between the sutures. The uterus is pushed to the left to place the right infundibulopelvic ligament on tension. Alternatively, the infundibulopelvic ligaments can be desiccated with bipolar forceps and divided. Figure 8 shows the right infundibulopelvic ligament being desiccated with Kleppinger bipolar forceps. The right ureter is seen below. For illustrative purposes the right ureter is being grasped with a ureteral dissector.

For women who want to preserve their ovaries, the uterine-ovarian ligaments and Fallopian tubes are sutured ligated adjacent to the Fallopian tube. Figure 9 shows ligation of the left uterine-ovarian ligament and Fallopian tube with 1-0 Vicyrl suture. Alternatively, the uterine-ovarian ligaments can be desiccated with bipolar forceps and divided with laparoscopic scissors.

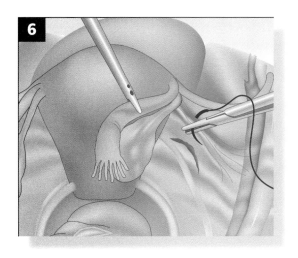

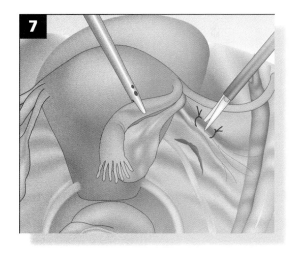

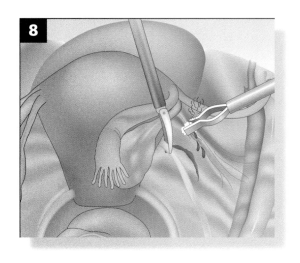

LIGATION OF THE ROUND LIGAMENTS

The round ligaments can easily be desiccated with bipolar forceps and divided with laparoscopic scissors. Figures 10 and 11 show desiccation of the left round ligament with bipolar Kleppinger forceps, followed by ligation with laparoscopic scissors. A grasper is used to place the round ligament on traction and to pull it away from the pelvic sidewall.

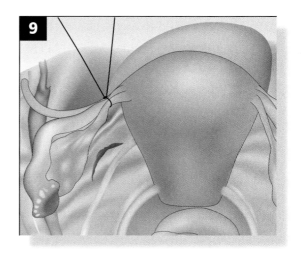

CREATION OF BLADDER FLAP

First identify the vesicouterine peritoneal fold. To facilitate identification of the vesicouterine fold, have an assistant retrovert the uterus and push it cephalad. The upper junction of the vesicouterine peritoneal fold is distinguished as a white line. Identification of the white line is important because above this demarcation the peritoneum is attached tightly to the uterus, while below this demarcation the peritoneum is loosely attached to the cervix. Dissection in the wrong tissue plane will lead to unnecessary bleeding. The dome of the bladder is approximately 2.0 cm to 2.5 cm below the white line. Using a grasper, place the vesicouterine fold on traction (Figure 12). Make a transverse incision just below the white line and dissect the bladder away from the lower uterine segment and cervix. If in the right tissue plane, the dissection should

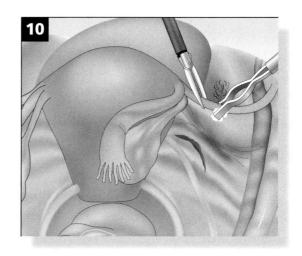

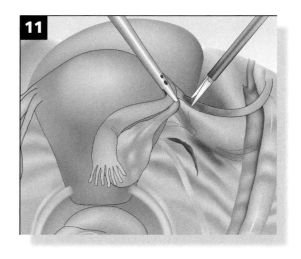

be relatively bloodless. The middle band of loose connective tissue is the vesico-cervical ligament (Figure 13). This ligament does not contain blood vessels and can be easily divided. The lateral bands of connection on both sides of the cervix are bladder pillars. The bladder pillars contain blood vessels and should be desiccated prior to ligation. Dissection of the bladder laterally helps pull the ureters away from the cervix. With meticulous dissection, the ureters can be seen as they approach the trigone of the bladder. In Figure 14, the bladder has been dissected laterally, away from the cervix, and down to the level of the vagina. Both ureters are seen lateral to the cervix as they approach the trigone of the bladder. Figure 14 shows the left uterine artery crossing above the left ureter and ascending from the cervix toward the uterus. If the demarcation of the bladder is obscured, instillation of 200 cc of fluid with or without dye is helpful in delineation of the limits of the bladder wall.

LIGATION OF THE UTERINE ARTERIES

The broad ligaments on both sides are opened downward and towards the cervix, skeletonizing the uterine vessels. Once the uterine vessels are skeletonized they can be ligated bilaterally incorporating part of the cardinal ligaments. Figure 15 shows ligation of the

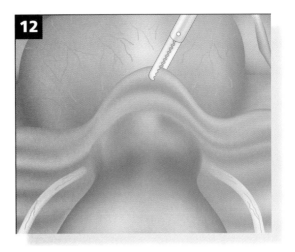

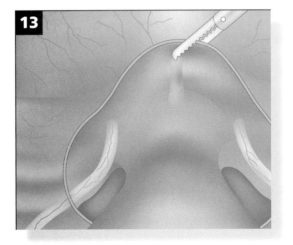

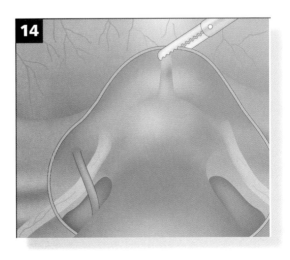

right uterine vessels with 1-0 Vicyrl suture on a CT-1 needle. The suture is placed immediately adjacent to the cervix and incorporates part of the cardinal ligaments. The suction irrigator is used to push the body of the uterus to the opposite side. The knot is tied extracorporeally with a knot pusher. With meticulous dissection, the uterine artery can be ligated at the level of the ureteric canal as it crosses above the ureter. Figure 16 shows ligation of the left uterine artery at the level of the ureteric canal with 1-0 Vicyrl suture on a CT-1 needle. The uterine artery is seen crossing above the ureter. Knowledge of the course of the ureter is essential at this point to avoid injury. Alternatively, the uterine artery can be desiccated with bipolar forceps and divided (Figure 17). Because of the close proximity of the ureter, we recommend ureteral dissection prior to desiccating or ligating the uterine artery.

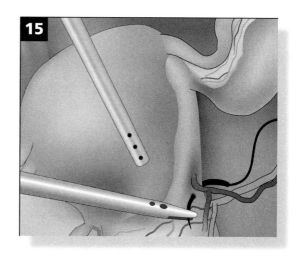

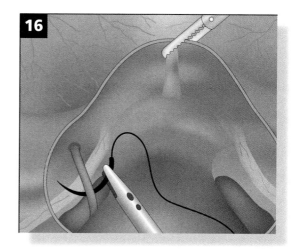

Supracervical hysterectomy may be an attractive alternative for the laparoscopic surgeon who is not comfortable with ureteral dissection. Routinely, the main trunk of the uterine artery is not skeletonized and the ureter is not dissected. Only the ascending branch of the uterine artery is ligated. This can be done far above the ureter at the uterocervical junction. Figure 18 shows the right uterine artery

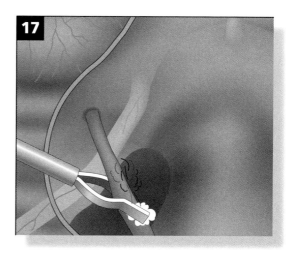

ascending across the lateral aspect of the cervix towards the uterus. Suture or bipolar coagulation can be used. The body of the uterus is then amputated from the upper portion of the cervix. We routinely desiccate the endocervical canal with electrocautery. The cardinal and uterosacral ligaments are left intact when performing a supracervical hysterectomy.

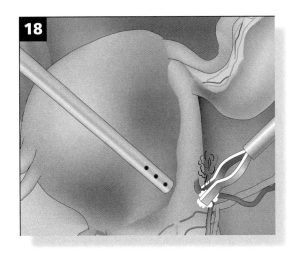

LIGATION OF THE UTEROSACRAL LIGAMENTS

With direct visualization of the ureters, both uterosacral ligaments are desiccated with bipolar forceps and divided. In Figure 19, bipolar Kleppinger forceps are used to desiccate the right uterosacral ligament. The peritoneum over the ureters has been dissected. In Figure 20, laparoscopic scissors are used to divide the right uterosacral ligament.

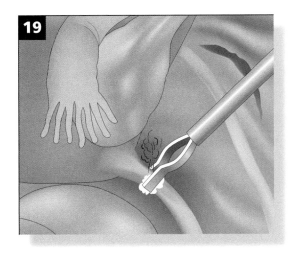

CULDOTOMY

By means of sponge forceps, a wet 4 x 4 sponge is placed into the anterior vaginal fornix and used to tent the vagina from below. An incision is made between the bladder and cervix, exposing the white fibers of the 4 x 4 sponge (Figure 21). We routinely use laparoscopic scissors or CO_2 laser. At this point, gas leaks rapidly from the peritoneal cavity. If a circumferential

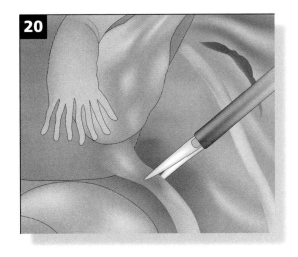

culdotomy can be easily and safely performed, it is reasonable to proceed. However, we have found it helpful to remove the uterine manipulator at this stage and place a sponge inside the vagina to maintain a pneumoperitoneum. We place a sponge inside a surgical glove and tie the open end of the glove. The glove with the enclosed sponge is then placed inside the vagina. After the pneumoperitoneum is recreated, circumferential culdotomy is performed by completely detaching the cervix from the vagina and cardinal ligaments. The anterior lip of the cervix is grasped with a single tooth tenaculum and with the cervix on traction, a circumferential culdotomy is performed with laparoscopic scissors. The sponge inside the vagina is removed and the uterus is removed vaginally.

There are a number of devices available commercially that can be applied vaginally around the cervix to better distinquish between the bladder and vagina. These instruments are also equipped with vaginal occluders to prevent failure of the pneumoperitoneum. Figure 22 shows the RUMI System™ (Cooper Surgical, Shelton, CT) with the Koh Colpotomizer and pneumo-occluder. The rim of the colpotomizer is easily visualized and palpated from above. Anterior colpotomy can be performed over the rim

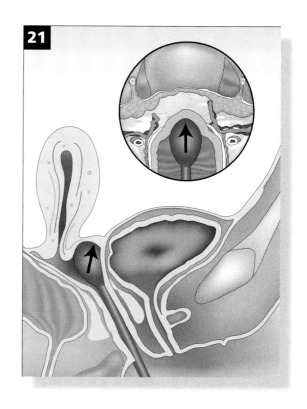

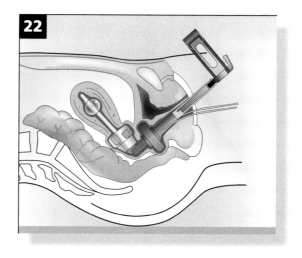

using unipolar scissors or the harmonic scalpel. Rotation of the RUMI's grip allows visualization of the posterior fornix and uterosacral ligaments.

Posterior colpotomy is then performed and carried around the cervix till the uterus is completely detached. Occasional cuff bleeders can be controlled with bipolar forceps. The uterus is then removed vaginally. If needed, the uterus can be morcellated vaginally to permit removal through the culdotomy incision. A surgical glove containing a sponge is placed vaginally to hold the pneumoperitoneum and it can be seen through the vaginal cuff in Figure 23.

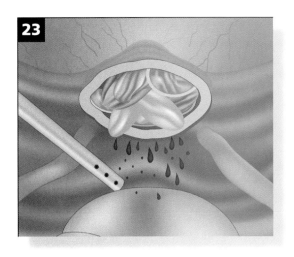

CLOSURE OF THE VAGINAL CUFF

After removal of the uterus, the surgical glove with the enclosed sponge is replaced inside the vagina to maintain a pneumoperitoneum. The vaginal cuff angles are sutured to their ipsilateral uterosacral and cardinal ligaments with figure of eight stitches. In Figure 24, the vaginal cuff angles have been sutured to their ipsilateral uterosacral and cardinal ligaments. Care is taken not to incorporate the ureters. The vaginal cuff is closed transversely laparoscopically. Alternatively, the vaginal cuff can be closed using a vaginal approach.

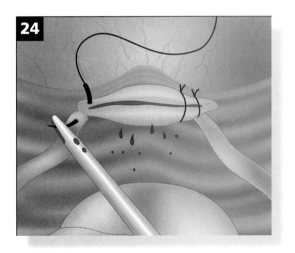

UNDERWATER EXAMINATION

To ensure hemostasis, the pelvis is partially filled with Ringer's lactate solution and the vaginal cuff is viewed by submerging the laparoscope underwater.

CYSTOSCOPY

We routinely perform cystoscopy to ensure ureteral patency. We ask the anesthesiologist to inject 5 mL of indigo carmine dye intravenously followed by 10 mg of furosemide (Lasix). Bilateral ureteral patency is confirmed by ejection of indigo carmine dye from the ureteral orifices. Cystoscope is connected to the endoscopic camera for better visualization and the entire surface area should also be inspected for signs of injury.

POSTOPERATIVE CARE

Patients are initially placed on a clear liquid diet when fully awake. The diet is advanced to 'regular' as tolerated. The majority of our patients go home within 24 hours of surgery. Patients are not discharged until they can ambulate well without assistance, void and tolerate a regular diet. Although it is feasible they could go home the same day, we recommend overnight hospitalization for observation and pain management. Although the procedure is performed laparoscopically, through small skin incisions, it still should be considered a major operation.

Patients who have undergone laparoscopic surgery should feel better each day during the postoperative period. In the event a patient does not progressively improve after surgery, operative complications should be considered. In addition to the standard blood tests and X-rays, a CT scan of the abdomen and pelvis may be indicated. To evaluate for ureteral injury, IV contrast should be given. To evaluate for intestinal injury, oral and rectal contrast should be given. Do not hesitate to perform a second look laparoscopy when there is doubt regarding the possibility of an operative complication. It is far better to error on the side of caution than to allow an operative complication to further go unrecognized and delay treatment.

SUGGESTED READING:

Garry R, Reich H, Liu CY. Laparoscopic hysterectomy–definitions and indications. Gynecol Endoscopy 1994; 3: 1-3

Sills ES, Saini J, Steiner CA, McGee M, Gretz HF. Abdominal hysterectomy practice patterns in the United States. Int J Gynaecol Obstet 1998;63(4):277-83

Kim DH, Bae DH, Hur M, Kim SH. Comparison of classic intrafascial supracervical hysterectomy with total laparoscopic and laparoscopic-assisted vaginal hysterectomy. J Am Assoc Gynecol Laparo 1998;5(3):253-260

Harkki-Siren P, Sjoberg J, Tiitinen A. Urinary tract injuries after hysterectomy. Obstet Gynecol 1998;92(1):113-8

Mettler L, Semm K. Subtotal versus total laparoscopic hysterectomy. Acta Obstet Gynecol Scand Suppl 1997;164:88-93

Parker WH. Total laparoscopic hysterectomy. Obstet Gynecol Clin North Am 2000;27(2):431-40

Chou DC, Rosen DM, Cario GM, Carlton MA, Lam AM, Chapman M, Johns C. Home within 24 hours of laparoscopic hysterectomy. Aust N Z J Obstet Gynaecol 1999;39(2):234-8

LAPAROSCOPIC SUPRACERVICAL HYSTERECTOMY (LSH)

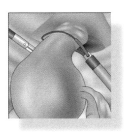

Thomas L. Lyons, M.D.

Hysterectomy is a very effective and efficient procedure with great benefit to those women requiring such surgery. All surgical procedures now in widespread use have undergone thorough clinical evaluation and meet the basic criteria required by ethical physicians for continued usage. As stated by Finley in 1943, hysterectomy must be used to:

1. Save life;

2. Correct deformity;

3. Eliminate suffering.

Historically, the procedure we now term hysterectomy dates only to the turn of the century when it was used predominately to treat large tumors of the uterus (usually fibroids) and catastrophic uterine bleeding. Most of these procedures were performed in a subtotal or supracervical manner and morbidity and mortality (M & M) were significant due to poor anesthesia techniques, absence of antibiotics, and lack of modern blood banking. Thus, if a patient had prolonged surgery, excessive bleeding, or infection, mortality was a major risk. Mortality rates decreased rapidly during the first half of the 20th century when progress was made in the techniques of surgery, anesthesia improved, and antibiotics became available.

Eventually, hysterectomy became safe enough to treat such benign conditions as pelvic floor prolapse. Another important influence at that time was the mortality rate from cervical carcinoma making it the third most common killer of women in the US. Between 1940 and 1955, the rate of total versus subtotal hysterectomy was reversed. In the early 1940s, the subtotal rate was 85%–95% but by 1955 it had decreased to less than 5%. The reason for this shift was to lower the death rate from cervical cancer. This goal was not accomplished until Papanicolaou smears became routine in the US in 1958. However, the wholesale extirpation of cervices continued for the next 40 years with over one million total hysterectomies performed in 1975.

By the late 1980s in the US, dramatic advances were introduced with laparoscopic cholecystectomy, rapid technological developments, and the concept of minimally invasive surgery to reduce morbidity. Although gynecologists were the leaders in this revolution, the movement into more advanced procedures by the generalist Ob/Gyn were stalled. Reich first reported laparoscopically assisted vaginal hysterectomy (LAVH) in 1989 and afterwards the use of the technique grew. It is imperative to emphasize that the goal of all minimally invasive procedures should be accomplishment of the surgical task in an efficient manner while lowering morbidity. This goal of LAVH has been studied carefully and has been accomplished. Reich, Liu, and others expanded the indications for this procedure to the point where even if a patient has indications for hysterectomy but cannot undergo a vaginal hysterectomy (TVH) then LAVH can be considered.

After carefully examining the use of LAVH to meet the needs of the patients and lower morbidity, I began a series of trials of laparoscopic supracervical hysterectomy (LSH) in 1990. We felt that the known lower morbidity of the supracervical procedure warranted its use. Further, maintaining hysterectomy as a totally laparoscopic procedure offered a potential simplification to the average surgeon. After completing a series of LSH and comparing them to a group of demographically similar patients undergoing LAVH, we found that LSH resulted in significantly lower morbidity. Over the next ten years we performed approximately 750 procedures with continued low morbidity while treating uteri up to 2400 g, stage IV endometriosis, severe PID, ovarian cancer, leiomyosarcoma, and total pelvic floor prolapse. These patients continued to have a remarkable recovery with lower than normal morbidity despite the increased complexity of the procedures. Of course, the learning curve played a role in these statistics but the clinical results were sufficient to warrant the continued use of LSH.

INDICATIONS

LSH is preferred for most patients in whom hysterectomy is indicated and include:

1) Dysfunctional uterine bleeding

2) Symptomatic uterine leiomyomata

3) Pelvic pain

4) Endometriosis

5) Pelvic floor prolapse

6) Ovarian cancer

7) Pelvic inflammatory disease

The absolute contraindications for LSH are:

1) Endometrial cancer

2) Invasive cervical cancer

3) Pelvic floor relaxation in a patient with a retroverted uterus and a short anterior wall (<7 cm)

4) Any patient who cannot be expected to continue cytologic surveillance

The real risk of cervical disease is no greater than in patients with an intact uterus but the patient should be counseled concerning the importance of continued PAP smears. The discussion should include an explanation of the potential benefits in maintaining the cervix as well as the possible liabilities of the cervix in situ.

TECHNIQUE

LSH is performed as described in Telinde, with the exception that laparoscopic incisions are substituted for the midline or Pfannenstiel incision. First, the patient is consented for LSH and laparotomy. Continued cytologic surveillance is emphasized and is documented in the chart. Bowel preparation with GoLYTELY™ or magnesium citrate is advised and preoperative antibiotics are prescribed (usually 1 g of cephalosporin intravenously 1 hour prior to surgery). Bowel prep and antibiotic use may vary but should correspond to the prep that is desired by the gynecologist's consulting general surgeon. Simplification of the procedure and emphasis on preoperative preparation must be stressed.

The room setup is critical to the efficiency of the procedure. The patient is placed in the modified dorsal lithotomy position in low stirrups (Figure 1). Allen stirrups or a similar device is recommended as positioning is critical for the safety and success of the procedure. The surgeon should monitor this positioning until he/she is comfortable that the OR team is totally competent in this preparation. Ultimately, it is the surgeon's responsibility medico-legally to ensure proper preparation and positioning of the patient. Thus, the importance for a team approach to this type of surgery is imperative. To become efficient, each member of the team should be well educated in the importance of his/her role in the procedure. This aspect has been addressed by Winer in other texts and cannot be overemphasized.

The devices used to complete LSH are the prerogatives of the surgeon. Vascular pedicles must be isolated and occluded. Laparoscopically, this may be

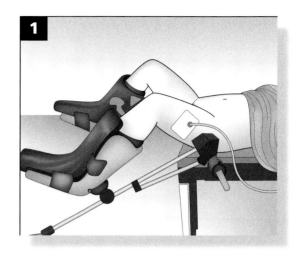

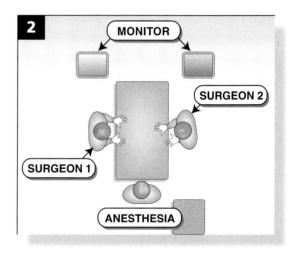

accomplished using suture, staples, clips, harmonic scalpel™ (Ethicon Endosurgery, Cincinnati, OH), bipolar electrosurgery, monopolar electrosurgery, or some form of laser energy. All of these energy forms have advantages and disadvantages, thus, the surgeon must have working knowledge of all these modalities and use those that best suit the particular style. In this chapter, we describe the use of bipolar energy for larger vessel occlusion and the contact Nd:YAG laser as a cutting device. We favor the harmonic scalpel™ as a cutter/coagulator and also have used monopolar electrosurgery as a primary cutting device. We also use suture in selected cases for large vessel occlusion. The procedure begins with careful positioning of the patient. The monitors are placed at or toward the foot of the table so the surgeon can eliminate the need to work in a 'mirror image' (Figure 2). Any time a surgeon works at an angle of 90° or greater (into or toward the laparoscope) a 'mirror image' is created reversing the directions needed within the operative field.

After the sterile prep is complete, the uterine manipulator is placed. The use of an effective manipulator is critical. We have used both the Valchev™ and the Pelosi™ (Apple Medical Corp., Bolton, MA) manipulators with success but we favor the Pelosi. The manipulator is critical as a retractor and definitely aids in efficient completion of this task. Whatever the uterine size, the manipulator is key. There are advantages to the use of either the Valchev™ or the Pelosi™ which enable both anteversion and retroflexion as well as rotation and lateral displacement all using only one hand. Further, the fact that the device is fixed to the

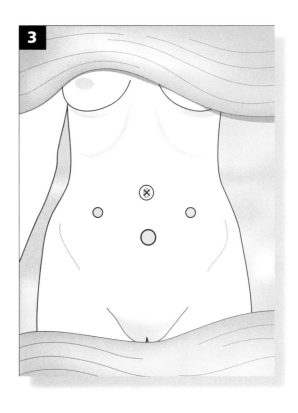

cervix is of critical importance in the physics of the task. The next step involves placement of trocars (Figure 3). We use a trocar scheme based upon experience from several thousand cases but it should not be considered the only effective technique. Several key points should, however, be noted. First, the subumbilical 10/12 mm trocar is placed using the open or Hasson technique. The open technique is used because of the frequent need to treat women with very large uteri and/or they have had multiple prior abdominal procedures. Other primary trocar techniques certainly can be considered but the surgeon should select a technique that he/she is familiar with and suits the clinical situation. Next, the distribution of the lateral trocars is well lateral on the abdominal wall. This lateral placement as well as the need to place the trocars above the pathology, particularly in the large uterus, is again helpful in facilitating adequate retraction and access to the vascular pedicles. When possible 5 mm trocars are used particularly in these lateral sites. The lower midline trocar is 10/11 mm and is used later for suturing and for morcellation of the specimen. In the very large uterus, the primary subumbilical trocar becomes the lower midline trocar and two 5-mm trocars are placed laterally on each side to accomplish this task. We currently use disposable trocars from Ethicon EndoSurgery™ but reusable devices are also available. The trocars should be threaded or gripped to the skin/fascia as otherwise unwanted pull out can occur which makes the procedure more difficult as well as lengthier. All secondary trocars should be placed under direct visualization with the laparoscope. A 10-mm operating laparoscope is placed through the upper midline port and the contact Nd:YAG laser scalpel (Surgical Laser Technologies, Philadelphia, PA) is passed through the operating channel of the laparoscope. A 45°

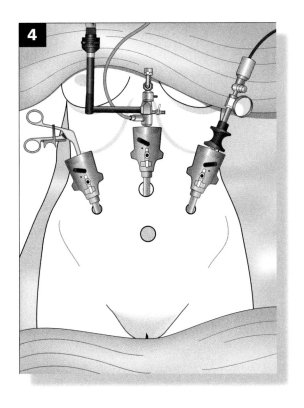

10-mm scope is also kept on hand particularly for the large uterus as this can be very helpful if the fibroid obscures a straight-on view of the operative field. The BiCoag™ bipolar dissector/ grasper (Everest Medical Corp, Minneapolis, MN) is used first through the left lower lateral port. An atraumatic grasper is used through the right lateral port and the suction irrigation device is placed in the midline lower portal (Figure 4). The procedure then proceeds by exploration, adhesiolysis, and restoration of anatomy. If possible, we then perform ureterolysis. In this procedure, an incision is made medial to the ureter beginning in the midpelvic area and is extended down to the level of the uterosacral ligaments (Figure 5). This serves two purposes. First the ureter is identified and marked so that it is easily found later. Therefore, if bleeding control is necessary the potential for injury to the ureter is decreased. Also, this allows for aggressive support of the vault using a high McCall's culdoplasty at termination of the procedure without ureteral kinking or compromise. Next, the round ligaments, tubes, and uteroovarian pedicle are desiccated on the specimen side to decrease back bleeding. The round ligament is divided and the anterior uterovesical fold is scored with the laser scalpel, and the bladder flap is developed (Figure 6). The posterior leaf of the broad ligament is also scored down the specimen side and the vasculature is skeletonized. If the adnexa are to be removed, the infundibulopelvic ligament is desiccated and divided in typical fashion (Figure 7). The ureter is constantly in view due to the ureterolysis incision. Once the uterine vessels are skeletonized these vascular pedicles can be removed with the bipolar placed in the ipsilateral lower lateral port while good countertraction is applied from the contralateral port and the uterine manipulator (Figure 8). The bipolar forceps is placed at a right angle perpendicular to the lateral uterus, which

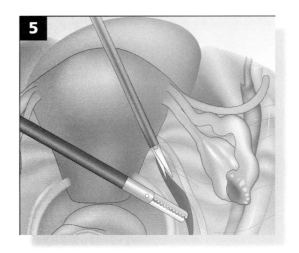

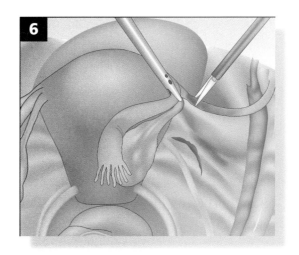

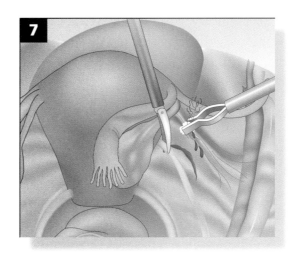

allows for better occlusion of the spiral uterine vascular pedicle and the heat energy from the bipolar to displace into the specimen rather than away from the uterus and toward the ureter. The manipulator is pushed inward toward the patient's contralateral shoulder thus increasing the distance from the lateral uterine wall and the ureter. The ureter will have been released by the ureterolysis incision further creating a safe margin for desiccation. Once these vascular pedicles are occluded, the uterus will become cyanotic indicating that it is devascularized. From this point the procedure is very straightforward with amputation of the cervix, coring well down into the endocervical canal. This amputation should begin at the level of the internal os or at the level of entry into the uterus of the uterine vessels. Aggressive coring downward into the cervix should be used while pushing upward with the manipulator (Figure 9). Endocervical mucous is almost always visualized during this amputation assuring that the surgeon is low enough and that no lower uterine segment is being left behind. Ablation of the remaining endocervical canal using bipolar is performed (Figure 10) and then the cervical stump is closed using a #0 Vicryl™ (Ethicon, Johnson & Johnson Co., Somerville, NJ) suture on a CT-2 needle. The vault is then sup-

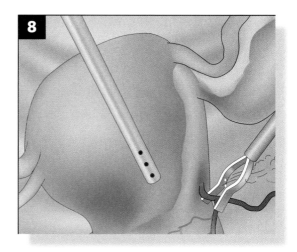

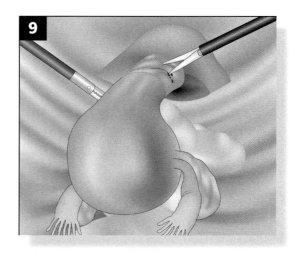

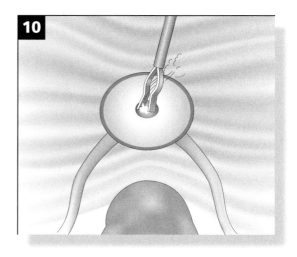

ported with ipsilateral McCall's sutures of #0 Ethibond™ (Ethicon, Johnson & Johnson Co., Somerville, NJ) suture. The amputation of the uterine corpus can be performed with blunt dissection with scissors, or using monopolar cutting current. Amputation can also be performed with the harmonic scalpel. Dr. Jacques Dequesne has introduced a monopolar loop electrode that can be placed around the cervix and tightened to facilitate fast and effective amputation of the uterine corpus. The Lap Loop System® (Circon, Santa Barbara, CA) is currently in an investigational phase in the United States and has not yet been FDA approved (Figures 11 and 12).

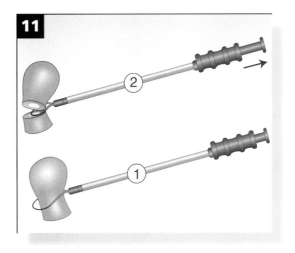

The final portion of the procedure is specimen removal. We use the mechanical morcellator from Gynecare, DIVA™, (Gynecare, Johnson & Johnson Co., Somerville, NJ) which requires a 10-mm single toothed tenaculum to work at maximum efficiency. The device will fit through the lower trocar site and requires minimal practice to obtain proficiency. Other morcellators (Storz, Culver City, CA; WISAP, Lenexa, KS) are available but the DIVA™ has been our preference (See Chapter 3) (Figure 13). Several safety steps should be considered when using the morcellator (Figure 14).

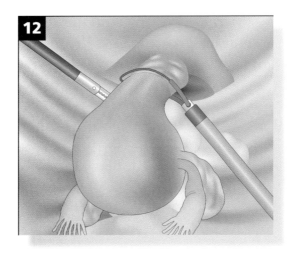

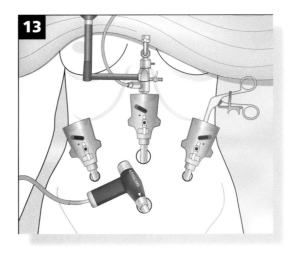

Following actions should not be performed while morcellating (Figure 15).

When the entire specimen is removed, the abdomen is thoroughly irrigated, the fluid is removed and the lower 10/11 mm site is closed using the Carter-Thomason fascial closure device. The larger sites receive a subcuticular closure and the 5-mm sites are steri-stripped. All sites are injected with 0.25% Marcaine with epinephrine and dressings are applied.

Postoperative care allows the patient to be discharged from the surgical facility within 24 hours. The Foley

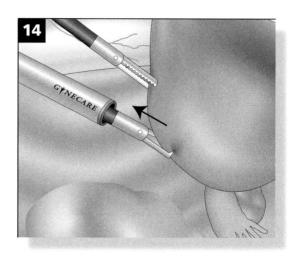

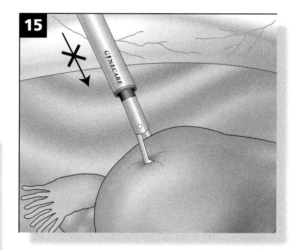

1. ALWAYS KEEP THE TIP OF THE MORCELLATOR IN THE MIDDLE OF THE VIEWING FIELD.

2. KEEP THE SHAFT OF THE MORCELLATOR IN A HORIZONTAL POSITION.

3. USE THE PORT ABOVE THE MORCELLATOR FOR THE CAMERA TO AVOID THE MIRROR IMAGING.

4. GRASP THE TISSUE, AND PULL IT INTO THE MORCELLATOR CANAL.

5. HOLD THE TISSUE WITH THE GRASPER TO PREVENT A ROTATION OF THE SPECIMEN.

6. MORCELLATE THE TISSUE TANGENTIALLY FROM THE SURFACE, LIKE PEALING AN APPLE.

7. DEACTIVATE THE PEDAL WHEN THE SHAFT HAS CUT THROUGH THE TISSUE

NEVER PUSH THE SHAFT OF THE MORCELLATOR INWARD WHILE MORCELLATING.

NEVER MORCELLATE THE TISSUE THAT HAS NOT BEEN DETACHED.

DO NOT HOLD THE MORCELLATOR IN A VERTICAL POSITION WHILE MORCELLATING.

AVOID PULLING THE MIDDLE OF THE MASS INTO THE MORCELLATOR SHAFT.

catheter is removed in the recovery room and ambulation is encouraged. The patient is allowed to perform all activities in which she is comfortable. Individuals are able to return to normal activity within a few days and may return to work within 1-2 weeks.

CLINICAL EXPERIENCE

Various authors have reported retrospective series of LSH. Donnez described the largest series with over 500 procedures. In these studies, as well as a 500 case series reported by Daniell, morbidity was extremely low again justifying the effectiveness of LSH. Our series is now at >750 procedures with continuing low morbidity and clinical outcomes based on patient satisfaction surveys and morbidity statistics (Table 1).

Semm first reported a form of supracervical hysterectomy called the CISH in 1991. Although technically a supracervical hysterectomy it differs sufficiently from LSH to separate the data from discussion of LSH. Data for this literature is seen in Table 2

LSH was proposed by the present author in 1990 as a possible alternative with further decreased morbidity and possible extended applications. Simon et al. have evaluated the economic morbidity of the LSH procedure as compared with total abdominal

Table 1

	PATIENTS	GRAMS	MINUTES	COMPLICATIONS
DONNEZ (1997)	500	60-810	30-135	0.6%
DANIELL (1999)	500	? SIZE	90 (MEAN)	<1%
LYONS (1995)	294	65-2180	55-224	< 1%

Table 2

	PATIENTS	GRAMS	MINUTES	COMPLICATIONS
SEMM (16) (1996)	90	? WGT.	90 (MEAN)	0%
METTLER (17) (1995)	200	50-250	120-240	"MINIMAL"
LEVINE (18) (1996)	100	27-950	105-240	3%
VIETZ (19) (1996)	60	? WGT.	90 (MEAN)	0%"MAJOR"

hysterectomy in a community hospital setting. This study concluded that LSH was a cost-effective alternative in those patients with indications for hysterectomy.

LSH has as its most positive attributes, decreased overall morbidity, application to virtually any size uterus, probable improved overall pelvic floor support secondary to the intact pericervical ring and intact neurovascular supply. In addition, the subtotal approach in virtually all cases adequately addresses the pathology associated with the admitting diagnosis.

Women today are concerned with destructive surgeries to the reproductive anatomy and the associated psychosocial effects. LSH is a viable alternative for these individuals offering a less invasive and less destructive procedure that can still eliminate their symptoms. Kilku addressed these concerns in a series of articles in the mid-1980s. Hasson also discussed this issue in an excellent review of subtotal hysterectomy in 1995.

The final factor is choice. Today's woman is an intelligent and well-informed consumer who desires and may demand medical alternatives based on the opinions and recommendations of her physicians. Those surgeons who are willing to discuss these options and apply them to appropriate patients may find greater success and a less litigious atmosphere than those who attempt to patronize their clientele.

Suggested Reading:

Thompson JD, Warsaw J. Hysterectomy. In Rock JA, Thompson JD (eds). Telinde's Operative Gynecology 8th Edition. New York, NY, Lippincott-Raven Publishers, 1996:771- 854.

Reich H, DeCaprio J, McGlynn F. Laparoscopic hysterectomy. J Gynecological Surgery 1989;5: 213-216

Lyons TL. Laparoscopic supracervical hysterectomy-A comparison of morbidity and mortality results with laparoscopically assisted vaginal hysterectomy. J Reprod Med 1993;38:763-767

Lyons TL. Subtotal Hysterectomy: In Diamond MP, Daniell JF, Jones HA (Eds). Hysterectomy. Cambridge, Mass., Blackwell Science, 1995:84-98

Lyons TL. Laparoscopic supracervical hysterectomy. In Wood C, Maher PJ (eds): Balliere's Clinical Obstetrics and Gynecology. London, UK, Balliere & Tindall, 1997,167-181

Winer WK: Operating Room Personnel. In Sanfilippo JS, Levine RL (eds). Operative Gynecologic Endoscopy 2nd Edition. New York, NY, Springer-Verlag, 1996:412-422

Liu CY. Laparoscopic hysterectomy. Report of 215 cases. Gynecol Endosc 1992;1:73-77

Donnez J, Nisolle M, Smets M, Polet R, Bassil S: Laparoscopic supracervical (subtotal) hysterectomy: a first series of 500 cases. Gynecol Endosc 1997;6:73-76

Anderson TL, Lindsay, JH, Daniell JF. Performing laparoscopic supracervical hysterectomy. OBG Management 1999;1:15-32

Semm K. Hysterectomy via laparotomy or pelviscopy. A new CASH method without culpotomy. Geburtshilfe Frauenheilkd 1991;51:996-1003

Simon NV, Laveran, RL, Cavanaugh S, Gerlach DH, Jackson JR. Laparoscopic supracervical hysterectomy vs. abdominal hysterectomy in a community hospital: A cost comparison. J Reprod Med1999;44(4):339-345

Kilkku P. Supravaginal amputation versus hysterectomy with reference to bladder symptoms and incontinence. Acta Obstet Gynecol Scand 1985;64:375-379

Kilkku P, Hirvonen T, Gronoos M. Supracervical uterine amputation vs. abdominal hysterectomy: The effects in urinary symptoms with special reference to pollakisuria, nocturia, and dysuria. Maturitas 1981;3:197

Kilkku P, Gronoos M, Hirvonen T, et al. Supravaginal uterine amputation vs. hysterectomy: Effects on libido and orgasm. Acta Obstet Gynecol Scand 1983;62:141-146

Hasson HM. Cervical removal at hysterectomy for benign disease. J Reprod Med 1993;38(10): 781-790

Semm K. Endoscopic subtotal hysterectomy without culpotomy, classic intrafascial SEMM hysterectomy. A new method of hysterectomy by pelviscopy, laparotomy, per vaginam or functionally by total uterine mucosal ablation. Int Surgery 1996;81(4): 362-370

Mettler L, et al. Comparative evaluation of classic intrafascial supracervical hysterectomy (CISH) with transuterine mucosal resection as performed by pelviscopy and laparotomy – our first 200 cases. Surg Endosc 1995;9(4):418-23

Levine DJ, Botney K. The classic intrafascial SEMM hysterectomy as an alternative to abdominal hysterectomy. J Am Assoc Gynecol Laparosc 1996;3(4):545-548

Vietz PF, Ahn TS. A new approach to hysterectomy without culpotomy: pelviscopic intrafascial hysterectomy. Am J Obstet Gynecol 1994;170(2):609-613

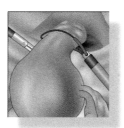

LAPAROSCOPIC MYOMECTOMY & LAPAROSCOPICALLY ASSISTED MYOMECTOMY

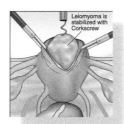

Ceana Nezhat, M.D.

Myomas are the most common uterine neoplasm, affecting 20-25% of women of reproductive age. Myomas develop from the benign transformation and proliferation of smooth muscle cells, and can develop in any area with smooth muscle cells of Müllerian origin. Uterine myomas can cause abnormal uterine bleeding, abdominal pressure, urinary frequency, and constipation. The severity of these symptoms is dependent on the number of tumors, their size, and location (Figure 1). Although not primarily the cause of infertility, myomas have been linked to fetal wastage and premature delivery. Indications for treatment are listed below. The number, size, and location of the tumors influence the technique used.

Preoperative evaluation should include assessment of anemia. The use of gonadotropin–releasing hormone (GnRH) is indicated for anemic patients as it may restore a normal hematocrit, decrease the size of the myoma, and reduce the need for transfusion. An intravenous pyelogram may be indicated to check for ureteral obstruction when there is a large broad ligament myoma. Pelvic ultrasound is another preoperative tool to monitor the growth rate of asymptomatic myomas and to check for submucous tumors.

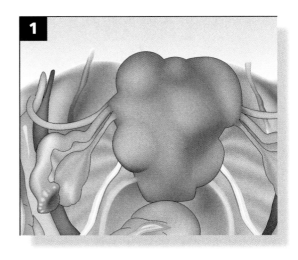

INDICATIONS FOR MYOMECTOMY

- MENOMETRORRHAGIA AND ANEMIA

- PELVIC PAIN AND PRESSURE

- ENLARGING LEIOMYOMA AND POSSIBILITY OF NEOPLASIA

- ASSOCIATED FETAL WASTAGE OR INFERTILITY

- GESTATIONAL SIZE MORE THAN 12 WEEKS AND INABILITY TO EVALUATE THE ADNEXA

- OBSTRUCTED URETER

Patients should always be counseled regarding the risk of intraoperative and postoperative bleeding, and autologous blood donation may be suggested. In addition, patients should be aware of the possible necessity for laparotomy and, although low, the potential chance of hysterectomy.

LAPAROSCOPIC MYOMECTOMY – TECHNIQUE

The necessary instruments include a CO_2 laser, unipolar electrode or harmonic scalpel, a bipolar Kleppinger forceps, clawed grasping forceps, myoma screw and suturing instruments.

Dilute Pitressin (vasopressin 20 units in 60-100 cc NaCl) is injected into the base of the stalk at the junction of the uterine fundus (Figure 2). Pedunculated leiomyomas are removed by coagulating and cutting the stalk, and bleeding areas controlled with bipolar forceps. For intramural myomas, dilute vasopressin is injected in multiple sites between the myometrium and the fibroid capsule.

An incision is made on the serosa overlying the leiomyoma using the

CO_2 laser, a monopolar electrode, a fiber laser, or harmonic scalpel. The incision is extended until it reaches the capsule, and the myometrium retracts as the incision is made, exposing the tumor. The suction–irrigator is used as a blunt probe to shell the leiomyoma from its capsule while two grasping, toothed forceps hold the edges of the myometrium. A myoma screw is inserted into the tumor to apply traction while the suction–irrigator is used as a blunt dissector (Figure 3). Vessels are electrocoagulated before being cut, and the uterine defect is irrigated after the myoma has been completely removed. If the defect is deep or large, the myometrium and serosa are approximated by using a 1-0 polydioxanone and 4-0 polyglactin suture in several layers. The repair mainly involves myometrium and the serosal and subserosal layers and may be accomplished in one layer, but we prefer two layers, if possible. The sutures should be applied in 1-cm increments using extracorporeal or intracorporeal knot tying (Figure 4). Once the repair is complete, the uterine surface is irrigated with warmed lactated Ringer's solution and Interceed™ (Johnson & Johnson Medical, Somerville, NJ) is applied over the suture line.

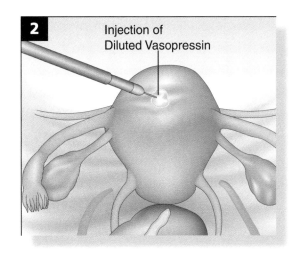

2 — Injection of Diluted Vasopressin

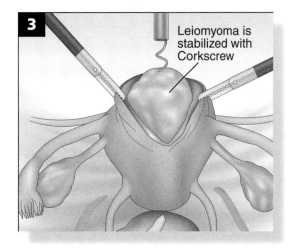

3 — Leiomyoma is stabilized with Corkscrew

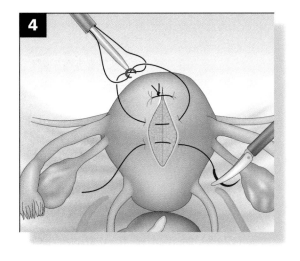

4

Spraying 10,000 IU of thrombin over the Interceed™ contributes to hemostasis (Figure 5). Suturing is limited because of the high incidence of postoperative adhesions. The defect will heal better and with less deformity when the edges are approximated. Even under ideal circumstances, laparoscopic microsurgical closure of the myometrial defect is difficult.

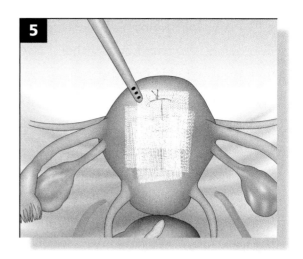

Ligamentous and broad ligament myomas require careful observation of the course of the ureters and large blood vessels. Depending on the location of the myoma, an incision is made on the anterior or posterior leaf of the broad ligament. The myoma is removed with the same techniques described for subserosal and intramural tumors. The location of the ureters is noted throughout the procedure. Hemostasis is obtained with sutures, clips, or bipolar forceps. None of the lasers can adequately coagulate bleeding myometrial vessels, however, a bipolar forceps or argon beam coagulator is excellent for this purpose. The broad ligament and peritoneum are not closed, but allowed to heal spontaneously. Drains are almost never used.

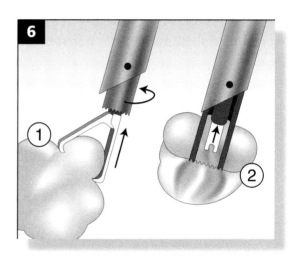

Removal of myomas from the abdominal cavity is a time-consuming procedure, and no methods or instruments are ideal for this purpose. A claw-toothed forceps is inserted through a 10-mm sleeve for myomas <5 cm. A long Kocher clamp is inserted through one suprapubic incision, which often has to be extended. The midline incision is preferred to avoid injury to the inferior epigastric vessels. This is a quick technique.

Larger myomas can be removed through a posterior colpotomy, however, this method may increase operative time, infectious morbidity, and add risk of bowel and ureteral injury. Colpotomy is not safe in women with concurrent posterior cul-de-sac abnormalities. Improvements in electronic morcellators have made this task easier (Figure 6).

LAPAROSCOPICALLY ASSISTED MYOMECTOMY

Laparoscopically assisted myomectomy (LAM) is a safe alternative to LM, and is less difficult and less time consuming. The criteria for LAM are: myoma greater than 8 cm, multiple myomas requiring extensive morcellation, and a deep, large, intramural or transmural myoma requiring uterine repair in multiple layers. Using a combination of laparoscopy and a 2-4 cm abdominal incision may enable more gynecologists to apply this technique (Figure 7). Uterine suturing in 2 or 3 layers reduces the chances of uterine dehiscence, fistulas, and adhesions.

The three major objectives of LAM are:

1. Reduction of blood loss,

2. Maintenance of myometrial integrity, and

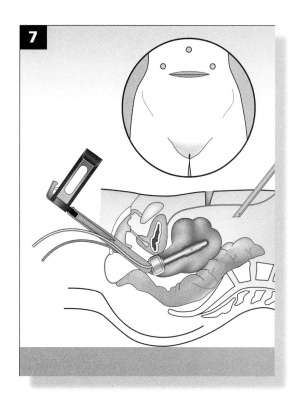

3. Decrease the chances of post-operative adhesions.

LAM reduces the duration of the operation and the need for extensive laparoscopic experience when performed with morcellation and conventional suturing.

LAM TECHNIQUE

When multiple myomas are encountered, the most prominent myoma is injected at the base with 10-15 mL of diluted vasopressin. A vertical incision is made over the uterine serosa on to the surface of the tumor. The incision

Chapter 16

230 | LAPAROSCOPIC MYOMECTOMY & LAPAROSCOPICALLY ASSISTED MYOMECTOMY . . . .

is extended until the capsule of the leiomyoma is reached (Figure 8). A corkscrew manipulator is inserted into the leiomyoma and used to move the uterus toward the midline suprapubic puncture and the puncture is enlarged to a 4-cm transverse skin incision. Once the incision of the fascia is made transversely, the rectus muscle is divided using a monopolar electrode. The inferior epigastric vessels, if found, are coagulated. This provides excellent access to the abdominal cavity (Figure 9).

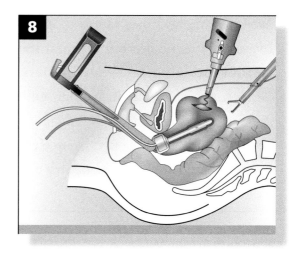

The peritoneum is entered transversely and the leiomyoma is observed. Using the corkscrew manipulator, the leiomyoma is brought to the mini-laparotomy incision. The corkscrew manipulator is replaced by two Lahey Tenacula (Figure 10). The tumor is shelled and morcellated (Figure 11). After complete removal, the uterine wall defect shows through the incision. If uterine size allows, the uterus is exteriorized to complete the repair. As many leiomyomas as possible should be removed through one uterine incision. When other leiomyomas are present and cannot be removed through the initial uterine incision, the abdominal opening is approximated with 2 or 3 Allis clamps or an inflated latex glove. The remaining leiomyomas are

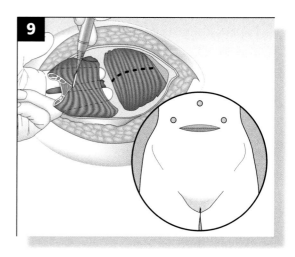

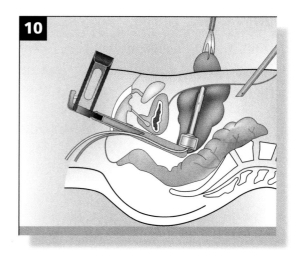

removed in the same manner under laparoscopic control. The uterus is then exteriorized through the 4-cm abdominal incision and the myometrium is closed in layers with 2-0 and 0 polydioxanone sutures (Figure 12). The uterus is palpated to ensure that no small intramural leiomyomas remain and it is returned to the peritoneal cavity. The fascia is closed with number 0 polyglactin suture and the skin is closed in a subcuticular manner. The laparoscope is used to evaluate hemostasis and the pelvis is observed to detect and treat any pathology that may have previously been obscured by myomas. Copious irrigation is used, blood clots are removed, and Interceed™ is applied over the uterus to help prevent adhesions.

Injections of dilute vasopressin into the myoma help reduce blood loss intraoperatively. In addition, vertical uterine incisions bleed less than transverse, and pneumoperitoneum seems to decrease intraoperative bleeding.

Most patients are observed in an outpatient unit and discharged the morning after the operation, and some can even leave on the day of the procedure. Women who desire future

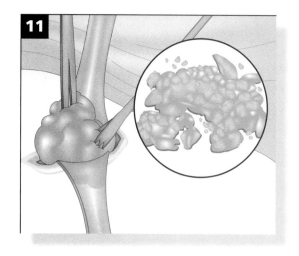

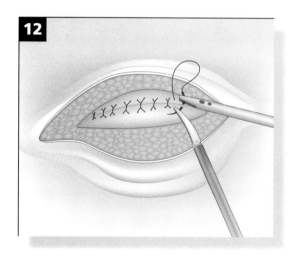

fertility and who require myomectomy for an intramural tumor may benefit from LAM to ensure proper closure of the myometrial incision. Cesarean delivery is safer in patients who had deep intramural myoma removed or who have had multiple myomectomies as well as penetration to the cavity.

SUGGESTED READING:

Buttram VC, Reiter RC. Uterine leiomyomata: etiology, symptomatology, and management. Fertil Steril 1981;36:433

Vollenhoven BJ, Lawrence AS, Healy DL. Uterine fibroids: a clinical review. Br J Obstet Gynaecol 1990;97:393

Freidman AJ, Rein NS, Harrison-Atlas D, et al. A randomized, placebo-controlled, double blind study evaluating leuprolide acetate depot treatment before myomectomy. Fertil Steril 1989;52:728

Nezhat C, Nezhat F, Silfen SL, Schaffer N, Evans D. Laparoscopic myomectomy. Int J Fertil 1991;36(5):275-280

Nezhat C, Nezhat F, Bess O, Nezhat CH, Mashiach R. Laparoscopically assisted myomectomy: a report of a new technique in 57 cases. Int J Fertil Menopausal Stud 1994;39(1)39-44

Melis GB, Ajossa S, Piras B, et al. A randomized trial to evaluate the prevention of de novo adhesion formation after laparoscopic myomectomy using oxidized regenerated cellulose (Interceed™) barrier. J Am Assoc Gynecol Laparosc 1995;2:S31

Nezhat C, Siegler AM, Nezhat F, Nezhat CH, Seidman D, Luciano AA. Operative Gynecologic Laparoscopy: Principles and Techniques. 2nd ed. New York: McGraw Hill, 2000

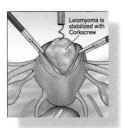

LAPAROSCOPIC TREATMENT OF STRESS URINE INCONTINENCE AND ANTERIOR VAGINAL WALL PROLAPSE

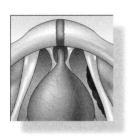

John R. Miklos, M.D.

Timothy B. McKinney, M.D.

INTRODUCTION

Since the introduction of the retropubic urethral suspension in 1910, over 100 different surgical techniques for the treatment of genuine stress urinary incontinence (GSUI) have been described. Many have been modifications of original procedures that attempt to improve clinical outcome, shorten operative time and/or reduce surgical morbidity. Despite the number of surgical procedures developed each year, the Burch colposuspension and pubovaginal sling operations have remained the mainstay of surgical correction for GSUI due to their high long-term cure rates. However, these procedures do not address the concurrent anterior vaginal wall prolapse often associated with GSUI secondary to urethral hypermobility. We use a laparoscopic approach to anterior vaginal wall reconstruction utilizing the paravaginal repair and Burch colposuspension for treatment of cystocele and stress urinary incontinence, respectively, due to lateral vaginal wall support defects.

Chapter 17

234 | LAPAROSCOPIC TREATMENT OF STRESS URINE INCONTINENCE AND ANTERIOR VAGINAL WALL PROLAPSE .....

Emphasizing the principles of minimally invasive surgery, the laparoscopic approach has been successfully adopted for many procedures that previously relied on an abdominal or transvaginal route. First described in 1991, the laparoscopic retropubic colposuspension has rapidly gained popularity due to its many reported advantages including: improved visualization, shorter hospital stay, faster recovery, and decreased blood loss.

OPERATIVE INDICATIONS

Laparoscopy should be considered only as a mode of abdominal access and not a change in the operative technique. Ideally the indications for a laparoscopic approach to retropubic colposuspension should be the same as an open (laparotomy) approach. This would include patients with genuine stress urinary incontinence and urethral hypermobility. We believe the laparoscopic Burch colposuspension can be substituted for an open Burch colposuspension in the majority of cases. If the patient demonstrates a cystocele secondary to a paravaginal defect diagnosed either pre- or intraoperatively, a paravaginal defect repair should be performed prior to the colposuspension. This approach combines the paravaginal repair with Burch

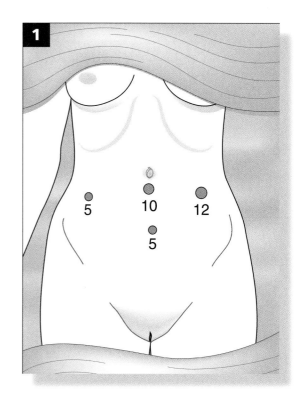

colposuspension for treatment of anterior vaginal prolapse secondary to paravaginal defects and stress urinary incontinence secondary to urethral hypermobility.

SURGICAL TECHNIQUE

LAPAROSCOPIC PARAVAGINAL REPAIR

We routinely perform open laparoscopy at the inferior margin of the umbilicus. A 10-mm access port is used at this site to introduce the laparoscope. The abdomen is insufflated with

CO_2 to 15 mmHg intraabdominal pressure. Even though this surgery can be performed using 5-mm trocar sleeves, we recommend two 5-mm ports and a 12-mm port (Figure 1). The 12-mm port allows for easier and faster access when passing the needle into the abdominal cavity for suturing. Choice of the individual port size depends on the surgeon and any concomitant surgery planned for each patient.

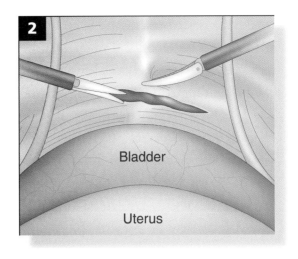

Bladder

Uterus

The bladder is filled in a retrograde fashion with 200–300 mL normal saline, allowing identification of the superior border of the bladder edge. Entrance into the space of Retzius is accomplished by a transperitoneal approach using a harmonic scalpel. The incision is made approximately 3 cm above the bladder reflection, beginning along the medial border of the right obliterated umbilical ligament (Figure 2). Immediate identification of loose areolar tissue at the point of incision confirms a proper plane of dissection.

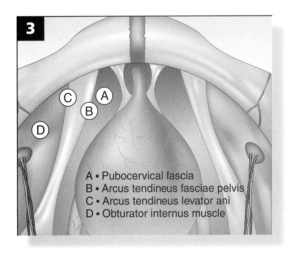

A • Pubocervical fascia
B • Arcus tendineus fasciae pelvis
C • Arcus tendineus levator ani
D • Obturator internus muscle

After the space of Retzius has been entered and the pubic ramus visualized, the bladder is drained to prevent injury. The retropubic space is developed by separating the loose areolar and fatty layers using blunt dissection. Blunt dissection is continued until the retropubic anatomy is visualized. The pubic symphysis and bladderneck are identified in the midline and the obturator neurovascular bundle, Cooper's ligament, and the arcus tendineus fascia pelvis are visualized bilaterally along the pelvic sidewall (Figure 3). The anterior vaginal wall and its point of lateral attachment from its origin at the pubic symphysis to its insertion at the ischial spine is identified. If paravaginal

Chapter 17

236 | LAPAROSCOPIC TREATMENT OF STRESS URINE INCONTINENCE AND ANTERIOR VAGINAL WALL PROLAPSE . . . . .

wall defects are present, the lateral margins of the pubocervical fascia will be detached from the pelvic sidewall at the arcus tendineus fascia pelvis (white line). The lateral margins of the detached pubocervical fascia and the broken edge of the white line can usually be clearly visualized confirming the paravaginal defect. Unilateral or bilateral defects may be present (Figure 4).

We recommend completion of the laparoscopic paravaginal repair prior to the colposuspension. After identification of the defect, the combined repair is begun by inserting the surgeon's nondominant hand into the vagina to elevate the anterior vaginal wall and the pubocervical fascia to their normal attachment along the arcus tendineus fascia pelvis. A 2-0 nonabsorbable suture with attached needle are introduced through the 12-mm port, and the needle is grasped using a laparoscopic needle driver.

The first suture is placed near the apex of the vagina through the paravesical portion of the pubocervical fascia. The needle is then passed through the ipsilateral obturator internus muscle and fascia around the arcus tendineus fascia at its origin 1–2 cm distal to the ischial spine. The suture is secured using an extracorporeal knot-tying technique. Good tissue

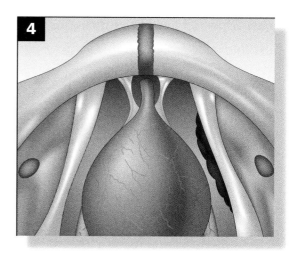

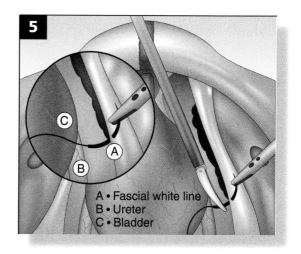

A • Fascial white line
B • Ureter
C • Bladder

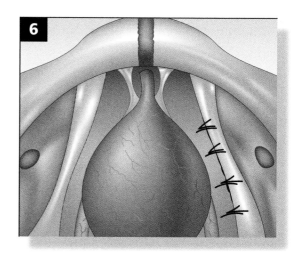

approximation is accomplished without a suture bridge (Figure 5). Sutures are placed sequentially along the paravaginal defects from the ischial spine toward the urethrovesical junction. Usually, a series of two to four sutures are placed between the ischial spine and a point 1-2 cm proximal to the urethrovesical junction (Figure 6). The laparoscopic colposuspension is performed distal to the urethrovesical junction. The surgical procedure is repeated on the patient's opposite side if bilateral defects are present. Upon completion of the bilateral paravaginal repair, the Burch colposuspension is performed. By performing the paravaginal defect repair first, normal anatomical support of the anterior vaginal segment is recreated, reducing the chance of over elevation of the paraurethral Burch sutures and subsequent voiding dysfunction.

LAPAROSCOPIC BURCH COLPOSUSPENSION

This laparoscopic technique parallels our open technique and has previously been described. The laparoscopic colposuspension is performed using nonabsorbable No. 0 sutures; we routinely use polytrifluoroethylene. The surgeon's nondominant hand is placed in the vagina and a finger is used to ele-

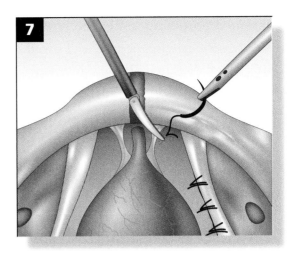

vate the vagina. The endopelvic fascia on both sides of the bladder neck and midurethra is exposed using an endoscopic Kitner. The first suture is placed 2 cm lateral to the urethra at the level of the midurethra. A figure of eight bite, incorporating the entire thickness of the anterior vaginal wall excluding the epithelium, is taken, and the suture is then passed through the ipsilateral Cooper's ligament (Figure 7).

With an assistant's fingers in the vagina to elevate the anterior vaginal wall toward Cooper's ligament, the suture is tied down with a series of extracorporeal knots using an endoscopic knot pusher. An additional suture is then placed in a similar fashion at the level of the urethrovesical junction, approximately 2 cm lateral to the bladder edge on the same side (Figure 8). The procedure is

Chapter 17

238 | LAPAROSCOPIC TREATMENT OF STRESS URINE INCONTINENCE AND ANTERIOR VAGINAL WALL PROLAPSE . . . . .

repeated on the opposite side. Excessive tension on the vaginal wall should be avoided when tying down the sutures. We routinely leave a suture bridge of approximately 2-3 cm (Figure 9).

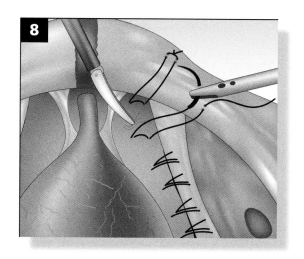

Upon completion of the paravaginal repair and Burch urethropexy, the intraabdominal pressure is reduced to 10-12 mmHg, and the retropubic space is inspected for hemostasis. Cystoscopy is performed to rule out urinary tract injury. The patient is given 5 mL of indigo carmine and 10 mL furosemide intravenously, and a 70° cystoscope is used to visualize the bladder lumen, assess for unintentional stitch penetration and confirm bilateral ureteral patency. After cystoscopy, attention is returned to laparoscopy. We recommend routine closure of the anterior peritoneal defect in a pursestring fashion using a 0-chromic suture on a CT-1 needle. All ancillary trocar sheaths are removed under direct vision to ensure hemostasis and exclude iatrogenic bowel herniation. Excess gas is expelled and fascial defects of 10 mm or more are closed

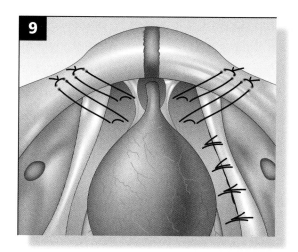

using delayed absorbable suture. Postoperative bladder drainage and voiding trials are accomplished using either a transurethral catheter, suprapubic tube, or intermittent self catheterization.

SUGGESTED READING:

Vancaille TG, Schussler W. Laparoscopic bladderneck suspension. J Laparoendo Surg 1991;1:169-73

Miklos JR, Kohli N. "Paravaginal Plus" Burch procedure: a laparoscopic approach. J Pelvic Surgery 1998;4:297-302

Kohli N, Miklos JR. Laparoscopic Burch colposuspension: a modern approach. Contemp Obstet Gynecol 1997;42:36-55

Miklos JR, Kohli N. Innovative Surgery for Stress Urinary Incontinenece. In: Urogynecologic Surgery. Lippincott Williams & Wilkins, Philadelphia, PA

Miklos JR, Kohli N. Laparoscopic paravaginal repair plus Burch colposuspension: review and descriptive technique. Urology 2000;56 (Suppl 6A): 64-9

Speights SE, Moore RD, Miklos JR. Frequency of lower urinary tract injury at laparoscopic Burch and paravaginal repair. J Am Assoc Gynecol Laparosc 2000;7(4):515-8

Liu CY. Laparoscopic treatment of genuine urinary stress incontinence. Clin Obstet Gyencol 1994;8:789-98

Ross JW. Laparoscopic Burch repair compared to laparotomy Burch for cure of urinary stress incontinence. Int Urogynecol 1995;6:323-328

Ross JW. Two techniques of laparoscopic Burch repair for stress incontinence: a prospective randomized study. J Am Assoc Gynecol Laparosc 1996;3:351-357

PELVIC FLOOR SURGERY

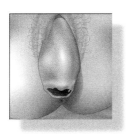

Timothy B. McKinney, M.D.

John Miklos, M.D.

Throughout hundreds of years of the earliest writings on operative gynecology, the problems of pelvic support have always been referred to as pelvic relaxation. Over the past 25 years, we have witnessed a major shift in our understanding of the concepts of pelvic floor support. Defects in these supports leads to a relationship which, if re-established, will generate the normal anatomical support of the internal pelvic viscera. Terms such as generalized stretching and attenuation have been employed commonly in almost all descriptions. The consensus has been that to repair all support tissue, it was necessary to correct the generalized stretching by way of plicating, resecting or shortening these attenuated tissues. The true causes of genital urinary prolapse are failures of the fibromuscular support system to confine the visceral organs within the pelvic cavity. When this fibromuscular support system of endopelvic fascia is damaged, visceral organ prolapse/herniation results. The anatomical proximity of all female genital organs to the lower urinary tract and alimentary tract predispose pelvic organ prolapse and can easily affect bladder, urethra and rectal function. This prolapse leads to voiding and defecating difficulties as well as sexual dysfunction in females (Figures 1 and 2).

Prior to 25 years ago the concepts of pelvic relaxation were rarely questioned. Cullen Richardson, in his manuscript "A New Look at Pelvic Relaxation" published in 1976 in the American Journal of Obstetrics and Gynecology, fostered a new understanding of pelvic floor defects. He stated that, "in all patients with cystoceles, there were isolated breaks in the pubocervical fascia". He proposed that breaks in the endopelvic fascial hammock of the pubocervical fascia, in one or more of four areas, would yield an anterior compartment hernia (cystocele/anterior enterocele) (Figures 3 and 4). It was further suggested and observed that isolated breaks in other areas of endopelvic fascia accounted for all other support defects. These findings of isolated breaks in the endopelvic fascia are the key to pelvic floor support and need to be addressed during any kind of reparative pelvic

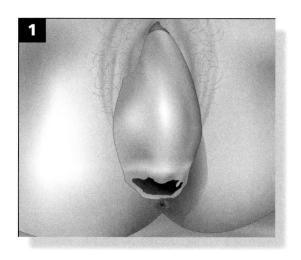

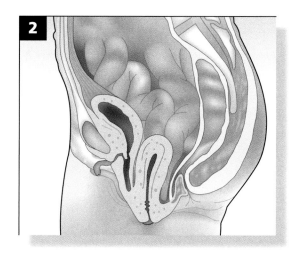

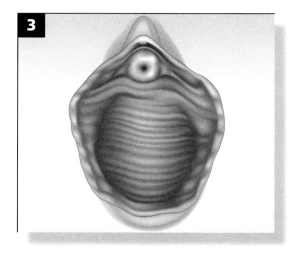

surgery. Isolated breaks in the recto-vaginal septum cause rectoceles as well as (Figures 5 and 6) breaks between the rectovaginal septum and pubocervical fascia, giving rise to enteroceles (Figure 7). It has been demonstrated that isolated breaks in the uterosacral ligament component of this network cause vaginal vault prolapse. This work was first performed extensively on cadaveric models, then moved to patients and, finally, was demonstrated on MRI studies. Today, it is generally accepted that essentially all support defects represent a break or breaks in the endopelvic fascial network. These breaks, as well as neuromuscular damage, combine to cause all pelvic support problems in the female patient. When these breaks in support have occurred and the normal anatomical relationships are disrupted, physiologic dysfunctions such as urinary and fecal incontinence and prolapse in the pelvic organs can ensue. The critical relationships of the pelvis rely heavily on the integrity of the structural elements, namely bones, ligaments, muscles and endopelvic fascia. It is imperative that in performing any reparative pelvic surgery that anatomical concepts are well understood before embarking on surgical correction of the problem.

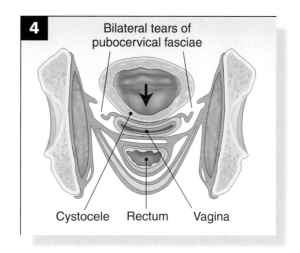

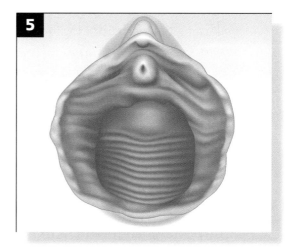

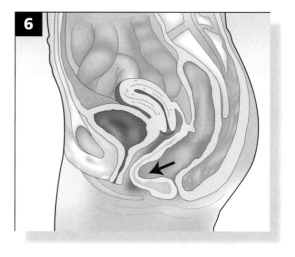

ANATOMY OF PELVIC SUPPORT

Various bulges we encounter in the vagina, cystoceles, urethroceles, uterine prolapse, enteroceles and rectoceles all represent some failure of the pelvic floor to support one or more of the visceral structures resting upon or contained within it. The pelvic floor acts as a unit and should be thought of that way. It is divided into three layers of support from the inside out: the endopelvic fascial network (Figure 8), the striated muscles of the pelvic diaphragm and, lastly, the urogenital diaphragm and bony pelvis (Figure 9). Although the bony superstructure surrounding the pelvis is in itself a great support for pelvic organs, it is truly the muscular and fascial structures that lie at the bottom that act as the strongest support layers. This combination of the connective tissue endopelvic fascia and the striated muscle pelvic diaphragm are responsible for the bulk of normal support. The mechanism of failure is always from the inside out in organ prolapse. Therefore, in all major prolapses there are isolated breaks in the innermost layer or endopelvic fascia.

Surgically we need to use these endopelvic fascial structures, the uterosacral ligament complex, pubocervical fascia and rectovaginal fascia in

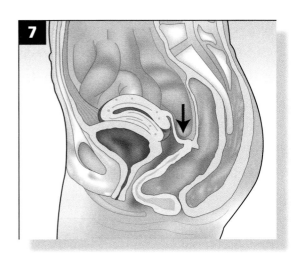

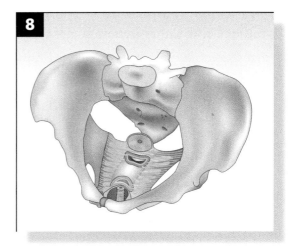

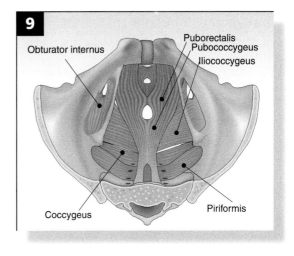

all of our repair procedures. The clinical identification of these defects allows for the appropriate repair. When contemplating the various supportive structures, it is helpful to consider the vagina as a flattened fibromuscular tube lined with vaginal epithelium. The top of the tube is supported by the pubocervical fascia. The bottom is the rectovaginal fascia or septum. The top of the tube, as well as the uterus, are supported above the pelvic diaphragm by structures identified as the cardinal/uterosacral ligament complex. The uterosacral ligaments represent the level one (1) support of endopelvic fascia as described by John DeLancey. The midportion of the endopelvic fascia support or level (2), attaches the vagina to the levator ani muscles from the ischial spines to the urogenital diaphragm. The anterior vaginal wall, pubocervical fascia, as well as the posterior vaginal wall, attach laterally at the same spot, the arcus tendineus ligament, and form a restraining layer that prevents the bladder and rectum from protruding into the vagina (Figure 10).

On the distal end of the tube, DeLancey level (3), there is a fusion with the urogenital diaphragm and perineal body (Figure 11). In the normally functioning pelvis, the levator ani muscles are always contracted keeping the pelvic floor closed and

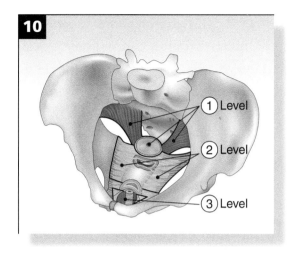

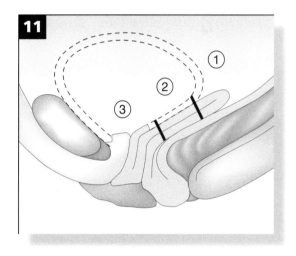

allowing for minimal exposure of pressure on the endopelvic fascia. The endopelvic fascia network simply suspends the organs in their proper position above the levator ani muscles. This interaction between the pelvic floor muscles and fascia is critical to the proper pelvic floor support and function. If the pelvic floor muscles are damaged or relaxed for prolonged periods of time, increases in intraabdominal pressure and gravity can damage the underlying endopelvic fascia or expose weaknesses in the fascia. It is these defects in the endopelvic fascia in conjunction with poorly functioning levator ani muscles that result in genital organ prolapse. In this chapter, we will describe surgical corrections that are geared at reconstruction of these endopelvic fascial defects. How we treat the levator ani problem greatly affects the long-term outcomes of our surgeries. Therefore, all patients that undergo pelvic floor reconstruction should be placed on some form of pelvic floor rehabilitation postoperatively much like the orthopedic surgeon would require after a knee replacement. We use biofeedback and good estrogenization to achieve this goal.

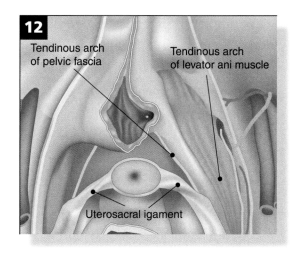

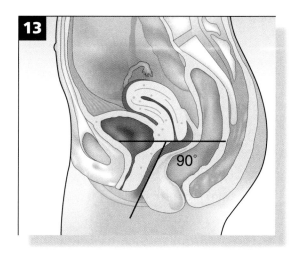

ENDOPELVIC FASCIA

Since the endopelvic fascia is the single most important element responsible for the maintenance of the normal anatomical relationship, it will be these layers that we emphasis most at this juncture. The endopelvic fascia is a skeletal matrix made up of a meshwork of collagen, elastin and smooth muscle. The endopelvic fascia serves two important purposes: first, to support the pelvic viscera in a proper orientation. In a standing female, the bladder, upper 2/3rds of the vagina and rectum lie in the horizontal axis thus, the endopelvic fascia (Figure 12) serve as support (Figure 13). This mechanism is critical in preventing prolapse of organs through the urogenital levator hiatus. The mechanism by which this works to maintain organ position is that during times of intraabdominal pressure, a perpendicular force is exerted against the vagina and pelvic viscera. Simultaneously, the contracting levator ani plate elevates the pelvic floor pinning organs and entrapping them in a flapper valve mechanism preventing organ prolapse. It is this mechanism that we aim to re-establish during our surgical reconstruction. The second purpose of the endopelvic fascia is to envelope and support blood vessels, visceral nerves and lymphatics as they course through the pelvis. The first support axis, DeLancey's level I, represents the upper vertical axis, and is delineated by the cardinal-uterosacral ligament complex holding the pelvic viscera horizontally over the levator plate. The uterosacral ligament does not contain any of the major blood supply or ureters. This structure represents a complex of endopelvic fascia beginning on the sacrum at the lateral aspect of S2, 3 and 4 and extends to fuse with the vagina and the levator ani muscles below. Clinically, they cannot be seen or palpated unless tension is applied to their distal margins. Therein lies the problem with their identification and utilization in repair of significant uterine and vaginal vault prolapse where the attachment has been ruptured. Cullen Richardson et al

demonstrated that the pelvic connective tissue is more likely to be damaged by rupture than by stretching. Richardson and Say presented a paper in 1996 at the Society of Gynecological Surgeons on the laparoscopic use of the uterosacral ligaments in the repair of uterine and vaginal vault prolapse in 46 consecutive patients. The uterosacral ligaments were identified in these patients with no evidence of uterosacral ligament attenuation appreciated. We utilize the uterosacral ligaments in all our surgical repairs whether it is laparoscopic, vaginal or abdominal for our level one support. The uterosacral ligaments provide bilateral attachment of the upper end of the vagina and uterus to prevent prolapse downward through the urogenital hiatus. The advantage to using these ligaments is that it allows free mobility of the attached vagina laterally and superiorly, which is so essential in proper sexual function. These ligaments suspend the vagina to the level of the ischial spine.

The second support axis or DeLancey's level II is a horizontal axis from the ischial spine to the posterior aspect of the pubic bone. The paravaginal or lateral supports of the bladder, upper 2/3rds of the vagina, and rectum are derived from this axis. They are supported by the pubocervical fascia anteriorly, and the recto-vaginal septum posteriorly which are attached laterally to the arcus tendineus ligament or white line (Figure 14). These levels can be approached quite readily laparoscopically both repairing the paravaginal defects anteriorly, as well as the rectovaginal septum posteriorly.

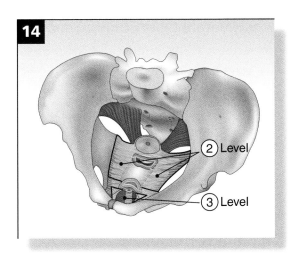

The third support axis, DeLancey's level III, is responsible for the almost vertical orientation of the urethra, lower third of the vagina, and anal canal. It travels perpendicularly to the urogenital triangles. The lower 1/3rd of the vagina passes through the levator hiatus, forming an almost 90° angle due to the puborectalis muscle posteriorly, and the pubocervical fascia hammock anteriorly. This allows for an almost 90° angle for the urethra to descend through and contributes greatly to the continence mechanism (Figure 15). Posterior level III defects are best handled vaginally and are extremely difficult to accomplish laparoscopically, although not impossible.

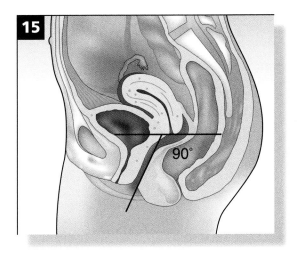

SURGICAL TECHNIQUE BY WAY OF LAPAROSCOPIC VAGINAL VAULT SUSPENSION

The patient is placed in the low semi-lithotomy position allowing laparoscopic instruments to be rotated 360° around the abdomen. Kendal boots and allen stirrups are used exclusively for patient's safety. Examination under anesthesia identifies all site-specific defects that need to be addressed. A low transverse defect, when noted on the perineal body of the recto-vaginal septal area, would be repaired first (Figure 16). The dissection of the rectovaginal septum free from the vaginal epithelium to the vaginal apex, allows for decreased work performed on the laparoscopic side to identify the rectovaginal septum. In the case of poor rectovaginal septal fascia, cadaveric fascia can be substituted and attached to the perineal body and the levator muscles laterally and the vaginal mucosa closed. When performing the laparoscopic posterior dissection we can then attach the high defect to the uterosacral ligament to complete the posterior repair. A three-way Foley catheter is placed into the bladder for drainage. We begin by making a vertical incision within the umbilicus and introducing a 10-12-mm optiview type of trocar which allows us to identify and count the layers entering into the abdominal cavity under direct visualization similar to open laparoscopy. Prior to making each incision, they are injected with 1% lidocaine with epinephrine. The abdomen is insufflated to a level of 15 mmHg of pressure with a humidified heated CO_2 insufflator. A series of three suprapubic ports are placed, one just in a suprapubic hairline area (5 mm), the other two just lateral to transversalis fascia and about the level of McBurney's point (1-12 mm and 1-5 mm) (Figure 17). The patient is then placed in a steep Trendelenburg position. A thorough bowel prep is used on all patients, thus, debulking the bowel for better

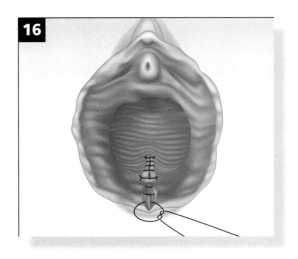

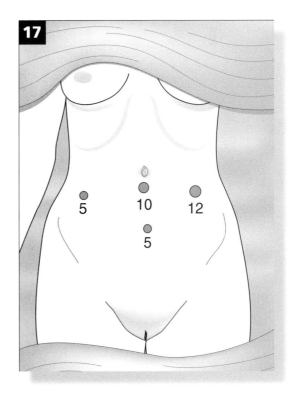

visualization and preparing for possible bowel injury. Importantly, nitrous oxide should not be used because it dilates/inflates the bowel. In a vaginal vault suspension, the first step should be to identify the ureters bilaterally, as in any surgical case. The vaginal vault is exposed and approximated by using either a vaginal blunt manipulator or an EEA rectal sizer. Identification of the uterosacral ligaments is accomplished by locating the ureter and making a releasing incision with the laparoscopic scissors or the harmonic scalpel just underneath the ureter and extending down the line of the ureter into the deep pelvis (Figure 18).

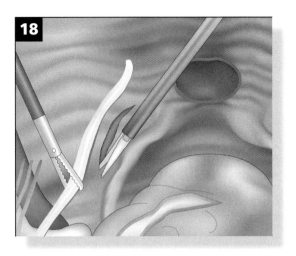

Palpation of the anatomy vaginally reveals where the ischial spine is found in relation to the ureter and will help locate the ureterosacral ligaments. A semi-traumatic grasper can be utilized to grab the uterosacral ligament structures including the peritoneal wall as well as all the tissue dissected free from the ureter downward towards the ischial spine area. The uterosacral ligament is then elevated towards the anterior abdominal wall and, with another instrument, you can actually palpate and pluck the tensed uterosacral ligaments (Figure 19). If this tissue stretches, you have not identified the ligament appropriately, and should continue to grasp the tissue until finding the true ligament. In my experience of performing well over 300 cases of vault suspension, the uterosacral ligaments were found in every patient, except one who had a

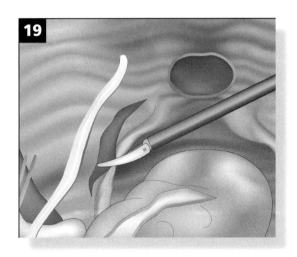

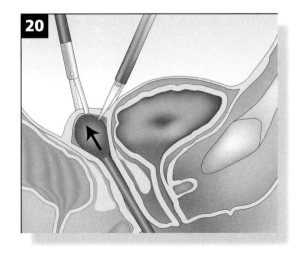

radical hysterectomy. Next, the bladder should be mobilized off the vagina. A three-way Foley catheter is then filled with 60–200 cc of saline expanding the bladder and noting the location of the vesical peritoneal fold. The bladder is mobilized all the way down to the pillars on either side exposing the pubocervical fascia at this level (Figure 20).

Attention is then directed posterior to the vagina where the peritoneum is entered and dissection is conducted to identify the rectovaginal septum (Figure 21). This layer should be avascular and, therefore, should separate fairly easily. The dissection is carried out laterally until you reach the levator muscles. Once again, it is often helpful to perform a vaginal or rectal exam at this time to identify the ischial spine as well as any particular site-specific defects that may exist. Once the dissection is completed and identification of a site-specific defect is identified, grab the actual rectovaginal septum and reapproximate it back to its normal support area. While holding it in the correct position, again perform a rectovaginal exam and identify whether this corrects the defect. With this accomplished, we repair the rectovaginal septal defects. We place interrupted stitches from the arcus tendineus ligament to the rectovaginal septum

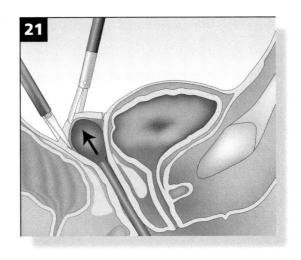

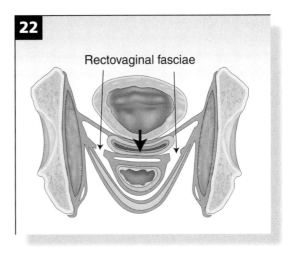

Rectovaginal fasciae

building the rectovaginal septum back to the ischial spine (Figure 22).

This needs to be performed bilaterally and can be tested again with a rectal exam. Once the rectovaginal septum is intact, a 2-0 ethibond is placed through the uterosacral ligament on the right side and then placed into the rectovaginal septum and then

Chapter 18

252 PELVIC FLOOR SURGERY . . . .

back to the uterosacral ligament and tied down securely (Figure 23).

We perform this again on the left side forming an individual attachment of the rectovaginal septum into the uterosacral ligament at the level of the ischial spine and the top of the uterosacral ligament. A stitch is then placed through the uterosacral ligament then back up anteriorly to the pubocervical fascia and then back posteriorly to the rectovaginal septum and then back to the uterosacral ligament (Figure 24).

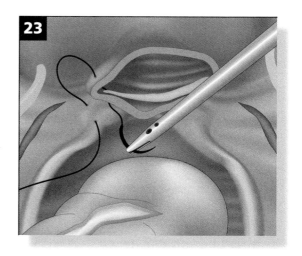

Before tying down the stitch a second stitch is placed on the left side through the uterosacral ligament, pubocervical fascia, rectovaginal septum, and back to the uterosacral ligament. These sutures are passed out through the opposite port on the right side once all throws have been made. This reduces the risk of entanglement while throwing the knots. At this time, a third stitch is placed through the pubocervical fascia and rectovaginal septum in the midline. The sutures are then tied down securely thus closing any of the enterocele defects (Figure 25). It is rare that any vaginal epithelium needs removing during the course of this technique and we find that most of the vaginal epithelium will remold itself into the exoskeleton of the vagina within 6 weeks. However, if concerns do exist, excess tissue may be excised from the

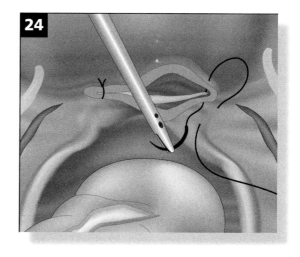

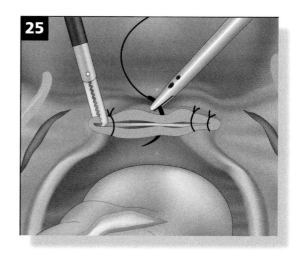

vaginal vault tissue prior to the previous suspension stitches, by using a glove in the vagina packed with a wet lap sponge to maintain the pneumoperitoneum and then removing the vaginal epithelium. The sutures are then tied securely closing the enterocele and creating the vault suspension.

A vaginal probe is then re-inserted to check if it can be pushed through the vaginal apex. If there are any further defects, sequential stitches are placed to gain the proper support. Never in the procedure are the uterosacral ligaments to be plicated across the midline. We feel that plicating the uterosacral ligaments will close down the cul-de-sac and will create an increased risk of problems in the future. These include a risk of the vaginal vault being torn down by the propulsion of bowel contents peristalsing and ramming into the suture anastomosis putting undue excess pressure on the vault. The cul-de-sac is designed to fill with stool and any compromise of this space will either cause pain, increased constipation, or increased risk of failure from the peristalsis pushing against the repair. Once the vault suspension is complete, sterile irrigation is performed. An underwater examination or decreasing the air pressure to approximately 6 mmHg, should identify any bleeders. Cystoscopy is usually performed at this point to ensure that ureters have not been com-

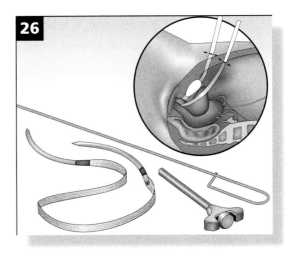

promised and that there have been no subsequent stitches placed into the bladder. At this time, if there are any paravaginal defects, an incision is then made in the peritoneum and the space of Retzius is opened and direct visualization of the ischial spine and the entire arcus tendineus ligament and pubocervical fascia defects are identified and repaired directly utilizing a 2-0 ethibond with interrupted stitches as described in the previous chapter. A retropubic urethropexy, TVT™ (Gynecare-Johnson & Johnson Inc., Somerville, NJ) (Figure 26) or other incontinence procedure of choice, can be accomplished as well if needed. The large ports are then closed with a 0 vicryl placed through the abdominal cavity utilizing a Carter Thompson needle-nosed grasper to pass the suture through the fascia, thus closing the port entry.

If the uterus is intended to remain in situ, this entire procedure is performed with interrupted stitches from the uterosacral ligament into the cervical ring at the level of attachment where uterosacral ligaments originate from the cervix (Figure 27). This would be accomplished bilaterally with sequential interrupted stitches into this high cervical ring area. A bladder flap is then developed and the bladder mobilized off the cervix and the vaginal area down to the level of the bladder pillars. The pubocervical fascia is identified and stitches placed through the pubocervical fascia and then reattached back into the cervical ring at the level of the transverse defect area (Figure 28). These are all tied off and secured. Any posterior repair of defects is performed laparoscopically as described in the complete vault prolapse section. Postoperatively, patients are sent to recovery with a Foley catheter in place and given analgesia by way of a PCA and then oral analgesia once a diet is tolerated. The patient's Foley catheter is usually removed on postoperative day 1 with a bladder trial. The bladder is filled with a known quantity of fluid, between 200–400 cc until the patient must void. The catheter is removed and the patient asked to walk to the bathroom to void. Knowing the volume of urine infused, we can measure the amount voided, and

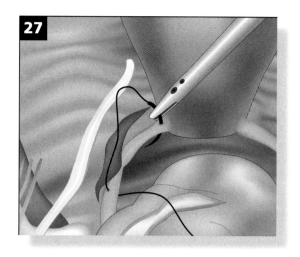

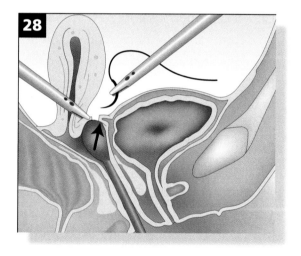

by simple subtraction, know the post-void residual urine. Once over 50% of the volume is voided, the catheter is left out. The majority of patients are discharged on day 0 or day 1. They are seen at follow-up 2 and 6 weeks postop and are sent home with pain meds, 3 days of a prophylactic antibiotic, and pyridium.

SUGGESTED READING:

Richardson AC, Lyon JB, Williams NL. A new look at pelvic relaxation. Am J Obstet Gynecol 1976;126:568

DeLancey JO. Anatomical aspects of vaginal aversion after hysterectomy. Am J Obstet Gynecol 1992;166:1717

Richardson AC. Transabdominal Paravaginal Repair. In Nichols DH; Gynecologic and Obstetrical Surgery. St. Louis, Moseby Yearbook Inc.1992:465-71

Youngblood JP. Paravaginal repair for cystourethrocele. Clin Obstet Gynecol 1993;36:960

Burgless B, Rubin IC. A study of supportive structures of the uterus by levator myelography. Surg Gynecol Obstet 1953;97:677

Richardson AC. The Rectovaginal Septum Revisited; Its Relationship to Rectocele and Its Importance in Rectocele Repair. Clinical Obstetrics and Gynecology. J B Lippincott Co. 1983;36(4):976-83

Uhlenhuth E, Nolley GW. Vaginal fascia: A myth? Obstet Gynecol 1957;10:349-58

Uhlenhuth E, Wolf WM, Smith EM, Middleton EB. The rectogenital septum. Surg Gynecol Obstet 1948;86:148-163

Goff BM. Histologic study of the paravaginal fascia in a nullipara. Surg Gynecol Obstet 1931;52:32-42

Richardson AC, Edmunds BP, Williams NL. Treatment of stress urinary incontinence due to paravaginal fascial defect. Obstet Gynecol 1981;57:357-63

Nichols DM. A correlative investigation of the human rectovaginal septum. Anatom Rec 1969;163:443-452

Krantz KE. The gross and microscopic anatomy of the human vagina. NY Acad Sci Ann 1959;83:89-104

Richardson DA, Bent AE, Ostragard DR. The effect of uterovaginal prolapse on urethrovesical pressure dynamics. Am J Obstet Gynecol 1983;146:901

Bergman A, Coonings PP, Bolard CA. Primary stress urinary incontinence and pelvic relaxation: prospective randomized comparison of three different operations. Am J Obstet Gynecol 1989;161:97

Frances WJA, Jeffcote TNA. Dyspareunia following vaginal operations. Br J Obstet Gynecol 1961;68:1

DeLancey, et al. Stress incontinence in cystoceles. J Urol 1991;145:1211

Haase P, Skibsted L. Influence of operations for stress incontinence and/or genital descensus on sexual life. Obstet Gynecol Scand 1988;67:659

Maser GA. Transabdominal repair of cystocele and 20 year experience compared with the traditional vaginal approach. Am J Obstet Gynecol 1978;131:203

VanGeelen JM, et al. The clinical and urodynamic effects of anterior vaginal repair and Burch colposuspension. Am J Obstet Gynecol 1988;159:137

Rogers B, Restsky S. The Evaluation of Urinary Incontinence. CIBA Series 1995

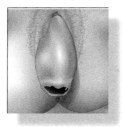

LAPAROSCOPIC PRESACRAL NEURECTOMY

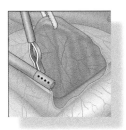

Ceana Nezhat, M.D.

In 1899, Jaboulay first described presacral neurectomy as the severance of sacral sympathetic afferent fibers using a posterior extraperitoneal approach. In the same year, Ruggi described resections of the utero-ovarian plexus. Leriche advocated periarterial sympathectomy of the internal iliac arteries. Perhaps the most fervent advocate of presacral neurectomy was Cotte, who in 1937 reported excellent results (98% success rate) after transection of the superior hypogastric plexus in 1500 patients. He emphasized that the only nerve tissue that should be resected is that within the interiliac triangle, and that resection of all nerve elements in the triangle is essential. Recent advances in endoscopic surgery have allowed surgeons to perform the technique via laparoscopy.

Twenty to twenty-five per cent of patients with central dysmenorrhea fail to respond to medical management and presacral neurectomy continues to be a useful alternative for these women. Presacral neurectomy is indicated in women who have disabling midline dysmenorrhea and pelvic pain, who have not responded to medication. It has been proven effective in the treatment of pelvic pain in women with endometriosis. Approximately 50-75% of patients will have pain relief. The procedure has also been as successful as laparotomy, with an apparently lower rate of postoperative morbidity. However, careful patient selection is a prerequisite to presacral neurectomy. The procedure should be done on women with deep, central pelvic pain that has been unresponsive to medical management.

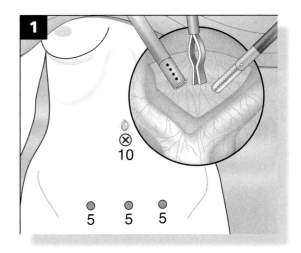

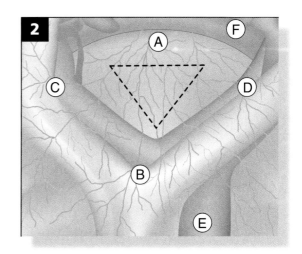

INSTRUMENTATION

An operating laser laparoscope is inserted through a 10-mm trocar placed through an umbilical incision. Two or three suprapubic 5-mm cannulas are inserted at about 5 cm mid-suprapubic and 7 cm left and right side for introduction of bipolar electrode, suction irrigator, and grasping forceps, respectively (Figure 1).

TECHNIQUE

The patient is placed in the steep Trendelenburg position and tilted slightly to the left. Identification of the aortic bifurcation, the common iliac arteries and veins, the ureters, and the sacral promontory, defined as the Triangle of Côte, is completed (Figure 2).

A Sacral promontory

B Bifurcation of the aorta

C Left common iliac vessels

D Right common iliac vessels

E Inferior vena cava

F Hollow of the sacrum

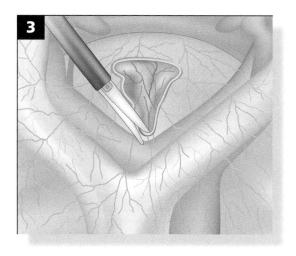

The peritoneum overlying the promontory is elevated with grasping forceps, and a small opening is made with the CO_2 laser or scissors (or any other cutting modality). The suction irrigator is inserted through this opening and the peritoneum is elevated by hydrodissection. The peritoneum is incised horizontally and vertically and the opening is extended cephalad to the aortic bifurcation (Figure 3). Bleeding from the peritoneal vessels is controlled with the bipolar electrocoagulator. Retroperitoneal lymphatic and fatty tissue is removed before the hypogastric plexus is reached. Hemostasis is obtained with bipolar electrocoagulation. The presacral tissue can now be identified.

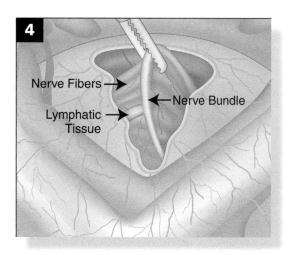

The nerve plexus is grasped with an atraumatic forceps (Figure 4), and using blunt and sharp dissection, the nerve fibers are skeletonized, desiccated, and excised. All the nerves that lie within the boundaries of the interiliac triangle are removed, including any fibers

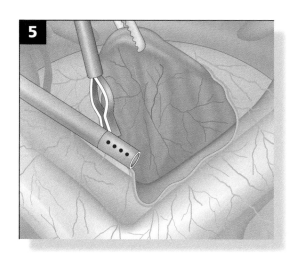

entering the area from under the common iliac arteries and over the left common iliac vein (Figures 4 and 5). The retroperitoneal space is irrigated, and bleeding points are coagulated. Sutures are not required to approximate the posterior peritoneum (Figure 6). Interceed (Johnson & Johnson Medical, Sommerville, NJ) can be applied over the incised area (Figure 7). The area heals completely on follow-up, and it is covered by the peritoneum. Excised tissue is sent for histologic confirmation.

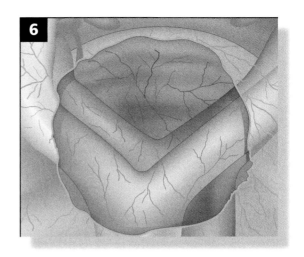

COMPLICATIONS

The most important intraoperative complication of presacral neurectomy is bleeding. An injury to the common iliac vein or vena cava can require an immediate laparotomy. Other complications of presacral neurectomy that have been reported are:

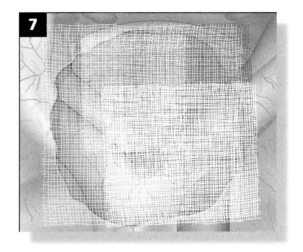

- Bleeding from midsacral to presacral vessels

- Ureteral injury

- Poor bladder emptying

- Urinary urgency

- Persistent constipation

- Painless labor

- Intermittent ileal obstruction due to adhesions

- Vaginal dryness

- Chylous ascites

Suggested Reading:

Jaboulay M. Le traitement e la navralgie pelvienne par a paralysie du sympathetique sacre. Lyon Med 1899;90:102

Ruggi G. Della sympathectamia al collo ed ale adome. Policinico 1899;1:193

Leriche R. Resultant eloigne cinq ans at deni d'une sympathectomie de deux ateres hypogastriques pour dysmenorrhee douloureuse. Lyon Ch 1927;24:360

Cotte MG. Sur le traitement des dysmenorrhees rebelles par la sympathectomie hypogastrique periaterielle ou la section du neuf presacre. Lyon Med 1925;135:153

Polan ML, DeCherney A. Presacral neurectomy for pelvic pain in infertility. Fertil Steril 1980;34:557

Fliegner JR, Umstac MP. Presacral neurectomy: A reappraisal. Aust N Z J Obstet Gynaecol 1991;31:76-80

Nezhat CH, Seidman D, Nezhat F, Nezhat C. Long-term outcome of laparoscopic presacral neurectomy for the treatment of central pelvic pain attributed to endometriosis. Obstet Gynecol 1998;91(5 pt 1):701-704

Metzger DA, Montanino-Olivia M, Davis GD, Redwine DB. Efficacy of presacral neurectomy for the relief of midline pelvic pain. J Am Assoc Gynecol Laparos 1991;1(4 pt 2):S22

Nezhat C, Siegler AM, Nezhat F, Nezhat CH, Seidman D, Luciano AA. Operative Gynecologic Laparoscopy: Principles and Techniques. 2nd ed. New York: McGraw Hill, 2000

Perez JJ. Laparoscopic presacral neurectomy. J Reprod Med 1990;35:625-30

Feste JR, Wilson EE, Presacral neurectomy. In: Adamson G, Martin DC, eds. Endoscopic management of gynecologic disease. Philadelphia: Lippincott-Raven Publishers, 1996:227

Nezhat C, Berger G, Nezhat F, Buttram V, Nezhat CH. Endometriosis: advanced management and surgical techniques. New York: Springer-Veralg, 1995

LAPAROSCOPY IN PEDIATRIC PATIENTS

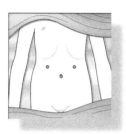

Claire Templeman, M.D.

INTRODUCTION

In adults, laparoscopy is an established alternative to open surgery. However, concerns regarding proven benefit and adequate equipment have, until recently, limited its use in pediatric patients. The advent of microendoscopic equipment has made pediatric endoscopy more practical but there are some important technical differences between it and adult laparoscopy and they will be the focus of this chapter.

INDICATIONS

There is now considerable experience with laparoscopy for appendectomy, cholecystectomy, exploration of non-palpable testis and trauma in children. Some relevant indications for gynecologists who treat young children and adolescents are listed below. Specific techniques for the management of ovarian masses and uterovaginal anomalies are detailed in Chapters 13 and 21, respectively.

GYNECOLOGICAL INDICATIONS FOR LAPAROSCOPY IN THE PEDIATRIC AND ADOLESCENT POPULATION

NEONATAL
- COMPLEX, ENLARGING OR SYMPTOMATIC OVARIAN MASS
- ABDOMINAL MASS OF UNCERTAIN ORIGIN

NEONATAL
- PERSISTENT OVARIAN CYST OR MASS
- PARATUBAL CYST
- OVARIAN TORSION
- OOPHOROPEXY

ADOLESCENT
- PERSISTENT OVARIAN CYST OR MASS
- OVARIAN TORSION
- PARATUBAL CYST
- SUSPECTED ENDOMETRIOSIS
- UTEROVAGINAL ANOMALIES
- OOPHOROPEXY
- PELVIC INFLAMMATORY DISEASE

ANESTHESIA

INSUFFLATION/WARMING/HUMIDIFYING CONSIDERATIONS

When contemplating laparoscopy in a pediatric patient, an experienced anesthetic team is essential. Insufflation of the abdomen with carbon dioxide gas (CO_2) increases intraabdominal and intrathoracic pressure with the potential for ventilation and perfusion abnormalities. Correct insufflation pressure is critical in infants because they rely on diaphragmatic excursion for adequate ventilation. Over insufflation may result in restricted diaphragmatic movement.

It has been demonstrated in animal models that intraabdominal pressures maintained between 0-10 mm Hg do not deleteriously affect ventilation or gas exchange. An insufflation pressure of 8 mmHg with a flow rate of 0.5 L/min is appropriate for neonates or infants with pressures of 10-12 mmHg appropriate for older children. Carbon dioxide insufflation may also result in hypercapnia and metabolic acidosis if the end tidal CO_2 and oxygen saturation are not monitored closely. A minute ventilatory rate that maintains the end tidal CO_2 in the range 30-45 mmHg is required and in neonatal patients undergoing laparoscopy this has been found to be 30%-40% more than that required at laparotomy (see Chapter 4). The use of humidified, heated gas (37°C) is advisable since it has also been shown to decrease the risk of hypothermia that may occur in pediatric patients undergoing laparoscopy. Intravenous fluids such as lactated Ringers solution should be administered to maintain urine output at 1 mL/kg/hour.

PATIENT POSITIONING

In pediatric patients, the supine position is used almost exclusively since there is no need to use instruments in the uterus (Figure 1). In older girls, where access to the vagina is required, proper use of padded stirrups that align the ipsilateral heel with the contralateral hip and shoulder are important. Stirrups that place the hips in hyperflexion are occasionally used in children because they give maximum access to the perineum, however, they place the patient at risk for femoral nerve damage, particularly if the case is lengthy.

Regardless of age, tucking the child's arms by their side also allows maximum flexibility while operating.

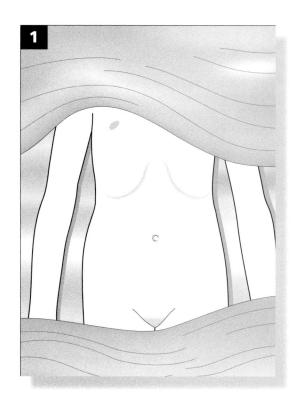

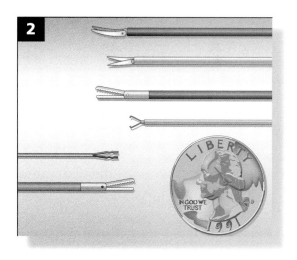

INSTRUMENTATION

There is now a range of instrumentation available that provides adequate optics for work in neonatal and pediatric patients including 3-5 mm trocars for 2.7-4.5 mm laparoscopes and instruments (Figure 2). It has been shown that the use of these smaller caliber instruments in pediatric patients is associated with greater postoperative comfort. Traditional 10 mm laparoscopes can be used in adolescents if required, but new optics and cameras allow 5 mm laparoscopes to be used.

Trocars are available as reusable metal, disposable plastic and newer radially expanding models. The choice of trocar is important since leakage from around these sites and compensatory rapid CO_2 insufflation into the abdomen may contribute to hypothermia, especially in neonates. A recent report suggests that the radially expanding trocars Inner-Dyne Medical™ (Sunnyvale, CA) may be the most effective in very young patients because they have a lower incidence of slippage from the abdominal wall (Figures 3 and 4).

Laparoscopes ranging from 2.7 to 10 mm in diameter with angles from 0° to 45° degrees allow the surgeon a wide choice of views depending upon the size of the patient. The newest cameras offer an autorotation feature maintaining an upright image regardless of

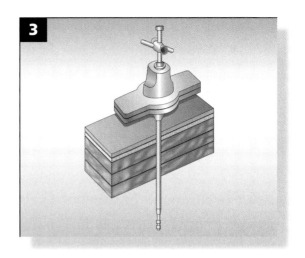

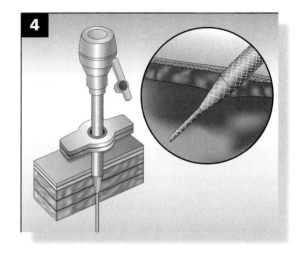

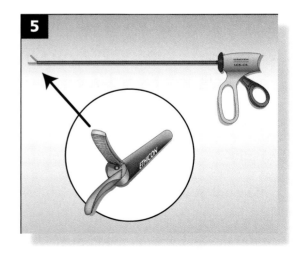

the angle of the camera. All these features are helpful when large masses or adhesions obscure the view within the abdomens of small infants.

In addition to conventional energy sources such as monopolar and bipolar cautery, the ultrasonically activated, harmonic scalpel can be a useful tool in pediatric laparoscopy (Figure 5). It uses mechanical energy, generated by a vibrating crystal in the hand piece, to cut and coagulate without the transmission of energy to structures out of immediate view. This instrument has been used to coagulate gonadal and bowel vessels in very small infants including neonates. The reported benefit of this dual action instrument in pediatric patients is a decrease in operating time resulting in a shorter time under anesthesia.

PORT PLACEMENT AND ENTRANCE INTO THE ABDOMEN

Surgical complications in pediatric laparoscopy are often related to the introduction of the Veress needle or the first trocar. In a large review of 5400 laparoscopic surgeries performed in patients ranging in age from 0 to 20 years, the significant predictors of

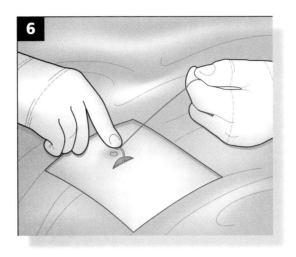

complications were operator experience and the method used to create a pneumoperitoneum. Specifically, the Veress needle was associated with a 2.6% major complication rate (viscus or major blood vessel injury) compared with 1.2% for the open technique. This difference continued even in experienced operators (>100 laparoscopic cases). This finding has lead to the suggestion that the open technique is the method of choice for the creation of the pneumoperitoneum in pediatric patients, however, the Veress needle is used by some practitioners.

In neonates, the umbilical vessels may still be patent at the time of surgery, therefore, correct identification and ligation of these is essential before proceeding with abdominal entry (Figure 6). This can be performed following skin incision at the umbilical site with the use of small claw retractors to retract the skin and fine hemostat clamps to dissect the superficial tissue away until the umbilical vessels are identified, clamped, and suture ligated. Due to the intraabdominal location of the bladder, there is a reduced margin of safety in children compared with adolescents or adults. Preoperative emptying is, therefore, very important in avoiding secondary trocar injury, especially if suprapubic trocars are used.

Port placement on the abdomen will depend upon the operation contemplated and surgeon preference. However, in prepubertal patients with large ovarian masses, the placement of secondary trocars that are high, typically 2 fingers above the umbilicus and lateral to the inferior epigastric artery, may assist with access to the pathology (Figure 7).

The fascia of all ports ≥ 5 mm in diameter should be closed with sutures in pediatric patients since there is a reported 2.7% incidence of port site hernia through open incisions. This can be achieved with claw retractors at the

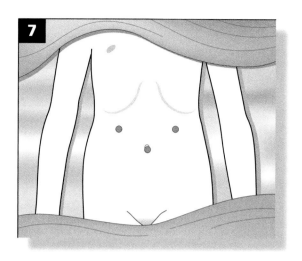

site of incision, identification of the fascia with kocher clamps and closure with an 0 Vicryl™ (Ethicon, Johnson & Johnson Inc, Somerville, NJ) suture on a UR5 needle.

OVARIAN MASSES

A young girl with a persistent or complex appearing ovarian mass presents a typical indication for surgery in the pediatric population and the likely ovarian pathology is dependent upon patient age. The techniques for removing ovarian masses including cystectomy, oophorectomy, and the use of an endobag are the same in children as adults and are described in the chapter on ovarian surgery. In neonates, ovarian cysts are usually functional as the result of maternal gonadotropin stimulation during the antenatal period. The indications for surgery, therefore, are complex, especially for enlarging or symptomatic masses where torsion is suspected or the diagnosis is in doubt. Since the incidence of ovarian malignancy in this age group approaches zero, laparoscopy is appropriate for surgeons experienced with neonatal surgery. In the prepubertal age group, approximately 11% of noninflammatory ovarian masses requiring surgery are malignant. Therefore, careful investigation on an individual basis is essential. If preoperative assessment suggests malignancy, laparotomy and staging is indicated unless the surgeon is proficient with laparoscopic oncologic surgery.

In conclusion, laparoscopy, when performed by experienced practitioners is a safe and practical approach to the surgical management of a variety of gynecological problems in children.

SUGGESTED READING:

Rubin SZ, Davis GM, Sehgal Y, Kaminski MJ. Does laparoscopy adversely affect gas exchange and pulmonary mechanics in the newborn? An experimental study. J Laparoendo Surg 1996;6(Suppl 1):S69-73

Fujimoto T, Segawa O, Lane GJ, et al. Laparoscopic surgery in newborn infants. Surg Endosc 1999;13:773-7

Fujimoto T, Segawa O, Kobayashi H, Lane G, Miyano T. Endosurgery in children: Prospects and problems - An analysis of 88 cases. Ped Endosurg Innov Tech 1997;1(3):189-95

Matsuda T, Ogura K, Uchida J, et al. Smaller ports result in a shorter convalescence after laparoscopic varicocelectomy. J Urol 1995;153:1175-7

Esposito C, Ascione G, Garipoli V, et al. Complications of pediatric laparoscopic surgery. Surg Endo 1997;11(6):655-7

Peters CA. Complications in pediatric urological laparoscopy: results of a survey. J Urol 1996;155(3):1070-3

Ure BM, Bax NM, van der Zee DC. Laparoscopy in infants and children: A prospective study on feasibility and the impact of routine surgery. J Ped Surg 2000; 35(8):1170-3

Templeman CL, Reynolds AJ, Hertweck SP, Nagaraj H. The laparoscopic management of neonatal ovarian cysts. J Am Assoc Gyn Laparosc 2000;7:401-404

Templeman CL, Fallat M, Blinchevsky A, Hertweck SP. Noninflammatory ovarian masses in girls and young women. Obstet Gynecol 2000; 96:229-223

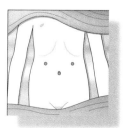

ENDOSCOPIC DIAGNOSIS AND CORRECTION OF MALFORMATIONS OF FEMALE GENITALIA

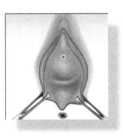

Leila V. Adamyan, M.D.

Ekaterina L. Iarotskaia, M.D

Congenital malformations of female genitalia comprise about 4% of all congenital anomalies. These malformations are associated with extragenital anomalies in about 74% of cases manifesting as skin marks and skeletal defects, as well as breast, heart, renal and digestive system anomalies. Diagnosis of malformations of the uterus, and/or vagina present significant difficulties that may confuse the character of the disease and cause incorrect, and sometimes, unwarranted or aggressive radical surgery in 24–34% of patients. The high rate of diagnostic mistakes may be due to absence of a universal classification of genital malformations. Suggested classifications do not reflect all clinical–anatomic features of malformations, which are essential for an optimal treatment strategy that will be beneficial for the patient's health, reproductive and sexual function, and general quality of life.

Chapter 21

272 | ENDOSCOPIC DIAGNOSIS AND CORRECTION OF MALFORMATIONS OF FEMALE GENITALIA ....

Presently, invasive diagnostic tools (ultrasonography, hysterosalpingography, magnetic resonance imaging and spiral computer tomography) together with endoscopic techniques may permit the determination of the real character of a malformation of the uterus and/or vagina, and reveal concomitant extragenital anomalies of the urinary and digestive systems. The correct diagnosis will allow the rational management of anomalies. Based on the results of clinical examination and treatment of 855 patients, using modern imaging techniques, hysteroscopy and laparoscopy, L.V. Adamyan and co-authors (1998) introduced a classification of genital malformations and outlined a paradigm of examination, surgical treatment and rehabilitation of patients with malformations. We suggest the original methods of reconstructive plastic surgery using an endoscopic approach, which we consider the methods of choice for this complicated pathology

CLASSIFICATION OF MALFORMATIONS OF UTERUS AND/OR VAGINA

CLASS I: VAGINAL APLASIA

1. Complete aplasia of vagina and uterus

a) one uterine myometrial rudiment (located laterally or in the center of the small pelvis)

b) two myometrial rudiments

c) absence of uterine rudiments

In this malformation:

- Uterine tubes are not connected with uterine rudiments.

- Uterine rudiments have no functional endometrium and no endometrial cavity

- Adnexa are located high on the lateral pelvic walls

2. Complete aplasia of vagina and functional rudimentary uterus

a) one or two functional uterine rudiments

b) functional rudimentary uterus with aplasia of the cervix

c) functional rudimentary uterus with aplasia of the cervical canal

- Uterine tubes are connected with rudimentary uterus

- The layers of uterine wall are differentiated

- In all variants hemato- or pyometra, chronic endo- and perimetritis, hemato- or pyosalpinx may be observed

3. Functional uterus and partial aplasia of vagina

a) aplasia of upper 1/3;
   a1) aplasia of upper 2/3

b) aplasia of middle 1/3 ;
   b1) aplasia of middle part of vagina comprising 2/3 of its length

c) aplasia of lower 1/3;
   c1) aplasia of lower 2/3 of vaginal length

- In a) and a1) hemato- and/or pyometra, hemato- and/or pyosalpinx

- In b) and b1) hemato- and/or pyocolpos

- In c) and c1) hemato- and/or pyocolpos

CLASS II: UNICORNUATE UTERUS

1. Unicornuate uterus with rudimentary horn communicating with the cavity of the main horn

2. Unicornuate uterus with noncommunicating rudimentary horn

- In both variants endometrium of the rudimentary horn may be functional or nonfunctional

3. Rudimentary horn without cavity

4. Absence of rudimentary horn

CLASS III: UTERUS AND VAGINA DUPLEX

1. Uterus and vagina duplex without obstruction to menstrual outflow

2. Uterus and vagina duplex without partial aplasia of one vagina

a) aplasia of upper 1/3;
   a1) aplasia of upper 2/3

b) aplasia of middle 1/3;
   b1) aplasia of middle part of vagina comprising 2/3of its length

c) aplasia of lower 1/3;
   c1) aplasia of lower 2/3 of vaginal length

- In a) and a1) hemato- and/or pyometra, hemato- and/or pyosalpinx

- In b) and b1) hemato- and/or pyocolpos

- In c) and c1) hemato- and/or pyocolpos, fistula in the vagina with partial aplasia

3. Uterus and vagina duplex with nonfunctional single uterus

CLASS IV: BICORNUATE UTERUS

1. Arcuate form
2. Incompletely bicornuate form
3. Complete bicornuate form

CLASS V: INTRAUTERINE SEPTUM

1. Complete intrauterine septum (reaching internal cervical os)

2. Incomplete intrauterine septum

- The septum may be thin or wide-based, one hemicavity may be longer than other

CLASS VI: MALFORMATIONS OF UTERINE TUBES AND OVARIES

1. Unilateral aplasia of adnexa

Chapter 21

274 | ENDOSCOPIC DIAGNOSIS AND CORRECTION OF MALFORMATIONS OF FEMALE GENITALIA ....

2. Aplasia of one or both uterine tubes

3. Accessory uterine tubes

4. Aplasia of ovaries

5. Hypoplasia of ovaries

6. Accessory ovaries

- These malformations may be isolated or associated with other uterine and/or vaginal malformations

CLASS VII: RARE FORMS OF GENITAL MALFORMATIONS

1. Genitourinary malformations: extrophy of the urinary bladder

2. Genitorectal malformations: recto-introital fistula associated with aplasia of uterus and vagina; recto-introital fistula associated with unicornuate uterus and functional rudimentary uterus

- These malformations may be isolated or associated with other uterine and/or vaginal malformations

CLASS I: APLASIA OF VAGINA

1.1. COMPLETE APLASIA OF VAGINA AND UTERUS

Aplasia of the vagina and uterus (Mayer-Rokitansky-Kuster-Hauser syndrome) is a malformation characterized by congenital absence of the uterus (usually presented by two muscular

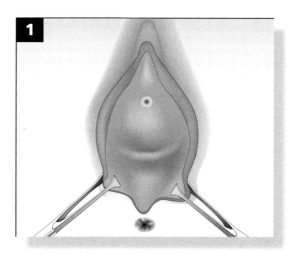

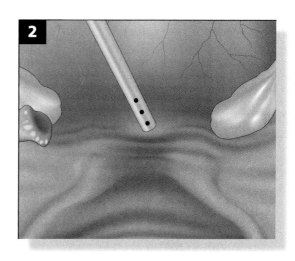

rudiments, but other variants can also be encountered: asymmetric muscular mounds, complete absence of rudiments, etc.), and vagina, normally functioning ovaries, female phenotype and karyotype (46,XX), and is often accompanied by other congenital anomalies (skeletal, urinary, digestive) (Figures 1-4). Figure 2 presents a laparoscopic view of aplasia of uterus and vagina: absence of uterine rudiments. Laparoscopic view of aplasia of uterus and vagina with symmetric uterine rudiments is shown on Figure 3, and a laparoscopic view of aplasia of uterus and vagina with asymmetric uterine rudiments is presented on Figure 4.

The main clinical features of uterine and vaginal aplasia are the absence of menstruation and inability to have vaginal sexual intercourse. The uterine rudiments may be affected by adenomyosis, causing pelvic pain.

The diagnosis is based on the patient's complaints, physical examination, ultrasonographic data and other methods of visualization (MRI, SCT), which are necessary to determine if associated malformations (especially of the urinary system which occur in almost 40% of cases) are present.

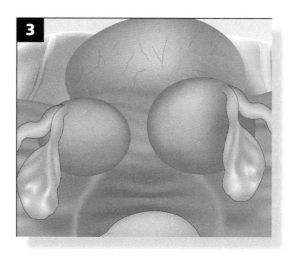

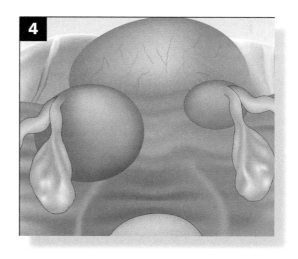

Surgical correction, although not absolutely necessary, is required if normal sexual activity is anticipated. Gynecologists have long discussed the ethics involved in creating an artificial vagina. Most surgeons are in agreement that safe and reliable methods are needed to achieve the goal of a functional vagina. Different methods of colpoelongation appear to be minimally invasive, but require considerable time and are not always effective. Another approach to correct this mal-

formation is based on techniques to create a canal between the urinary bladder and rectum. In this case, subsequent tamponade and dilatation with various prosthetic appliances is required. Another possibility is creating a lining with skin flaps or segments of rectum, sigmoid, small intestine, or pelvic peritoneum. One-stage colpopoiesis from pelvic peritoneum has proved to be the most simple and at the same time the most safe and effective. This method supplies a better quality of neovagina with rapid epithelization and sufficient capacity and depth. In 1993 L.V. Adamyan introduced a method of colpopoiesis incorporating pelvic peritoneum using laparoscopy in all the main steps of the operation, confirming diagnosis, identification and opening of the peritoneum, and creation of a vaginal vault, which we consider to be a method of choice for correction of this anomaly.

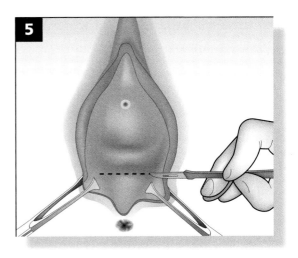

Surgical technique

Surgery is performed by a combined laparoscopic-perineal approach. The patient is placed in the lithotomy position with legs wide apart. Under general (endotracheal) anesthesia, diagnostic laparoscopy is carried out to specify the character of malformation and to evaluate the mobility of the peritoneum. The number and location of muscular rudiments, and their status are noted. Enlarged uterine rudiments, causing pelvic pain and possibly affected by adenomyosis, should be removed laparoscopically with subsequent restoration of peritoneum.

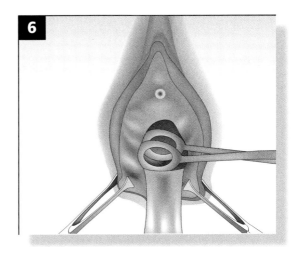

After laparoscopy, the perineal step is initiated: the skin is incised 3-3.5 cm transversally between the rectum and

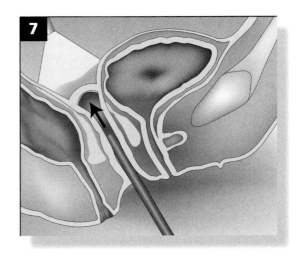

urinary bladder at the level of the lower border of the labia minora (Figure 5). By sharp and/or blunt dissection in a strictly horizontal direction along the urinary bladder, the canal is created (Figure 6). This step is the most difficult because of the high risk of possible injury to the bladder and rectum. Most difficulties occur in the case of atypical (low) location of the urethra and when scarring is present at the site of the potential introitus. Scarring may be caused by repeated courses of colpoelongation, attempts at sexual intercourse or perineal surgery, which may lead to formation of a false passage directed toward the rectum. The canal is formed up to the pelvic peritoneum. The most crucial step of the operation – identification of peritoneum – is performed using the laparoscope (Figure 7). The most mobile part of the peritoneum is between the bladder and the rectum and is often divided by the transverse fold between two muscular rudiments. It is identified, then marked with an atraumatic laparoscopic instrument (a manipulator or forceps) and is brought down into the created canal. The peritoneal fold is grasped in the canal by the forceps and transected either laparoscopically or from below (Figure 8). The edges of peritoneal incision are brought down and sutured to the edges

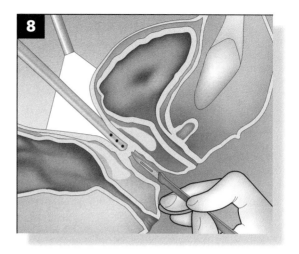

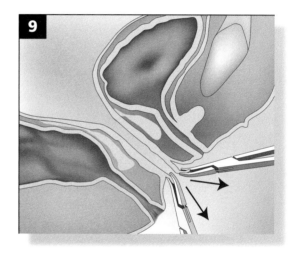

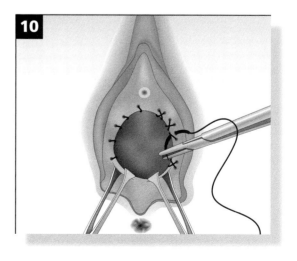

of the skin incision with separate vicryl stitches, forming the introitus (Figures 9 and 10). In case of previous scarring and excessive bleeding in the canal, fibrin glue made from the patient's blood may be applied for better attachment of the peritoneum to the canal walls. However, this is not available in the United States. A moist sponge or vaginal probe is then placed at the introitus of the neovagina, to re-establish the pneumoperitoneum.

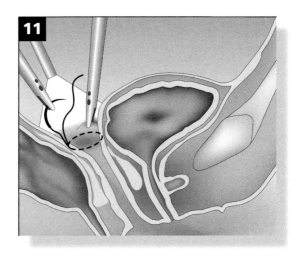

Formation of the neovaginal vault – the final step of the operation – is performed by laparoscopic placement of one purse-string or two semipurse-string sutures on a curved needle, incorporating the bladder peritoneum, muscular uterine rudiments, and peritoneum lining the pelvic sidewall and sigmoid colon (Figure 11). The suture is tied with an extracorporeal knot. In case there is too much tension in the tissues the vault can be formed by separate sutures, connecting the transverse peritoneal fold with muscular rudiments and peritoneum of the backside pelvic walls (Figure 12). When muscular rudiments are absent (for example, in patients with testicular feminization) and there is a shortage of peritoneum, the neovaginal vault can be formed using biologically compatible polymeric material, (e.g. copolymer of glycolid and lactid

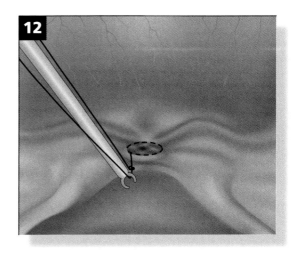

(vicryl mesh) or polyglycolic acid (dexon mesh). The mesh is sutured endoscopically to the anterior, posterior and lateral aspects of the pelvic end of the neovaginal tunnel to provide the barrier between the pelvic cavity and the neovagina.

Laparoscopically assisted colpopoiesis takes approximately 25–45 min, and the operation itself is almost bloodless. Antibiotics are introduced intraoperatively for prophylaxis. Subsequent anti-bacterial therapy for 24-36 hours is considered only if there is a high risk of infectious complications. A Foley catheter is placed into the bladder immediately after the operation to facilitate urination which may be difficult in the early postoperative period due to a displacement of the urethral orifice by tension of the anterior neo-vaginal wall. A gauze sponge moistened with an antiseptic solution and Vaseline is introduced into the neo-vagina for 1-2 days. The patients are allowed to sit and stand 5-6 hours after surgery. Gynecologic examination is performed on the 5-7th postoperative day to assess the reaction and patency of the tissues of the neovagina. The neovagina usually permits insertion of two fingers and its length varies from 11-12.5 cm. The patient is asked to wear a sterile glove and to insert her index finger lubricated with KY Jelly into the neovagina. This manipulation is necessary to acquaint the patient with her new anatomy, and for maintenance of the neovaginal caliber until she starts regular sexual activity, which is allowed 2-4 weeks after this procedure. Most patients do not feel any discomfort during coitus and appear to be satisfied with their sexual activity which significantly contributes to their psychological well-being.

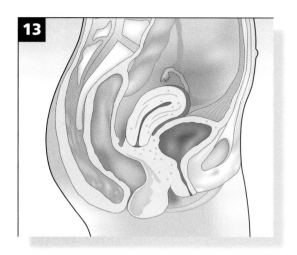

The main features of the neovagina (the ability to perform a vaginal examination and to permit intercourse) are assessed 3-4 months after the operation. On examination the border between the introitus and neovagina itself is absent; the vagina is about 11-12 cm long with sufficient caliber. The walls are moderately folded, producing some mucus. Morphologic and electron-microscopic examination of the neovaginal wall reveals that 3 months after colpopoiesis the neovaginal epithelium is similar to the stratified squamous epithelium of a normal vagina, most likely due to metaplasia.

1.2. APLASIA OF VAGINA IN CASE OF FUNCTIONAL UTERUS

Aplasia of the vagina can be complete or partial and associated with a functional normal or functional rudimen-

Chapter 21

280 | ENDOSCOPIC DIAGNOSIS AND CORRECTION OF MALFORMATIONS OF FEMALE GENITALIA ....

tary uterus (Figure 13). The main clinical features in this malformation are absence of menstruation, cyclic or permanent pelvic pain from menarche, and inability to have vaginal sexual intercourse.

Diagnosis is based on the patient's complaints, physical examination, ultrasonographic data and other methods of visualization (MRI, SCT). Diagnostic difficulties may lead to unjustified surgery (in 24-65 % of cases). In most of the patients hemato- and/or pyometra, chronic endometritis and perimetritis, hemato- and pyosalpinx and in patients with partial vaginal aplasia hemato- and/or pyocolpos, are found.

Surgical correction is necessary and should be undertaken as soon as the diagnosis is established. One should remember that this malformation usually manifests itself in adolescence and may result in a distortion of the reproductive organs' anatomy. Definitive surgery is essential for the further reproductive health of these patients.

METHODS OF
SURGICAL CORRECTION

The patients with partial vaginal aplasia and a normal functional uterus, accompanied by hematocolpos, need conventional vaginoplasty. Laparoscopy in this malformation is

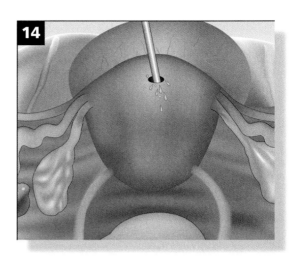

absolutely necessary to evaluate the status of the internal genitalia (the character of the malformation, damage caused by menstrual reflux) and for correction of pathology (pelvic irrigation, drainage of the hematosalpinx, adhesiolysis, endometriosis elimination, etc.).

In patients with complete aplasia of the vagina and a functional uterus, the first crucial aspect to be determined in order to choose the correct surgical modality, is absence or presence of a cervical canal. For this purpose, we have introduced a method of retrograde hysteroscopy (by laparoscopic approach) by perforating the uterine fundus (Figure 14). The correction, which may be attempted to preserve a functional rudimentary uterus in patients with cervical and vaginal aplasia, is the creation of a tunnel between the uterus and neovagina, which can be performed as follows:

Operative technique

- Transverse incision of perineal skin between the urethra and lower border of labia minora;

- Creation of a canal between the urinary bladder and rectum;

- Simultaneous laparoscopy, pelvic revison, final diagnosis;

- Laparoscopic grasping and opening of peritoneum of rectouterine pouch;

- Bringing down the peritoneal incision edges and suturing to the introital skin;

- Laparoscopic hysterotomy and retrograde hysteroscopy for identification of a site for further tunnel creation between the uterine cavity and neovagina;

- Canalization of the uterine wall towards the created tunnel;

- Fixation of the uterus at the tunnel, introduction of the dilator into the neocanal.

If such correction appears impossible or ineffective, resulting in atresia of the previously created tunnel, the method of choice is total laparoscopic hysterectomy and laparoscopically assisted colpopoiesis from pelvic peritoneum. Total laparoscopic extirpation of a functional uterus in case of cervical and vaginal aplasia is performed according to our technique of laparoscopic hysterectomy applied for other uterine pathology, and includes the following steps:

- Coagulation and transection of round ligaments with simultaneous dissection of the plica vesical-utero fold, downward bladder dissection and anterior dissection of uterine vessels;

- Fenestration of posterior leaves of broad ligaments and dissection to the uterosacral ligaments with their partial transection and simultaneous exposition of the uterine vessels;

- Ligation of ovarian ligaments and proximal uterine tubes;

- Suturing of ascendent uterine vessels;

- Transection of ovarian ligaments and uterine tubes (if technically advisable);

- Transection of uterine vessels and circular dissection of posterior aspect of the uterus from the pelvic fascia with transection of rudiments of cardinal and uterosacral ligaments. The specificity of this step of the operation is substantiated by abnormal development of the uterus (absence of cervix and normal cardinal and uterosacral ligaments).

Another peculiarity of this operation is the inability to use a uterine manipulator. Therefore, this requires the manipulation of the uterus with laparoscopic graspers introduced through secondary abdominal punctures. The uterus is removed from the abdominal cavity by electro-mechanical morcellation. Colpopoiesis is performed according to the technique described above, with particular care of the peritoneum, which can be damaged by hysterectomy, adhesiolysis, and removal of endometriosis and when forming the neovaginal vault. Average operating time is 1.5 hours with minimal blood loss. Average hospital stay is 4.5 days.

CLASS II: UNICORNUATE UTERUS

Unicornuate uterus is an anomaly caused by formation of only one para-mesonephric duct, whereas, the other has remained undeveloped. From an embryologic view, a unicornuate uterus is half of a normal uterus. The variants of the horn, or unicornuate uterus with a supplementary rudimentary horn may be encountered. Some-

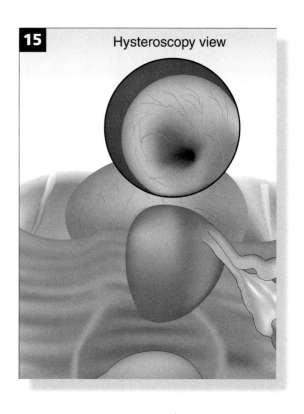

15 Hysteroscopy view

times the rudimentary horn is embedded in the wall of the main horn.

Unicornuate uterus without a supplementary horn usually does not cause any gynecologic or obstetric problems. On the contrary, the patients with a supplementary non-communicating (or obstructed) rudimentary horn with functioning endometrium complain of painful menses from menarche or of perimenstrual pain due to the formation of hematometra. One of the potential dangers in this malformation is the possibility of an ectopic pregnancy in the rudimentary horn, as well as a high rate (over 50%) of endometriosis. Thus, the removal of a rudimentary horn is substantiated by a range of indications.

Preliminary diagnosis is based on the patient's complaints, physical examination (pelvic mass), and information provided by imaging techniques – ultrasonography, MRI, SCT. Definite diagnosis, however, is possible only during laparoscopy and hysteroscopy (Figure 15), which allows the differentiation of four variants of this malformation: 1) unicornuate uterus with supplementary rudimentary horn communicating with principal horn; 2) unicornuate uterus with supplementary non-communicating horn (sometimes embedded in the wall of the main uterine horn); 3) unicornuate uterus with supplementary horn without endometrial cavity; 4) unicornuate uterus without supplementary rudimentary horn

SURGICAL CORRECTION

Laparoscopic removal of the rudimentary horn is performed according to the hysterectomy technique.

- The horn is grasped, and round ligament, proximal tube, and ovarian ligament are coagulated and transected;

- Broad ligaments and utero vesical-fold are dissected up to the level of junction between the principal and rudimentary horn, exposing uterine vessels supplying rudimentary horn;

- Securing of the vessels by extracorporeal suturing or bipolar coagulation (as the diameter of vessels is rather small);

- Transection of the rudimentary horn by monopolar cutter or ultrasonic scalpel;

- Endosutures are placed at the uterine wound;

- Rudimentary horn is removed from the abdominal cavity by electric morcellation or through a colpotomy.

Our technique of resection of the rudimentary horn when incorporated in the uterine wall, allows preservation of the uterine wall due to minimal resection of myometrium:

1. The wall is opened over the rudimentary horn cavity;

2. The cavity lining is ablated by CO_2 laser;

3. The uterine wall is restored by suturing.

These techniques are usually free from complications. The patients may stand up and walk 2–3 hours after surgery, and are discharged on the 2nd or 3rd postoperative day. Pregnancy is allowed 2-3 months after operation, and a vaginal delivery may be performed.

CLASS III: UTERUS DUPLEX

Uterus duplex is characterized by presence of two uteri and one or two vaginas. The following variants of this malformation are differentiated: uterus duplex without obstruction to menstrual outflow; uterus and vagina duplex with partial vaginal aplasia; uterus and vagina duplex where one uterus is non-functional.

Clinical manifestation depends upon the malformation variant. The first variant (uterus duplex without obstruction to menstrual outflow) in most cases does not cause any problems and is often an occasional discovery, but, if not previously diagnosed, there may be difficulty in choosing the mode of delivery in a pregnant patient. Uterus and vagina duplex with partial aplasia of one hemivagina is accompanied by pelvic pain, caused by hematocolpos. Sometimes the diagnosis presents difficulties when one uterus is normally menstruating. Patients in whom one uterus is non-functional may appear infertile if intercourse involves the vagina of the non-functional uterus.

Patient's complaints, physical examination, ultrasonographic data and other methods of visualization (MRI, SCT) contribute to the preliminary diagnosis but only simultaneous hysteroscopy and laparoscopy provide the final differentiation between uterus duplex and other symmetric malformations (complete intrauterine septum and bicornuate uterus).

SURGICAL CORRECTION

Uterus duplex without obstruction to menstrual outflow itself does not necessitate surgical correction. In patients with uterine and vagina duplex with complete or partial aplasia of one of the hemivaginas, laparoscopy is used for final diagnosis, correction of associated gynecologic disease and control after resection of the wall of the obstructed hemivagina which must provide a wide communication between the latter and the functional vagina. Laparoscopy with simultaneous correction of gynecologic disease during vaginoplasty in patients aged 12-15 years provides normal reproductive function.

CLASS IV: BICORNUATE UTERUS

Bicornuate uterus is a malformation where the upper part of the uterine body is divided into two horns. In some patients the bicornuate uterus is found during routine examinations or treatment for other gynecologic diseases. In some patients this malformation may be a cause of miscarriage, isthmical–cervical insufficiency, and abnormal labor. Various anomalies are presented on Figure 16.

None of the available diagnostic tools (ultrasonography, CT, MRI, HSG, hysteroscopy or laparoscopy alone) is adequate to provide 100% accuracy in differentiation between bicornuate and septate uterus. The hysteroscopic picture may look like that of an intrauterine septum. Laparoscopic examination performed together with hysteroscopy is crucial because the definitive diagnosis is possible only after visual evaluation of the external shape of corpus uteri.

SURGICAL CORRECTION

The only indication for surgical correction of this malformation is miscarriage. We use our own methods of combined laparoscopic–hysteroscopic metroplasty based on the principles of the conventional Strassman technique, comprising creation of a united cavity that includes:

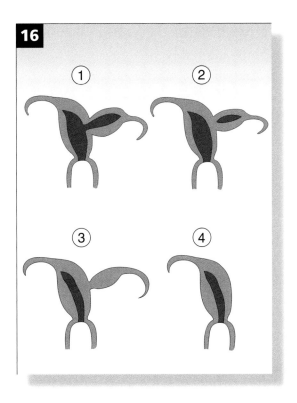

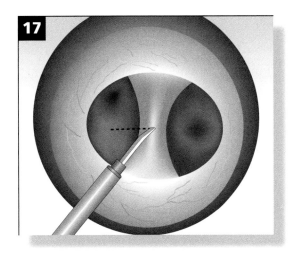

1. Dissection of the uterine fundus in the frontal plane with opening of both hemicavities;

2. Suturing of the uterine wound in the sagittal plane.

In case of incomplete bicornuate uterus, and if simultaneous distension of both hemicavities is possible, the operation is started by hysteroscopy. Five per cent mannitol or 5% glucose solution may be used as the distension media. The mucosal-muscular layer of the uterine wall is dissected by the hook electrode of the resectoscope up to the serosa in the frontal plane, avoiding the tubal ostia. The depth of dissection is visually controlled hysteroscopically and laparoscopically by transillumination of the uterine wall (Figures 17 and 18). The hysteroscopic step is terminated by planned perforation of the uterus, which is necessary to determine the direction of the incision of the serosa. Further steps are performed laparoscopically.

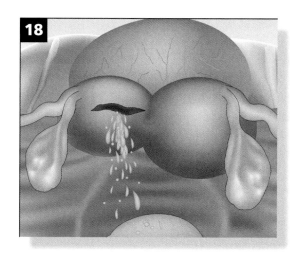

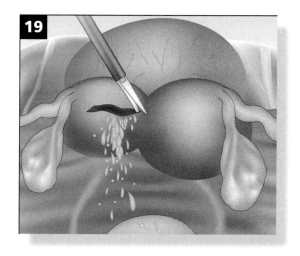

Laparoscopy is performed through four punctures of the anterior abdominal wall. The uterine serosa is transected in the frontal plane by a monopolar electrode or ultrasonic scalpel (Figure 19). Hemostasis is achieved by bipolar coagulation (Figure 20). Two layers (mucosal-muscular and muscular-serosal) of absorbable sutures are placed at the uterine wound in the sagittal direction (Figure 21 and 22). The ends of the first

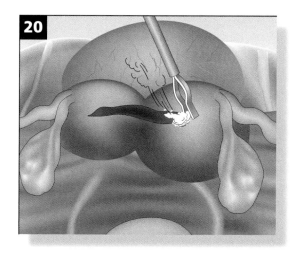

layer of sutures are withdrawn from the abdominal cavity through a central puncture outside the trocar sleeve, and are left untied until the last suture is placed. The ligatures are then consecutively introduced into the trocar sleeve and tied extracorporeally. To avoid excessive tension and tissue sawing during knot-tying, both halves of the uterus are brought to the midline with the manipulators. The serosal-muscular suture may be placed continuously. Second-look laparoscopy and hysteroscopy performed 3 months after endoscopic metroplasty show no evidence of adhesions either in the pelvis, or in the uterine cavity. Satisfactory results of endoscopic metroplasty lead us to believe that minimally invasive approaches are more effective than conventional laparotomy techniques.

CLASS V: INTRAUTERINE SEPTUM

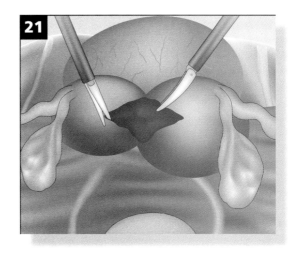

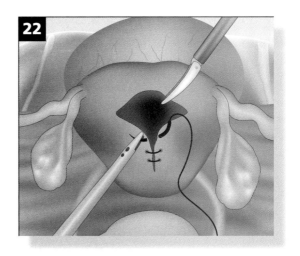

Intrauterine septum is a symmetric malformation in which the uterine cavity is divided into two hemicavities by a longitudinal septum of varying length. The patients with intrauterine septum often suffer from reproductive failures (miscarriages or infertility). Final diagnosis is possible only under simultaneous hysteroscopy and laparoscopy. Laparoscopy shows united corpus uteri. Hysteroscopy is necessary to evaluate the volume of the uterine cavity, and the length and thickness of the septum. Two variants of malformation exist:

1. Complete septum;

2. Partial septum (not reaching internal ostium).

This intervention is incomparably less invasive than laparotomic metroplasty using the Jones or Tompkins techniques. Our method provides excellent anatomic effectiveness and is almost free from complications and disadvantages such as formation of pelvic adhesions and the necessity of subsequent Cesarean section.

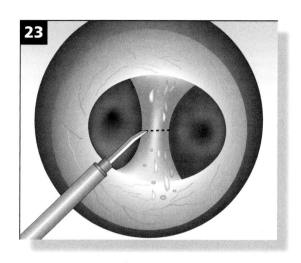

Hysteroscopic resection is performed in the early follicular phase of the menstrual cycle (preferably immediately after menstruation) or after medical preparation of the endometrium (for reduction of its thickness, operative blood loss, and for better visualization) with 2 months of GnRH agonists, according to the following technique (Figure 23):

- Cervical canal is dilated up to 10.5–11.5 Hegar;

- Resectoscope is inserted into uterine cavity; intrauterine septum is consecutively transected in its middle part from the summit to the base with the small movements of the hook electrode, and by monopolar pure cutting current of 100-130 W, until the uterine cavity assumes a normal triangular shape;

- Bleeding is controlled by coagulating current of 40-60 W.

For distension, 5% glucose solution or other non-electrolytes are used. The fluid (2-6 L, depending on the septum length and thickness) is delivered at a rate of 150–400 mL/min, average pressure in the cavity is maintained at 60–80 mmHg. If the procedure duration exceeds 20 min, 20 mg of Lasix can be given intravenously for prevention of complications associated with possible fluid overload. Laparoscopic control after hysteroscopic resection of the intrauterine septum is advisable, considering the risk of perforation of the uterus, and for simultaneous evaluation and correction of associated pelvic disease.

The operation rarely lasts longer than 15 min. The patient is allowed to stand up 2 hours after surgery, and to leave the hospital on the same day. Contraception is recommended for 2-3 months. Reproductive function is restored in about 64% of patients who have undergone hysteroscopic resection, and they usually deliver vaginally, provided there are no obstetric indications for operative delivery.

To conclude, laparoscopy and hysteroscopy not only provide the definitive diagnosis of the full spectrum of malformations of the genitalia, but are the most rational and minimally invasive operative approaches to the majority of surgically correctable anomalies.

SUGGESTED READING:

Buttram VC, Jr. Mullerian anomalies and their management. Fertil Steril 1983;40:159

Adamyan LV. Additional international perspectives: colpopoiesis in vaginal and uterine aplasias In: Gynecologic and obstetric surgery (ed) David Nichols, Mosby, 1993:1167-1182

Adamyan LV. Laparoscopic management of vaginal aplasia with or without functional noncommunicating uterus. In: Principles of laparoscopic surgery: basic and advanced techniques. (ed) Maurice E.Arregui, et al., Springer-Verlag, 1995:652-671

Adamyan LV. Laparoscopy in surgical treatment of vaginal aplasia: laparoscopy assisted colpopoiesis and perineal hysterectomy with colpopoiesis. Int J Fertil, 41(1);1996:40-45

Adamyan LV. Therapeutic and endoscopic perspectives: colpopoiesis in vaginal and uterine aplasias. In: Gynecologic and obstetric surgery (ed) David Nichols, Mosby, 1999:187-195

Monks P. Uterus didelphys associated with unilateral cervical atresia and renal agenesis. Aust NZJ Obstet Gynaecol 1979;19:245-6

Jones HJ, Wheeless C. Salvage of the reproductive potential of women with anomalous development of the Mullerian ducts: 1868-1968-2068. A J Obstet Gynecol 1969; 104:348-64

Frank RT. The formation of artificial vagina without operation. Am J Obstet Gynecol 1938;35:1053-5

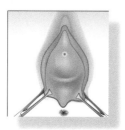

LAPAROSCOPIC BOWEL SURGERY

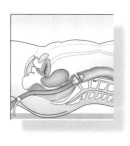

Jeff W. Allen, M.D.

Benjamin D. Tanner, M.D.

After mastering basic laparoscopic techniques such as tissue handling, intracorporeal suturing, and optical facility with 0° and 30° telescopes, operations that are more difficult can be performed using a minimal access approach. This includes many operations on the small and large bowel. This chapter will review some advanced laparoscopic procedures such as colon resection and also some of the problems encountered during operations such as closure of iatrogenic enterotomy.

COLON RESECTION

The laparoscopic approach to colon resection for benign disease is now preferred over the open operation in many circumstances. With malignant disease, there are unanswered issues of port site recurrences, inadequate oncologic resections, and intraperitoneal tumor spread with pneumoperitoneum. Benign diseases treated by laparoscopic partial colectomy include diverticular disease, some polyps, arterial venous malformations, endometriosis, benign strictures, and certain cases of colitis. Most patients benefit from the laparoscopic approach to colon resection because there is a decrease in postoperative pain, wound infections, and delayed bowel function, along with improvements in pulmonary function and cosmesis.

SIGMOID COLECTOMY

With sigmoid colon resections, the patient is positioned in stirrups. Care is taken to adequately pad the legs in the stirrups to prevent neuropraxia. The patient is placed in the Trendelenburg position, and the operating table is rolled so that the patient's left side is elevated. Some surgeons advocate a full lateral position with the use of beanbags. Pneumoperitoneum is obtained and 5-mm working trocars in the left upper quadrant, left lower quadrant, and right lower quadrant are placed (Figure 1). Since the extended incision of the left lower quadrant port is often the site for specimen extraction, this port can be 10 mm in size. A 10-mm camera port is placed below the umbilicus. A 30° laparoscope enables maximum viewing.

After port placement, the sigmoid colon is grasped using atraumatic bowel graspers or a Babcock and retracted medially. The line of Toldt is incised

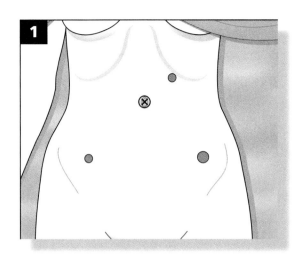

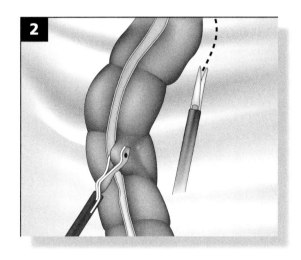

using scissors equipped with electrocautery passing through the port in the left lower quadrant (Figure 2). Retroperitoneal structures including the ureter are identified. This dissection is continued cephalad to the splenic flexure. In some instances, the splenic flexure must be fully mobilized to ensure an adequate length of colon for a tension-free anastomosis.

After the colon is completely mobilized and the ureter identified, the major terminal portion of the inferior mesenteric artery is identified and ligated. The vessel is most easily located by visualizing the arterial pulsations in the mesentery, while the colon is retracted toward the anterior abdominal wall. Ligation of this vessel includes creating a mesenteric window on either side of the artery and transecting it either with a linear laparoscopic stapler or large clips (Figure 3). In most patients, this vessel is too large for safe division with the harmonic scalpel.

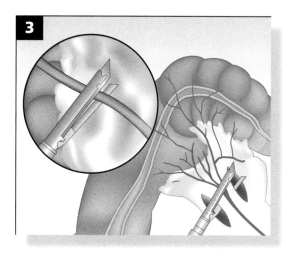

Next, the remainder of the sigmoid colon mesentery is divided using the harmonic scalpel. It is important not to divide too far into the mesentery of the descending colon because this can decrease the length of viable bowel available for anastomosis. After the mesentery has been divided, a linear laparoscopic stapler is fired across the distal sigmoid colon at the rectosigmoid junction, below the area of pathology (Figure 4). It is important to re-identify the ureter prior to transecting the bowel.

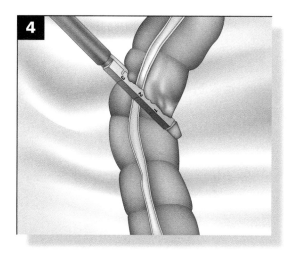

The incision of either the left lower quadrant or the infraumbilical port site is extended, and the specimen with attached proximal colon is delivered (Figure 5). The proximal end is transected with a reload of the laparoscopic stapler and opened. The anvil of an end-

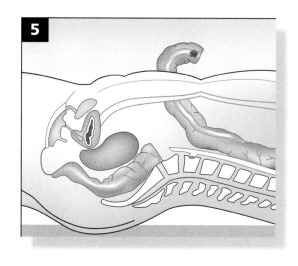

to-end (EEA) stapler is placed in this colotomy and secured with a pursestring suture of 0 Prolene (Figure 6). The descending colon with anvil in place is then returned intraabdominally and the extended excision closed. It is important to make this closure airtight because pneumoperitoneum is then re-established.

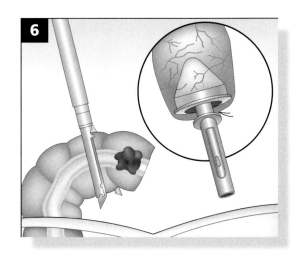

The EEA stapler is introduced per rectum, and the spike deployed through the rectal stump. The proximal colon with anvil in place is stretched into the pelvis to the spike (Figure 7). If the anastomosis appears to be under tension, it is best to further mobilize the splenic flexure before performing the intracorporeal anastomosis. The EEA stapler spike is then interfaced with its anvil, closed, and fired. The entire stapling apparatus is removed.

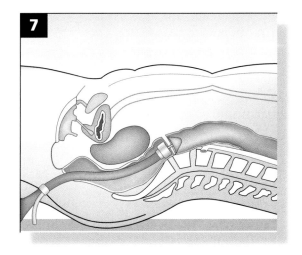

It is important to test this anastomosis by clamping the colon proximal to the anastomosis with a non-crushing grasper, filling the pelvis with sterile saline or water, and insufflating with air (Figure 8). A rigid sigmoidoscope can further test the anastomosis. The pneumoperitoneum is decompressed and the skin incisions are closed.

RIGHT HEMICOLECTOMY

The patient is placed supine on the operating room table. No stirrups are

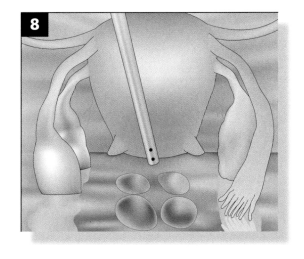

used and the arms are tucked at the patient's side. Maximal exposure is provided by rotating into the left lateral position. Open pneumoperitoneum is obtained via a 10-mm infraumbilical trocar. Working ports of 5 mm are placed in the right lower, the right upper, and left lower quadrants (Figure 9). The table is rolled toward the patient's left. The terminal ileum, appendix, and cecum are located, and the right line of Toldt is identified and incised as previously described. This mobilization continues so that the cecum is free from its retroperitoneal attachments (Figure 10). Often, the dissection is continued around the hepatic flexure, and the harmonic scalpel is used to prevent bleeding. At this point, the ureter is identified by many surgeons.

Medial and inferior traction on the right and transverse colon is applied and the duodenum is visualized and bluntly dissected away from the transverse mesocolon. Once the duodenum is completely freed, the pathologic process identified, and an adequate margin obtained, the distal colon is transected using a linear laparoscopic stapler. The mesentery is divided using the harmonic scalpel, and the laparoscopic stapler is used to divide the right colic artery (Figure 11). Alternatively, large clips may be used. The specimen is delivered through one of the port sites, which has been extended. In our

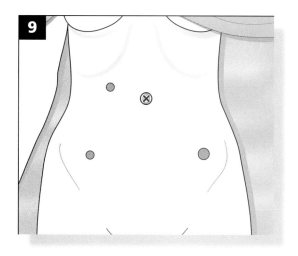

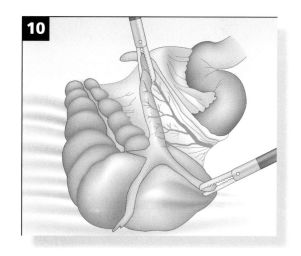

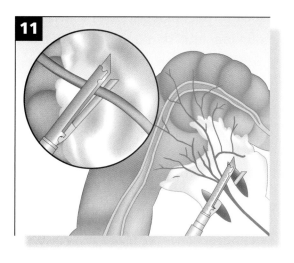

experience, either the infraumbilical or right lower quadrant incision may be used for this purpose. Note the ileum is still attached to the right colon and, given its freedom, it too is delivered extraabdominally and transected. The ileum is transected with the linear stapler and then either a hand-sewn end-to-end or side-to-side stapled anastomosis is performed extracorporeally (Figure 12). The ileocolic segment is returned to the abdomen and the incisions closed.

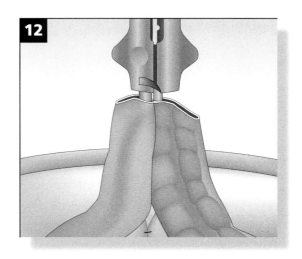

Alternatively, this may be performed entirely intracorporeally with a side-to-side stapled anastomosis and closure of the common stoma with running sutures tied intracorporeally. The specimen may then be delivered through an extended incision.

COLOSTOMY CREATION

Sigmoid or transverse colostomy is easily created laparoscopically. First, obtain pneumoperitoneum via an infraumbilical skin incision and place working ports in the right upper and left lower quadrant. The large bowel is identified and a sling is placed around it for easy manipulation (Figure 13). This is helpful because the colostomy site can be located based on how easily the colon reaches to the skin site, as opposed to vice versa. After the colostomy site is identified, any needed mobilization

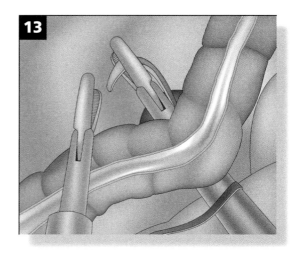

along the line of Toldt is undertaken as previously described. Once the loop will reach freely, an incision is made, and the colon is pulled through and matured in the usual fashion. A colostomy bar may replace the sling through the same aperture.

An end colostomy, with or without colon resection, entails identifying the site for the colostomy and dividing the colon and mesentery for proper length. The colon proximal to the colostomy is stretched to the site for the colostomy, a skin incision made, and the colon delivered. The colostomy is matured in a standard fashion (Figure 14).

COLOSTOMY CLOSURE

The takedown of a colostomy is often a more morbid procedure than colostomy creation because of the large adhesion lysis that often is necessary and the occasional difficulty in identifying the distal colon for anastomosis.

With the laparoscopic approach, the patient is placed in the supine position in stirrups. Care is taken to pad the legs to prevent neuropraxia. Port placement is based on previous incisions and the assumption that generally there will be fewer adhesions under unscarred skin. During the lysis of adhesions, the peristomal area is cleared, and the colon that is proximal to the colostomy is mobilized. This often involves mobilizing the splenic flexure in the case of a descending colostomy.

Next, the colonic stump is identified. At this point, the pneumoperitoneum is decompressed and a peristomal incision is made with dissection of the colon off the fat and skin (Figure 15). The colostomy is then equipped with the anvil of an EEA stapler secured with a

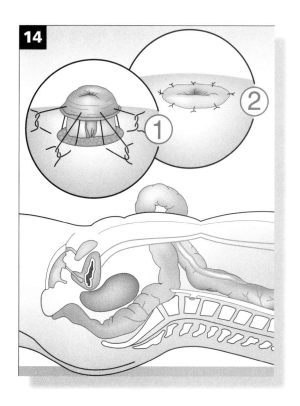

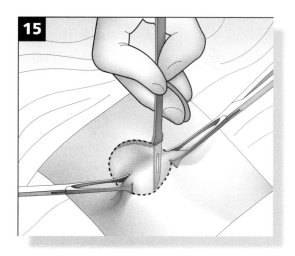

pursestring suture and the colon delivered intraabdominally (Figure 16). The colostomy incision is closed in an airtight fashion. The skin may be closed over drains or left open based on the preference of the surgeon.

Next, the pneumoperitoneum is re-established and the colon with anvil is directed into the pelvis. The EEA stapler is passed per rectum following the curve of the sacrum. Once the EEA stapler is observed in the rectal stump, the sharp spike is deployed and the anvil and spike are interfaced. The stapler is fired after the appropriate pressure is obtained by closing the stapler (Figure 17). The anastomosis is checked as previously described.

APPENDECTOMY

The laparoscopic approach to appendectomy is a controversial subject. We believe it is most beneficial for patients when the diagnosis is uncertain. This is often the case in obese patients, in children and adolescents, and especially in women when the possibility of adnexal pathology mimicking appendicitis is present.

For maximum cosmesis, an infraumbilical incision is made for the camera port and two lower 5-mm incisions in the hairline are placed (Figure 18). The technique involves creation of a pneumoperitoneum, establishing a diagnosis requiring appendectomy, and isolating the appendix from its surrounding structures. Occasionally, the appendix is

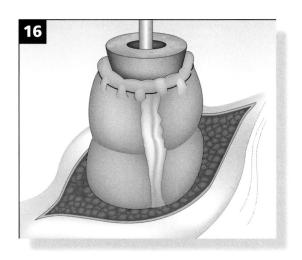

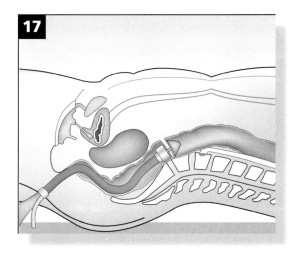

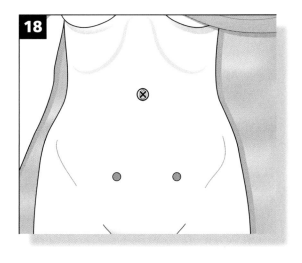

adherent to the retroperitoneal structures through filmy adhesions, and these must be incised.

After freeing the appendix, the mesoappendix is divided with clips and scissors, or alternatively bipolar electrocautery (Figure 19), the harmonic scalpel, or a linear stapler (Figure 20). Once the appendix is free from its mesoappendix, it is divided with the linear stapler. This step may also be safely and cost-efficiently performed using a series of endoloops (Figure 21). The appendix is delivered through the largest port. To minimize contamination, a prepackaged laparoscopic plastic bag is used. Alternatively, to decrease costs, the thumb of a large powderless glove may be used.

MECKEL'S RESECTION

Asymptomatic Meckel's diverticuli are probably best treated without an operation. However, in cases when a symptomatic Meckel's is discovered or in the instance when an operation is performed for abdominal pain with no clear cause, a Meckel's resection is indicated. The surgery for Meckel's diverticulum is either a simple diverticulectomy or a small bowel resection with enteroenterostomy.

A diverticulectomy is performed most commonly in the laparoscopic realm

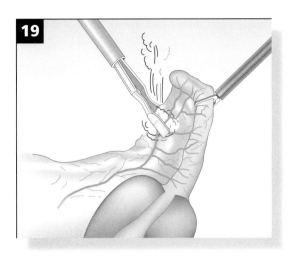

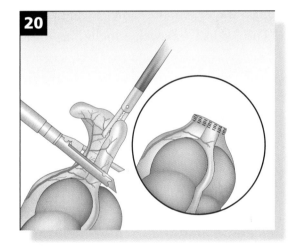

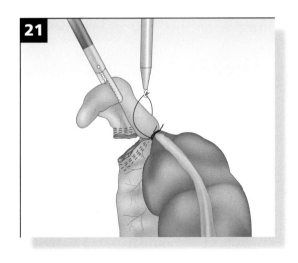

with a laparoscopic linear stapler fired at the base of the diverticulum (Figure 22). This is performed after proper alignment and identification of the Meckel's. It is important not to excessively impinge on the lumen of the small bowel, and equally important not to leave heterotopic mucosa behind.

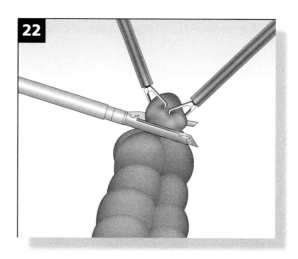

In cases when the Meckel's is causing gastrointestinal hemorrhage, the diverticulum is large (>5 cm), or when an associated omphalomesenteric band is present, an enterectomy is indicated. The small bowel, including the Meckel's, may be delivered extracorporeally through an extended port site incision. The excision and subsequent anastomosis are performed extracorporeally and then returned intraabdominally (Figure 23). This may also be performed intracorporeally, by firing a linear stapler across the bowel proximal and distal to the Meckel's and then fashioning a side-to-side stapled anastomosis. It is imperative to have generous margins, because in a case of hemorrhage, the small bowel mucosa is likely to be the source of the bleeding, due to the heterotrophic gastric acid-producing mucosa upstream. After firing a stapler proximal and distal to the Meckel's, the mesentery is transected either with an ultrasonic sheer or with an additional load of the linear stapler. A side-to-side anastomosis is then fashioned using the stapler. The common stoma is closed

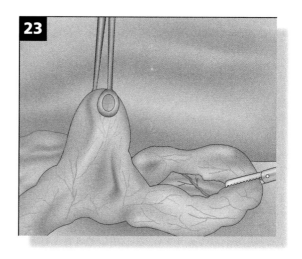

with a running intracorporeally tied suture. The specimen is then delivered through the largest port in a protective bag.

INCIDENTAL ENTEROTOMY

In the past, the expected management of a recognized iatrogenic enterotomy at the time of laparoscopy was unquestionable. This would include conversion to a laparotomy, consultation with a general surgeon, if indicated, and repair of the enterotomy. When the enterotomy involves heavily contaminated fecal material, the possibility of a diverting colostomy is entertained. Just as less conservative approaches to the management of penetrating colon injuries are becoming more readily accepted, so too are the approaches to management of laparoscopic enterotomies.

As the skills of laparoscopic surgeons increase, their ability to laparoscopically manage a complication such as an enterotomy is improved. Iatrogenic enterotomies in prepped bowel may be safely repaired by a surgeon with intracorporeal suturing skills. Contraindications to this management would include: heavy spillage, hypotension, inadequate exposure, or the belief that additional unrecognized enterotomies exist. A review of 26 laparoscopic closures of enterotomies was performed by Nezhat et al., with no appreciable morbidity or mortality associated with the technique.

In cases of left colon injuries, the management is even more controversial because high luminal levels of bacteria portend a high rate of wound infection, sepsis, and possible leakage. A review of the recommendations for colon injuries caused by penetrating trauma may be

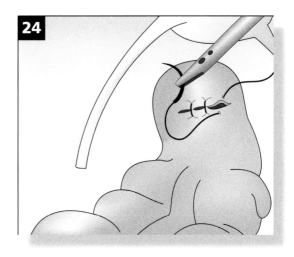

insightful. There is sufficient evidence in the trauma literature to support primary repair for non-destructive colon wounds when the patient has no peritonitis, significant underlying disease, or evidence of shock. These same basic recommendations can be applied to laparoscopic surgery.

A colotomy may be oversewn; we recommend that this be done in two layers (Figure 24). It is helpful to check the colotomy for leakage in left colon injuries by insufflating air and methylene blue or povidone-iodine (Betadine) transrectally. It is probably best to leave a drain in as well. Whenever there is a question about the appropriate management, the exposure, or the ability of the surgeon to repair the injury, consultation with a general surgeon and/or conversion to an open procedure are indicated.

SUGGESTED READING:

Muckleroy SK, Ratzer ER, Fenoglio ME. Laparoscopic colon surgery for benign disease: A comparison to open surgery. JSLS 1999;3:33-37

Jager RM. Laparoscopic right hemicolectomy in left lateral decubitus position. Surg Laparosc Endosc 1994;4:348-352

Berne JD, Velmahos BG, Chan LS, Asensio JA, Demetriades D. The high morbidity of colostomy closure after trauma: further support for the primary repair of colon injuries. Surgery 1998;123:157-164

George SM, Fabian TC, Voeller GR, Kudsk KA, Mangiante EC, Britt LG. Primary repair of colon wounds: A prospective trial in nonselected patients. Ann Surg 1989;209:728-734

Sasaki LS, Allaben RD, Golwala R, Mittal VK. Primary repair of colon injuries: A prospective randomized study. J Trauma 1995;39:895-901

Gonzalez RP, Merlotti GJ, Holevar MR. Colostomy in penetrating colon injury. Is it necessary? J Trauma 1996;41:271-275

Nezhat C, Nezhat F, Ambroze W, Pennington E. Laparoscopic repair of small bowel and colon. Surg Endosc 1993;7:88-89

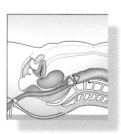

GASLESS LAPAROSCOPY

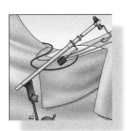

Daniel Kruschinski, M.D.

Bernd Bojahr, M.D.

Miroslav Kopjar, M.D.

PREFACE

Gasless laparoscopy is a system that does not require a pneumoperitoneum. Instead, it uses an abdominal wall lifting system. One such system is the AbdoLift® (Karl Storz Endoscopy, Tuttlingen, Germany). With a special design of the retractors, the AbdoLift® mechanical elevation of the abdominal wall provides the surgeon with the necessary space comparable with that of pneumoperitoneum laparoscopy. As no gas is needed, flexible and valveless trocars can be used. This technique avoids several typical intraoperative problems of pneumoperitoneum laparoscopy such as gas leakage, rinsing and suction as well as removal of tumors and organs out of the abdominal cavity.

By utilizing conventional instruments and standard surgical techniques and avoiding disposables, gasless laparoscopy is a cost effective procedure with benefits for the patients, surgeons, hospitals, and the health system. Gasless laparoscopy is a simple, effective, and economical introduction to operative laparoscopy and extends the indications of minimal invasive surgery. It combines minimal invasive surgery and modern magnification with endoscopic imaging systems, opening the possibility of using standard techniques and conventional instruments, which have been developed and modified for a very long time. They allow the surgeon, in contrast to laparoscopic instruments, to use tactile sense and palpation, as they are very short and have only one link. Performing surgery with short instruments means that the hand is close to the area of operation and the fulcrum is short so that accuracy is relatively higher than that of laparoscopic instruments where the surgeon's hand is very far from the area of the operation.

Via flexible trocars, conventional and/or laparoscopic instruments can be used. It is also possible to introduce several instruments simultaneously through the same trocar. The insertion and the change of instruments, as well as suturing and tying, can be performed easier through the flexible valveless trocars. Gasless laparoscopy has the advantage of performing laparo-vaginal procedures more extensively than with gas laparoscopy.

Complications during the blind Veress needle or trocar insertion such as vascular lesions or intestinal injury are virtually excluded by this technique. Problems and complications of the iatrogenic insufflation of CO_2 (pneumothorax, pneumomediastinum,

MAIN INDICATIONS FOR GASLESS LAPAROSCOPY ACCORDING TO TECHNICAL OPERATIVE ABILITIES AND ADVANTAGES ARE:

- ENUCLEATION OF MYOMAS (SUFFICIENT CONVENTIONAL SUTURING OF THE MYOMETRIUM)

- OTHER ORGAN PRESERVING SURGERY AS ENUCLEATION OF OVARIAN TUMORS (AVOIDANCE OF RUPTURE AND CELL SPILLAGE)

- ORGAN RECONSTRUCTIVE SURGERY SUCH AS TUBAL SURGERY

- TOTAL LAPAROSCOPIC HYSTERECTOMY

- SUPRACERVICAL HYSTERECTOMY

- LAPAROSCOPIC ASSISTED VAGINAL HYSTERECTOMY

- COMBINED LAPARO-VAGINAL SURGERY AS THE EXCISION OF RECTOVAGINAL ENDOMETRIOSIS

- OPERATIVE AND DIAGNOSTIC PROCEDURES IN RISK PATIENTS AND IN PREGNANT WOMEN UNDER GENERAL, REGIONAL, OR LOCAL ANESTHESIA

- OPERATIVE AND DIAGNOSTIC PROCEDURES FOR CANCERS OR SUSPICIOUS TUMORS (OVARIAN TUMORS, PELVIC/PARAAORTIC LYMPHADENECTOMY)

pneumopericardium, air embolism, massive subcutaneous empholism) are completely excluded. Physiologically, gasless laparoscopy is less invasive than pneuomoperitoneum insufflation and allows the use of laparoscopic surgery in high-risk patients, e.g. those with heart insufficiency or lung obstruction as well as in pregnancy. The ability to utilize operative laparoscopy under regional anesthesia as the combination of minimal invasive surgery and minimal invasive anesthesia (MIS MIA) will become a new challenge.

In case of oncologic surgery gasless laparoscopy might have some advantages over pneumoperitoneum laparoscopy as experimental studies indicate that utilizing CO_2 could possibly lead to a more aggressive spreading of tumor cells and progressive tumor cell implantation in the abdominal cavity.

Lift-laparoscopy offers the concept of laparopscopy as a minimally invasive surgery, and is simpler, cost–effective, and extends the range of application.

PATIENT POSITIONING, PREPARATION AND ANESTHESIA

It is advisable and also mandatory that both arms should be tucked along the body and shoulder braces must be used to allow a steep Trendelenburg position (up to 30°). If a diagnostic procedure along with an operative surgery is going to be performed, it is recommended that the bowel should be prepared as for laparotomy.

ANESTHESIA

If general anesthesia is chosen, it should be performed without the use of N_2O, as nitrogen oxide distends into the bowel after 90-120 minutes with the consequence that the distended bowel is placed in the pouch of Douglas and might disturb parts of the operation. A bladder catheter can be inserted into the rectum during the procedure to evacuate air from the bowel if necessary. In cases of spinal, epidural, or combined spinal/epidural anesthesia the patient should have both hands free due to the psychological stress of being unable to move any part of the body. For the patient's convenience, a CD-player or a DVD-player is very helpful. To prevent intraoperative pain or nausea, especially in anxious patients, sedative drugs can be administered.

CREATION OF THE ABDOMINAL WALL ELEVATION

The patient is placed in the lithotomy position and covered with a sterile drape. The fixing stand has to be attached to the right rail of the operating table by the fixation device, usually at the height of the patient's shoulder (Figure 1). The vertical arm of the AbdoLift is attached on top of the fixing stand, the spring balance and the retractor can be inserted and the system can be adjusted to the anatomical position of the patient by using all joints to correct the position of the components (Figure 2).

APPROACHING
THE ABDOMINAL CAVITY

The technique is similar to the Hasson open procedure, however, the skin incision in the lower umbilical fold is only 12-15 mm (Figure 3). With the help of special S-shaped hooks one can reach the fascia layer by layer, displacing the subcutaneous and fatty tissue by blunt dissection (Figure 4). After reaching the fascia, a small incision (2-3 mm) is made with a number 11 scalpel followed by insertion of blunt scissors and opening of the fascia up to 15 mm. By using the S-hooks, the rectus muscle is pushed aside and the peritoneum can be visualized. The light of the endoscope is used for transilluminating the abdominal cavity to visualize adhesions if present. At an adhesion-free area, the incision of the superficial layer of the peritoneum can

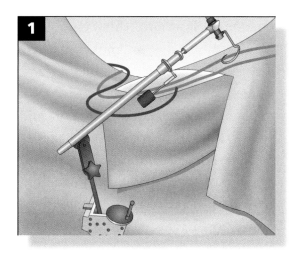

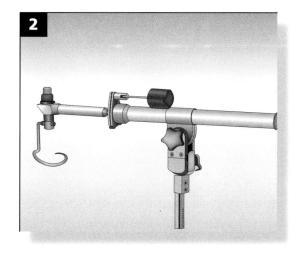

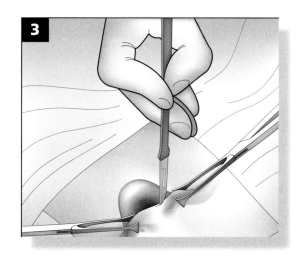

be performed either by a number 11 scalpel or scissors and then widened by spreading the scissor arms. After reaching the abdominal cavity, the left and the right S-hook are inserted into the abdomen under vision and the abdominal wall is elevated. Introducing the endoscope, the entire periumbilical area can be visualized to detect adhesions that would prevent insertion of the retractor. Sometimes, a digital palpation of the anterior abdominal wall is useful in detecting any adhesions. Under elevation of the abdominal wall with the S-hooks by the assistant, the retractor is then inserted under vision rotating into the abdominal cavity (Figure 5). Behind the retractor, a trocar for the endoscope is introduced. Following this step, the endoscope is inserted for inspection. The purpose of this inspection is mainly to examine whether the omentum or the bowel have become pinched between the retractor and the abdominal wall. If so, it is necessary to remove the retractor and to start the procedure for reposition of the retractor.

Gasless laparoscopy is more difficult than pneumoperitoneum laparoscopy when severe adhesions are present around the periumbilical area. If adhesions in the lower abdominal quadrant are found, the retractor can be inserted first in the direction of the upper

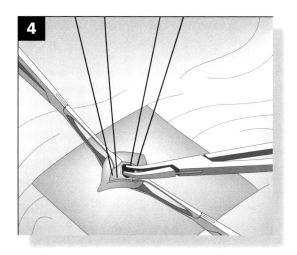

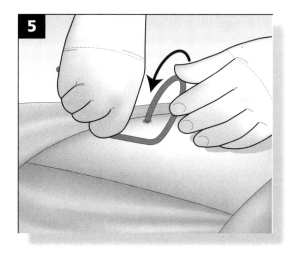

abdominal cavity or in a direction where no adhesions are present. After inspecting the abdominal cavity with the endoscope, an area free of adhesions must be found to introduce a trocar and perform an adhesiolysis. Sometimes a low-pressure (8–10 mmHg) pneumoperitoneum is necessary to perform adhesiolysis, prior to insertion of the abdominal wall retractor.

Checking the appropriate position of the retractor, the abdominal wall can be elevated by the height adjusting wheel (Figure 6) to the level of the mark 'Max' on the spring balance, which gives the level of approximately 1.5 Kg. This mark can be higher or lower according to the weight of the abdominal wall and the size of the patient. After the abdominal wall is elevated, the upper abdominal quadrant can be visualized with the endoscope in the same manner as in pneumoperitoneum laparoscopy. In some corpulent patients, it might be necessary to change the position of the retractor to the upper abdomen for visualization of the organs from the upper abdominal quadrant. When changing the retractor and the optic back to the pelvis the patient has to be placed in steep Trendelenburg position (up to 30°) which allows the bowel to slide to the upper abdominal quadrant that serves as a 'reservoir' for the intestine. Routinely, two ancillary ports can be introduced in the suprapubic region. In contrast to gas laparoscopy, these ports might be placed very close to each other (both trocars are medial from the epigastric vessels!) and about 1 cm under the pubic hairline, since using conventional instruments that are curved, makes it possible to reach all pelvic organs and structures (Figure 7). After

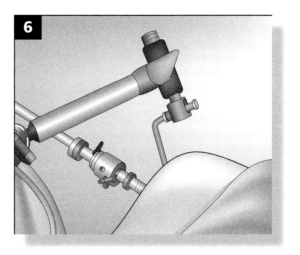

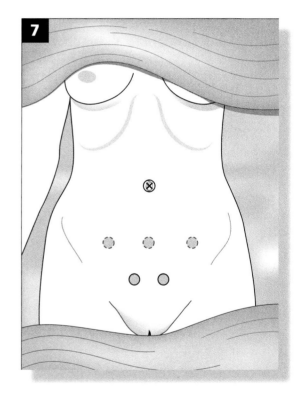

a few weeks the pubic hair covers the incisions and the cosmetic results obtained by this technique are better than in pneumoperitoneum laparoscopy, where the incisions have to be placed above the hairline (as marked in Figures 8 and 9) in order to reach the area behind the uterus with the long and straight laparoscopic instruments.

Recent applications show that it is possible to perform surgery even with one incision where two instruments can be introduced at the same time (Figure 8). This incision can be widened as required and a laparoscopic assisted

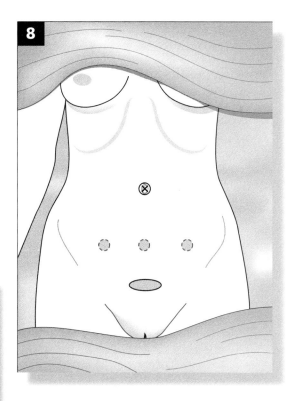

CREATION OF THE ABDOMINAL WALL ELEVATION:

1. MAKE A 12-15 MM SKIN INCISION IN THE LOWER UMBILICAL FOLD

2. ATTACH AND FIX THE ABDOLIFT TO THE OPERATING TABLE

3. DISSECT FAT, SUBCUTANEOUS TISSUE, FASCIA AND MUSCLE UNTIL REACHING THE PERITONEUM

4. DETECT ADHESIONS BY TRANSILLUMINATION

5. MAKE A 2-3 MM INCISION IN THE PERITONEAL LAYER AND SPREAD IT WITH BLUNT SCISSORS

6. INSERT THE RETRACTOR AND THE SCOPE AND CHECK FOR VESSEL OR BOWEL INJURIES

7. PLACE THE PATIENT IN STEEP TRENDELENBURG POSITION AFTER AN OVERVIEW

8. INTRODUCE TWO ANCILLARY PORTS IN THE SUPRAPUBIC REGION

9. BEGIN PROCEDURE

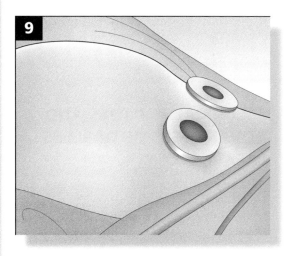

mini-laparotomy can be performed, allowing extension possibilities and principles from open surgery, like palpation and grasping of tissue or applying a ligature knot with two fingers.

To introduce the ports, one can use the same technique as in gas laparoscopy. Through a skin incision of 10 mm, a round sharp obturator with a rubber sheath that has a thread on the external site, can be introduced with a little force and turned clockwise through the abdominal wall. The abdominal wall may be transilluminated by the endoscope to avoid injury to epigastric vessels. The obturator is removed after insertion, leaving the trocar sheath in place (Figure 9).

If the bowel is still in the posterior cul-de-sac, it can be displaced to the upper abdomen with the help of two sponges. Then examination of the pelvic organs can take place exactly in the same manner as in pneumoperitoneum laparoscopy and the operative procedure can begin.

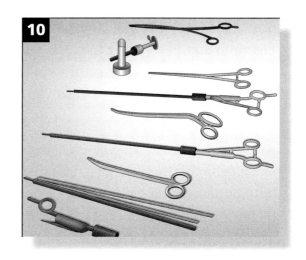

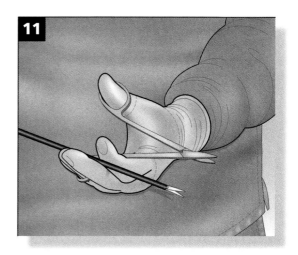

TECHNICAL ABILITIES AND ADVANTAGES OF GASLESS LAPAROSCOPY

The new concept of gasless laparoscopy allows identical exposure and vision as in pneumoperitoneum laparoscopy, but the operative procedure is technically less difficult to perform. By means of Lift-laparoscopy it is not only possible to manage all operative procedures performed under gas laparoscopy, but additionally to extend the range of application to more complex procedures and advanced surgery.

Conventional instruments are used. The grasping parts or the cutting edge of a conventional instrument is ergonomic with the ability to grasp or to cut tissue very precisely (Figures 10 and 11). With sponges for blunt dissection the procedures become easy and rapid (Figure 12). Where necessary, one can introduce a finger for palpation or dissection. It is also very easy to control bleeding by suction with a conventional plastic tube, irrigation, or sponges and to grasp the vessel with a clamp to apply a ligature or to coagulate it with the bipolar forceps.

Suturing can be performed very easily and fast using conventional suture material with curved needles as in open surgery (Figure 13). Tying the thread extracorporeally and pushing the knot with a knot pusher makes suturing as easy as in open surgery.

As no gas leakage occurs, Lift-laparoscopy allows extraction and removal of tissue from the abdominal cavity in a less problematic manner than in gas laparoscopy. Small myoma or morcellated pieces can be extracted directly through the flexible trocar. Ovarian tumors and other tissue samples should be extracted via an endobag. Conventional instruments allow open endobags for use inside the abdominal cavity and inserting the tissue sample is easy.

Despite all advantages of open surgery, Lift-laparoscopy still remains laparoscopy and it is logical to use special instruments which allow multifunctionality and multimodality. For example, one of these instruments is the bipolar diathermic scissors,

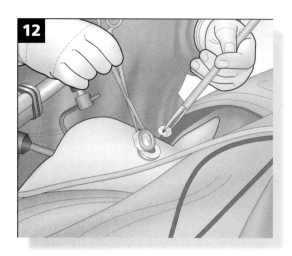

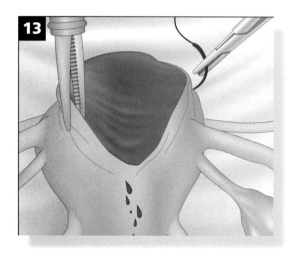

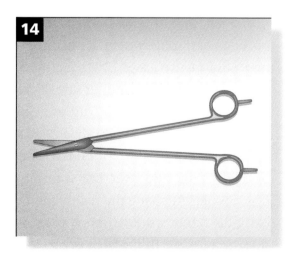

PowerStar™, (Ethicon, Cincinnati, OH) (Figure 14). These are like Metzenbaum scissors (originally developed for open surgery) covered with special ceramics so that the energy is applied only on the tip of the scissors and between the scissor blades.

ADNEXAL TUMORS

In case of enucleation of an ovarian cyst, it should be removed from the ovary without rupture and spillage of the cystic contents, especially in case of suspicious findings. Conventional surgical methods, which are very easy to apply using gasless laparoscopy, avoid spillage. In Figures 15 and 16, the procedure of a blunt dissection of an endometrioma by traction with a sponge and countertraction with a forceps is shown. With the help of conventional instruments and surgical techniques it is possible to avoid spillage in most ovarian tumors. For example, in our series of 102 gasless laparoscopic operated dermoids, we had a microrupture only in two cases (2%). In these cases, it was easy to continue surgery as one was able to grasp the rupture site with a long forceps longitudinally and continue the procedure of enucleation or apply a ligature over the ruptured cyst capsule. Applying the technique of blunt dissection spares as much ovarian tissue as possible. In lift-laparoscopy the

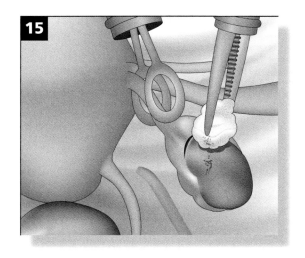

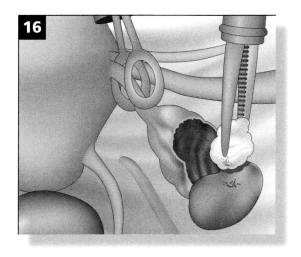

removal of tissue specimens is less problematic as there is no interaction with gas leakage and the endobag can be grasped with conventional curved instruments, allowing the bag to be held open around the instruments. The closure of the ovarian capsule is performed with ordinary suture material and a curved needle as used in laparotomy.

ENUCLEATION OF FIBROIDS

Fibroids, which are located intramurally are sometimes difficult to enucleate. After an incision is made through the myometrium with the bipolar scissors, the enucleation of the myoma can begin by grasping the myoma with forceps (Figure 17). The enucleation procedure must be performed using bipolar forceps or bipolar scissors. In case of bleeding, conventional plastic suction tubes from open surgery can be used to evacuate blood clots, and rinse out water and smoke. After removing the fibroid, the myometrium must be sutured. In case of intramural fibroids, an adequate closure of the myometrium is necessary.

In contrast to gas laparoscopy, conventional needle drivers can be used (Figure 18) to manipulate suture material with a curved needle for an adequate closure of the myometrial tissue. We perform closure of all layers with as few stitches as necessary (Figure 19) to achieve an adequate and functional closure of the myometrial wound. With this technique, we avoid wound healing problems due to infections and necrosis that may occur with numerous stitches. With this technique, we have performed more than 200 myomectomies in infertile patients with 77% pregnancy rate. There have

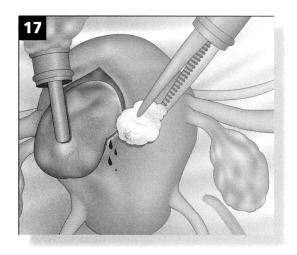

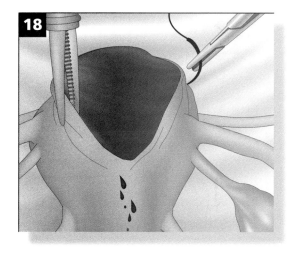

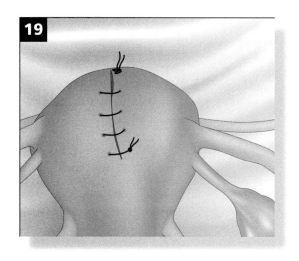

been no uterine ruptures during pregnancy or during delivery.

Lift–laparoscopy extends organ preserving operations for fibroid removal of any size according to the skill of the surgeon. Even myomatous uteri with a size of about 1.5 kg can be managed. For morcellation of such huge fibroids, an electrical morcellator should be used, however, small myomas can be morcellated without difficulties with a scalpel or scissors.

HYSTERECTOMY

The most difficult problem for hysterectomy is how to divide vessels, especially the uterine artery. Gasless laparoscopy allows plenty of variations for this procedure. Without these problems, one can apply a ligature around the uterine vessel (Figure 20). With a knot pusher the vessels are ligated and after applying a ligature contralaterally, the uterine vessels can be cut.

The coagulation with the bipolar forceps or other energy sources is, of course, also possible in gasless laparoscopy. An additional positive effect is that the open abdomen prevents smoke from accumulating and avoids the fogging of the laparoscope.

Using the bipolar scissors, coagulation and cutting can be securely

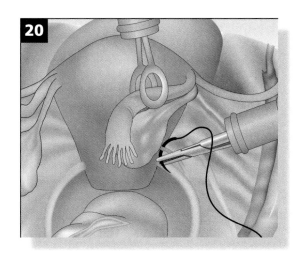

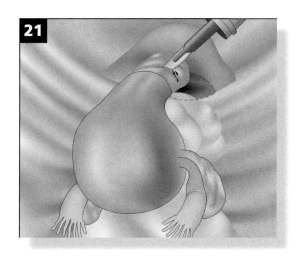

performed in one step without carbonization and with less of a coagulation edge to avoid injury to other structures like the ureter. With one-step coagulation and cutting, the laparoscopic procedure becomes very fast as there is no change of instruments during the vessel ligations. To open the vaginal cuff, one can use the scalpel (Figure 21) or the bipolar scissors.

PELVIC AND PARAAORTIC LYMPHADENECTOMY

Even though a magnified vision extends the ability of laparoscopic surgery for cancer, in general, abdominal cancer operations are not performed laparoscopically. However, laparoscopy may even obtain a better surgical result and reduce morbidity, the duration of hospitalization, and recovery time associated with conventional surgery. The feasibility of diagnostic or therapeutic laparoscopic pelvic and/or paraaortic lymphadenectomy is described in a growing number of publications (see Chapter 24). Importantly, increasing numbers of reports concerning laparoscopic approaches for cancer patients have discussed the possible role of CO_2 in spreading cancer cells, tumor dissemination, implantation, and trocar site metastasis. Clinical reports and the results of experimental animal studies suggest that CO_2 pneumoperitoneum should be avoided for malignant or suspicious tumors. Further studies are needed to compare conventional abdominal methods with the approach of gasless laparoscopy.

The results of our pilot study show that gasless laparoscopy allows similar surgical results to those obtained by the conventional abdominal route. During

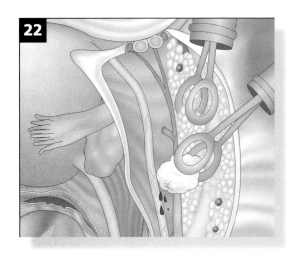

the operative procedure, Lift-laparoscopy can be used for a number of surgical maneuvers as in open surgery. Using cotton swabs, for example, fatty tissue lateral to the iliac vessels can be dissected and extracted using conventional grasping forceps (Figure 22). Thus the external iliac artery and vein can be easily identified. After incising and opening the perivascular sheath along the external iliac artery, the lymph nodes and the fatty tissue can be removed from this area while sparing the genitofemoral nerve.

The outstanding technical possibilities using gasless laparoscopy may contribute to increased safety compared with CO_2 laparoscopy. Through the valveless trocars, conventional instruments can be introduced and changing instruments is rapid and without gas loss. In case of severe bleeding, a hemostat or a conventional clamp can be placed during constant irrigation and/or suction without affecting visibility. Suturing or placement of clips is easier due to the lack of valves in the trocar sleeves. The introduction of curved needles is less problematic via the 10-mm flexible trocars than through the metal trocars used with pneumoperitoneum laparoscopy. Using conventional needle drivers and clamps, suturing is as easy as in open surgery.

Isolated lymph nodes or lymph node groups can be separated by simply pulling them bluntly using a fenestrated clamp and dissecting the lymph nodes out of fatty and surrounding tissue (Figure 22). Coagulation is used only in case of hemorrhage. To remove the lymphatic tissue, one can simply extract the specimen through the flexible trocars without contamination of the trocar incision.

Moreover, the lack of pneumoperitoneum has a positive effect on the iliac vessels as they are filled with blood and do not collapse as in pneumoperitoneum laparoscopy. This improves the process of isolating vessels and dissecting lymph nodes. Using a finger, one can also palpate tissue, vessels, lymph nodes, or suspicious findings (Figure 23).

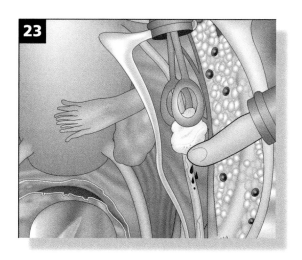

TERMINATION OF THE GASLESS-LAPAROSCOPIC PROCEDURE

When the procedure is completed, the entire abdominal cavity is checked for hemostasis. Then, the ancillary trocars should be withdrawn under vision. To prevent hernia formation, the fascia of the umbilical and the ancillary ports should be closed. Closure of ancillary ports should be performed under endoscopic vision. Afterwards, the retractor can be removed out of the abdominal cavity turning it counter-clockwise. The abdominal cavity can then be elevated by one hand while the other hand is holding the endoscope. The trocar sheath is removed from the incision while the scope remains in the abdomen. Withdrawing the endoscope slowly out of the abdominal cavity ensures that no bowel or omentum is pinched in the incision. The fascia is sutured, and, after approximating subcutaneous tissue, the skin is adapted by sutures. The AbdoLift® is then removed piece by piece from the operating table and prepared for cleaning and sterilization.

SUGGESTED READING:

Nezhat CR, Burrell MO, Nezhat FR, Benigno BB, Welander CE. Laparoscopic radical hysterectomy with paraaortic and pelvic node dissection. Am J Obstet Gynecol 1992;166:864-865

Melendez TD, Childers JM. Laparoscopic lymphadenectomy. Curr Opin Obstet Gynecol 1995;7:307-310

Possover M, Krause N, Plaul K, Kuhne-Heid R, Schneider A. Laparoscopic para-aortic and pelvic lymphadenectomy: experience with 150 patients and review of the literature. Gynecol Oncol 1998;1:19-28

Dargent DF. Laparoscopic techniques for gynecologic cancer: description and indications. Hematol Oncol Clin North Am1999;13:1-19

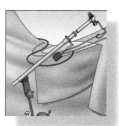

LAPAROSCOPIC LYMPHADENECTOMY IN GYNECOLOGIC ONCOLOGY

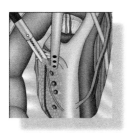

Farr Nezhat, M.D., FACOG

Tanja Pejovic, M.D.

In patients with gynecologic cancer, prognosis correlates with the extent of the disease according to the established FIGO classification systems. Surgical staging is superior because it provides histologic verification of tumor extent. Lymph node status is the most important prognostic factor in gynecologic cancer and surgical removal of pelvic and/or paraaortic lymph nodes for histologic assessment, is a part of staging of gynecologic malignancies. Additionally, removal of bulky lymph nodes may have therapeutic benefit.

Lymphadenectomy has generally been performed via laparotomy, leading to large incisions and significant intra- and perioperative morbidity. Dargent and Salvat were the first to describe laparoscopic lymphadenectomy for the management of gynecologic malignances in 1989. In 1991, Querleu et al. reported transperitoneal pelvic lymphadenectomy in 39 patients with cervical cancer. Nezhat et al. reported the first laparoscopic paraaortic lymphadenectomy in 1992. Since that time a number of other reports have described the safety and accuracy of laparoscopic lymphadenectomy for cervical, endometrial, and ovarian cancer. Numerous reports describe better magnification, fewer complications, and superior visualization of the anatomy provided by the video laparoscope in comparison with conventional techniques (Figures 1-3).

> PLACING THE PATIENT IN STEEP TRENDELENBURG POSITION DISPLACES THE BOWEL CEPHALAD AND EXPOSES THE AREA OF THE PERITONEUM WHERE THE INCISION IS MADE FOR LYMPH NODE RETRIEVAL.

PELVIC LYMPHADENECTOMY

Pelvic and paraaortic lymphadenectomy is accomplished before or after hysterectomy and bilateral oophorectomy. The initial approach is to expose the anterior and posterior leaves of the broad ligament by incising the round ligament and cutting the broad ligament in a cephalad fashion lateral and parallel to the infundibulopelvic ligament (Figures 4-6).

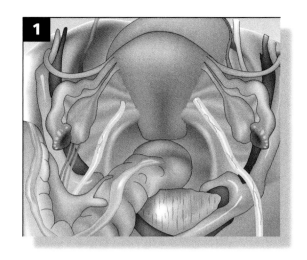

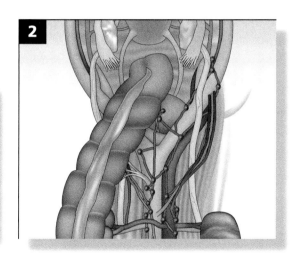

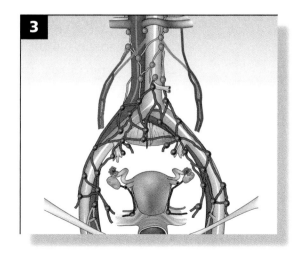

An incision is made in the broad ligament lateral or parallel to the infundibulopelvic ligament to develop the paravesical space. The round ligament can be coagulated and cut either before or after this space is developed (Figure 5).

Using the suction-irrigation probe, grasper and scissors, paravesical space is created. It is bordered medially by the obliterated hypogastric artery bladder and vagina and laterally by the pelvic sidewall.

Creating the avascular paravesical space helps identify the ureter, obturator nerve and vessels, and pelvic vessels (Figure 6). The obliterated hypogastric artery and external iliac vein are landmarks to get to the paravesical space. The spaces lateral to this vessel and medial to the external iliac vein and obturator internus muscle are created with blunt and sharp dissection. Electrocoagulation should not be necessary as this space is generally avascular. Once this space is created, the bony lateral sidewall, the levator plate

THE NODES ALONG THE EXTERNAL ILIAC ARTERY AND VEIN ARE REMOVED TO THE LEVEL OF THE DEEP CIRCUMFLEX VEIN.

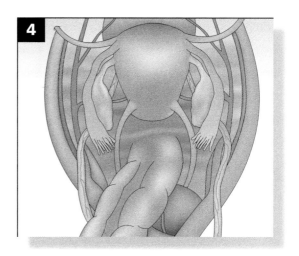

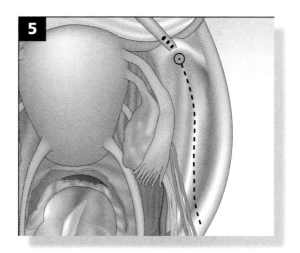

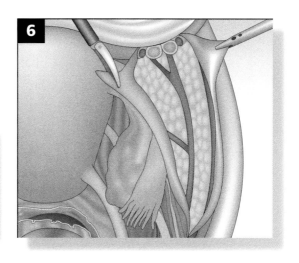

laterally, and the obturator nerve and vessels anteriorly should be visible. The pelvic lymph nodes can now be safely removed. Starting laterally over the psoas muscle and proceeding medially provide a safe approach that avoids the genitofemoral nerve. The external iliac nodes along the external iliac artery and vein are excised caudally to the level of the deep circumflex iliac vein seen crossing over the distal portion of the external iliac artery (Figure 7).

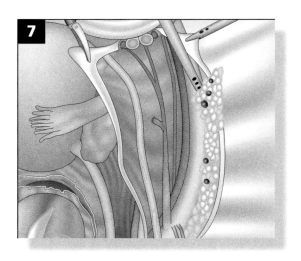

The obturator nerve is identified by blunt dissection below and between the obliterated umbilical artery and the external iliac vein. Of note is that although the obturator vessels are usually posterior to the nerve, sometimes an aberrant obturator vein may enter the midpoint of the external iliac vein and is anterior to the nerve. The nodal tissue anterior and lateral to the nerve and medial and inferior to the external iliac vein is removed by blunt and sharp dissection. Venous anastomosis between the obturator and the external iliac veins are saved from injury. The obturator nerve nodes are excised caudally to the pelvic sidewall where the obturator nerve exits the pelvis through the obturator canal and cephalad up to the bifurcation of the common iliac artery. Before the removal of each nodal bundle, each pedicle is ligated by electrocoagulation, endoscopic hemoclips, or an Endoloop to prevent lymphocyst formation. The lymph node packets are removed in a bag through the largest trocar to avoid any contact between potentially malignant lymph node tissue and the abdominal wall. Using sharp and blunt dissection, the nodes between the external iliac vessels and the obliterated hypogastric artery are removed. Hemoclips can be used as needed. The nodes along the hypogastric vessels are excised up to the bifurcation of the common iliac vessels. Caution is necessary to avoid injury to the obturator nerve and hypogastric vein (Figures 8 and 9).

To excise the lymph nodes around the common iliac artery, a plane is created between the posterior peritoneum and the adventitia overlying the common iliac artery. Another option is to extend the dissection over the common iliac vessels when removing the proximal portion of the external iliac nodes. Before the nodes are detached, the orientation of the ureter and ovarian vessels crossing the common iliac artery is identified. When one is performing a left pelvic lymph node dissection, it may be necessary to take down rectosigmoid colon from the left pelvic sidewall to allow visualization of the pelvic vessels.

PARAAORTIC LYMPHADENECTOMY

There are several ways to begin the dissection: incising the peritoneum overlying the aorta, opening the peritoneum over sacral promontory, and extending the incision overlying the common iliac artery toward the aorta. The peritoneum over the sacral promontory or lower aorta is incised. The underlying retroperitoneum is developed by using hydrodissection, or blunt and sharp dissection (Figure 10). Next, the retroperitoneal space is created by infusing this space with lactated Ringer's solution, or by using sharp and blunt dissection, to develop the space lateral to the aorta. Before cutting, it is essential to identify the ureter, separate it from underlying tissue, and retract it laterally. The nodal tissue

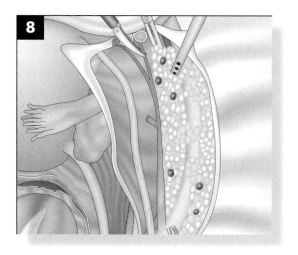

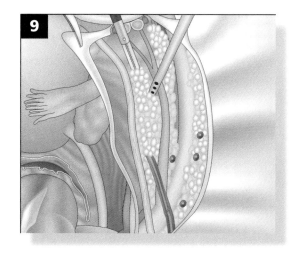

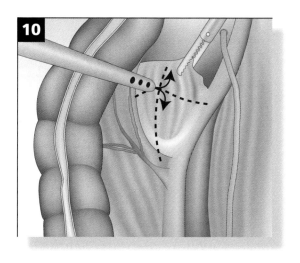

overlying the aorta, right common iliac artery, and sacral promontory is removed laterally toward the psoas muscle. Fatty and nodal tissue overlying the sacral promontory are removed. This tissue may contain hypogastric nerves. The left common iliac vein must be observed before starting this dissection (Figure 11). This maneuver allows the nodal tissue anterior to the vena cava to be detached. The dissection is continued cephalad to the level of the inferior mesenteric artery, removing all lymphatic tissue anterior to and between the aorta and inferior vena cava (Figure 12). Again, it

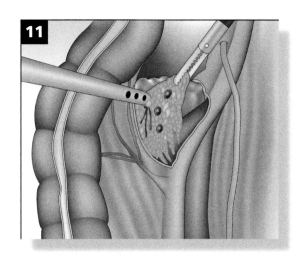

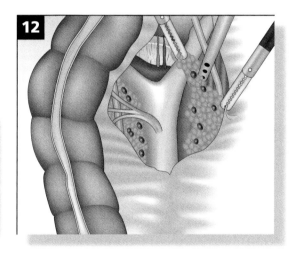

> THE NODAL TISSUE ALONG VENA CAVA IS REMOVED ABOVE THE LEVEL OF THE INFERIOR MESENTERIC ARTERY. THE RIGHT URETER MUST BE SEEN AND CONSTANTLY RETRACTED LATERALLY.

is essential to identify the ureter along the inferior border of the dissection and the transverse duodenum along the superior margin of the dissection. Perforating vessels from vena cava are electrocoagulated or ligated with hemoclips.

The removal of the left paraaortic nodes may be more difficult because of the location of the sigmoid colon.

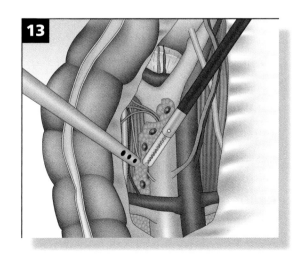

Attention is necessary to avoid injury to the inferior mesenteric artery, ovarian vessels, and the ureter. The left common iliac vein lies at the bifurcation of the aorta. The dissection proceeds from the aorta laterally toward the psoas muscle, excising the lymph nodes from above the inferior mesenteric artery to below the left common iliac artery (Figure 13). This allows the surgeon to dissect laterally in a plane

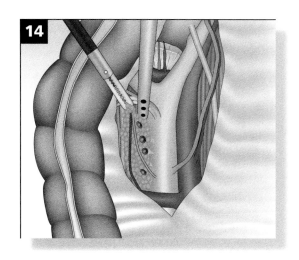

THE LYMPH NODES ALONG THE LEFT SIDE OF THE AORTA ARE REMOVED FROM ABOVE THE INFERIOR MESENTERIC ARTERY TO BELOW THE LEFT COMMON ILIAC ARTERY.

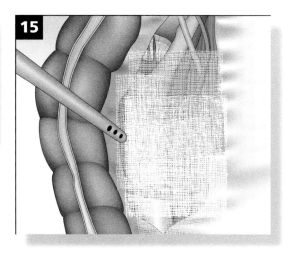

that is beneath the inferior mesenteric artery and the mesentery of the sigmoid colon. It is important not to dissect laterally until the adventitia of the aorta is incised to prevent entering the wrong plane.

In ovarian cancer, the paraaortic lymphadenectomy is extended to the level

IN PATIENTS WITH OVARIAN CANCER, THE PARAAORTIC NODES ARE EXCISED TO THE LEVEL OF THE LEFT RENAL VEIN AND RIGHT OVARIAN VEIN

of the left renal vein and right ovarian vein (Figure 14). The ovarian vessels are ligated, if necessary, to prevent bleeding. After the lymphadenectomy is completed, evaluation of the area under decreased pneumoperitoneal pressure is done to ensure hemostasis.

As with pelvic lymphadenectomy, the peritoneum is not closed and the drains are not placed. Interceed can be applied to decrease postoperative adhesions (Figure 15).

Data published in the literature suggest that the mean number of pelvic lymph nodes retrieved laparoscopically was 23, and that the mean number of paraaortic nodes was seven. This number is similar to that of lymph nodes retrieved by laparotomy. One report addressed the fact that 25% of the pelvic lymph nodes were still present at laparotomy after laparoscopic lymphadenectomy; however, no patient with negative nodes at laparoscopy had positive nodes at laparotomy. Along with this the objective that must be remembered is to remove the significant nodes, not the high number of nodes. The rarity of pelvic sidewall recurrences in node-negative patients managed without a complete lymphadenectomy indicates that laparoscopy may enable us to remove the significant nodes even when the total number of nodes removed is low. If the requirement of clearly identifying the dorsal part of the obturator nerve and lumbosacral nerve is fulfilled, the risk of missing a positive pelvic lymph node is very low.

Despite the degree of caution used, complications do occur during laparoscopic lymphadenectomy. In a series by Passover et al. (1998) ten major vessel injuries were identified among 150 procedures. These included four vena cava, two right renal vein, two external iliac vein, one internal iliac artery, and one internal iliac vein injuries. A conversion to laparotomy was necessary in four cases. The mean hospital stay for patients undergoing laparoscopic lymphadenectomy was 3.2 days. In other studies, the length of hospital stay, and recovery time were significantly shorter for patients managed laparoscopically. If continuing reports reveal the feasibility, safety, diagnostic accuracy, and treatment equivalence of laparoscopic and open retroperitoneal lymph node dissection, wide acceptance of this surgical approach in gynecologic oncology should result.

SUGGESTED READING:

Nezhat CR, Burrell MO, Nezhat FR, Benigno BB, Welander CE. Laparoscopic radical hysterectomy with paraaortic and pelvic node dissection. Am J Obstet Gynecol 1992;166:864–865

Melendez TD, Childers JM. Laparoscopic lymphadenectomy. Curr Opin Obstet Gynecol 1995;7:307–310

Possover M, Krause N, Plaul K, Kuhne-Heid R, Schneider A. Laparoscopic para-aortic and pelvic lymphadenectomy: experience with 150 patients and review of the literature. Gynecol Oncol 1998;1:19-28

Dargent DF. Laparoscopic techniques for gynecologic cancer: description and indications. Hematol Oncol Clin North Am 1999;13:1-19

COMPLICATIONS OF LAPAROSCOPY

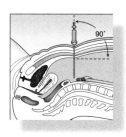

Barbara Levy, M.D.

Complications are inherent in any surgical encounter. Unfortunately, the only way to avoid all complications is to become a writer or editor and never enter the operating room as either a surgeon or a patient. It is easy to write about those circumstances which tend to predispose to surgical mishaps, however, the art of surgery is a clinical one that requires acute attention to detail, a lot of practice and the experience to sense trouble before it happens. These are not things any of us can teach.

Successful surgical outcomes depend on the anatomy of the patient, the severity of the abnormality to be corrected, the overall health status of the patient, and most particularly, the goals established by surgeon and patient together prior to undertaking the procedure. Many times patients pursue laparoscopic surgery in the misguided view that it is not really surgery – that it carries a lower risk of adverse events than 'open' surgery. Their expectations may be unrealistic and their tolerance for complications quite low.

I will try to outline the most common complications of laparoscopic surgery in this chapter. My goal is to provide some insight into those circumstances in which complications are more likely to occur in an effort to inform both surgeons and patients of the potential hazards of laparoscopic surgery.

PATIENT POSITIONING

While not unique to laparoscopic surgery, nerve injuries are more common after long, difficult procedures. Patient positioning is key to preventing many of these problems (Figure 1). Steep Trendelenburg position and hyperextension of the arm may cause brachial plexus traction and damage. The peroneal nerve on the outer side of the knee may be at risk when there is pressure between the knee and some fixed object. Femoral neuropathy may occur, particularly in very thin patients, when this large, relatively avascular nerve is stretched around the sciatic notch. This may

---

LAPAROSCOPIC COMPLICATIONS

POSITIONAL

EQUIPMENT

INSUFFLATION

TROCAR PLACEMENT

ELECTRICAL ENERGY

VASCULAR INJURY

BOWEL INJURY

GENITOURINARY

WOUND HERNIA

INCIDENCE OF LAPAROSCOPIC COMPLICATIONS

VASCULAR	1.2%
URINARY TRACT	2.7%
BLADDER	1.5%
URETER	1.2%
BOWEL	0.4%

N = 1165 HYSTERECTOMIES

FINNISH NATIONAL REGISTRY

happen when the hips and knees are flexed. Padding the sacrum and keeping the hips as flat as possible will help to avoid this problem.

ALWAYS CHECK
PATIENT POSITIONING AND THE
INSTRUMENTS BEFORE EACH
PROCEDURE

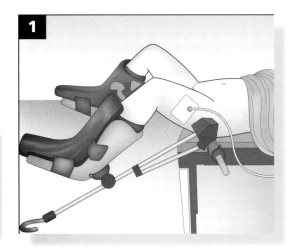

ABDOMINAL ENTRY

Gaining access to the peritoneal cavity for laparoscopy is hazardous. Even with open laparoscopy, the surgeon's view is extremely limited placing intraabdominal structures at risk for injury. There are many techniques for entering the abdomen – none of which are uniformly safe. Both the anatomy of the patient and the surgeon must be considered when determining the appropriate method of access for any procedure. Thin, nulliparous patients may require a different technique than the morbidly obese. Patients with previous abdominal surgery – either laparoscopic or open – present additional challenges. I do not believe that any one technique, angle or instrument is appropriate for all surgeons or all procedures. The experience, training and the judgment of the surgeon must combine to choose the instruments in any given circumstance.

POSITIONAL COMPLICATIONS

BRACHIAL PLEXUS –
ARM EXTENSION > 90°

PERONEAL NERVE –
LATERAL PRESSURE

FEMORAL & SCIATIC NERVE –
COMPRESSION

SHOULDER BRACE

RETURN ELECTRODE POSITIONING

FOLEY CATHETER

There are, however, certain principles that may help us avoid injuries most of the time. A knowledge of the three dimensional anatomy of the abdomen and pelvis will prompt us to 'map out' the hazardous regions for each patient prior to making the first incision. While in obese patients the aortic bifurcation may be as deep as 6 cm or more below the umbilicus, it may be as close as 1.5 cm in a thin woman. Trocar insertion at 90° may be quite reasonable for the obese patient, but extreme caution would be required in using that technique in the thin patient (Figure 2).

In general, there are a few tricks that provide some measure of safety in gaining access to the abdomen:

1) Avoid the Trendelenburg position. This rotates the sacral promontory closer to the umbilicus (Figure 3). Keep the patient flat and centered on the operating table.

2) Use standard length instruments. If the anatomy is considered and the appropriate access site and angle are chosen, there should be no need to use long needles or trocars.

3) In patients with difficult access – either very thin or obese patients, or those who have had prior abdominal surgery, consider alternate sites for needle and trocar insertion. An alternate site should be chosen in patients with failed insufflation attempt since preperitoneal insufflation pushes the peritoneum away making it difficult to

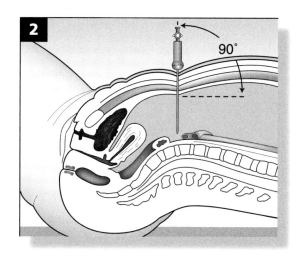

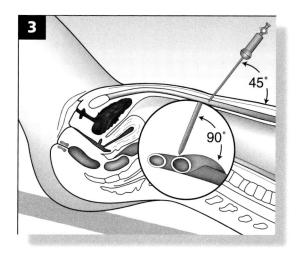

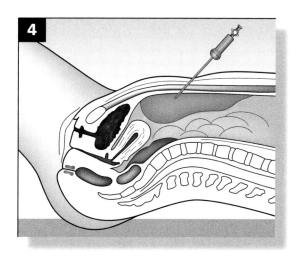

enter the peritoneal cavity in the same place (Figure 4). The left upper quadrant location is usually adhesion-free and easy to access.

4) Use a spinal needle with a syringe filled with saline or local anesthetic to explore the region underlying your intended insertion site. Inject and then aspirate, looking for either bowel contents or blood (Figure 5). A sufficient volume must be injected to permit aspiration of thick material such as fecal matter.

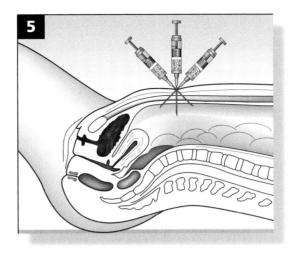

5) Insufflate the abdomen to a relatively high pressure (e.g. 25 mmHg) for a short period of time to permit maximal counter pressure while inserting the trocar (Figure 6).

6) Determine the estimated depth of the peritoneal cavity and note it on the trocar or needle, then use slow steady pressure on the instrument to insert it just to the predetermined depth. In general, it is not so much the angle of insertion that creates retroperitoneal injuries as it is the depth of insertion of the instruments. It is advisable to hold the trocar shaft with the non-dominant hand or to hold the index finger along the trocar shaft to prevent excessive insertion of the trocar, and retroperitoneal injuries shown on Figure 7. If resistance is felt during

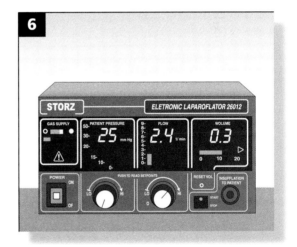

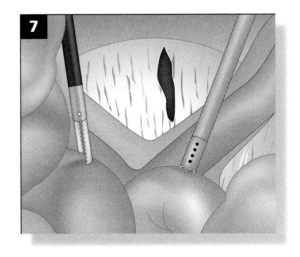

the trocar insertion, as if the trocar is hitting against a hard surface after the laparoscopic camera is introduced, the patient should be placed in a steep Trendelenburg and the bowel moved away in order to inspect the retroperitoneal space underneath the primary trocar.

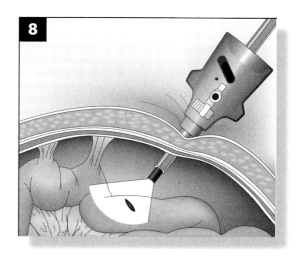

7) Avoid multiple passes with the needle or the trocar.

WC Fields said, "If at first you don't succeed, try again. Then quit. There's no use being a damn fool about it." This is reasonable advice for the laparoscopic surgeon. If abdominal access is difficult at one location, consider alternate sites or methods rather than risking injury with repeated attempts at insertion in a tough place.

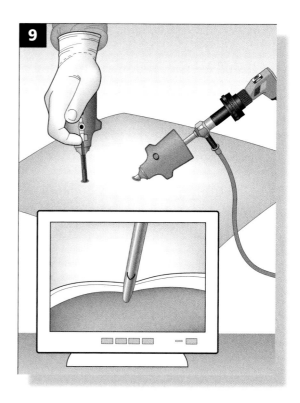

8) Inspect the region underneath the insertion site immediately upon placement of the laparoscope. Look for blood, debris or bowel contents (Figure 8). Bleeding may be an ominous sign and mandates careful inspection of the retroperitoneum for hematoma formation. Similarly, damage to bowel is most easily identified early in the procedure before the patient has been placed into steep Trendelenburg position and the bowel contents swept out of the visual field. This step will not avoid

a complication, but it may permit early recognition and treatment.

9) Place all secondary ports under direct vision (Figure 9). Consider placement carefully in order to

avoid the inferior epigastric vessels as well as the pelvic sidewall and the bladder. I like to use a 22-gauge needle with local anesthetic to explore the areas of secondary trocar placement as well. That way I can be sure the region of entry is in my visual field and I can determine the angle and depth of trocar insertion. For patients with prior pelvic surgery, the bladder may have been advanced as the peritoneum was closed. Sometimes filling the bladder may help to identify its borders before midline insertion of a trocar.

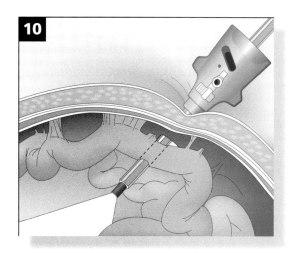

10) Finally, at the conclusion of the procedure, remove the laparoscope under direct vision, looking at each layer of the abdominal wall as the trocar sleeve is removed. With a through and through injury to a loop of bowel, this maneuver may be the only way to recognize the perforation (Figure 10).

There are a few late complications related to abdominal entry that should be discussed. Hematoma formation in the abdominal wall is not particularly uncommon. In complicated cases however, these hematomas may become infected. Necrotizing fasciitis has resulted in destruction of the abdominal wall and fascia requiring months of treatment and multiple

THINGS TO KEEP IN MIND

- ATTENTION TO ANATOMY AND PATIENT'S SIZE
- AVOID TRENDELENBURG POSITION DURING INSERTION
- USE STANDARD SIZE INSTRUMENTS
- INSUFFLATE TO HIGH PRESSURES FOR TROCAR INSERTION
- AVOID MULTIPLE PASSES
- CONSIDER ALTERNATIVE SITES
- INSPECT THE SITE UNDERNEATH THE INSERTION SITE
- PLACE ANCILLARY TROCARS UNDER DIRECT VISION
- REMOVE THE LAPAROSCOPE UNDER DIRECT VISION

reconstruction procedures. Pressure dressings may help to avoid hematomas as it is often difficult to isolate and control oozing from small, deep trocar sites.

Complex laparoscopic procedures often require multiple 10-12 mm ports for instrumentation. Several factors may predispose patients to hernia formation in these areas (Figure 11). Although there are many instruments available to help us close these port sites, none will be uniformly successful in avoiding hernias. Just as with open surgery, the most meticulous closure may still break down. Infection, hematoma formation, poor nutrition, and abdominal distension will all predispose the patient to wound breakdown. In addition, several technical issues may predispose to hernias. The anchoring threads on many trocars may cause pressure necrosis of the fascia during long operative procedures. This compromised tissue may break down early allowing sutures to pull through. Pyramidal or knife-blade trocars, if inserted with a twisting motion, may shred the fascial fibers making it difficult for sutures to hold. Finally, multiple passes through the abdominal wall in any one site may compromise the strength and viability of tissue in that location, once again compromising suture placement and security.

One last complication of abdominal entry sites must be mentioned. Tumor seeding at laparoscopic port sites has been reported in our literature as well as the general surgery literature. Oper-

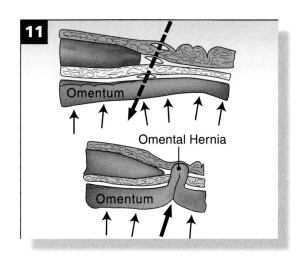

ating laparoscopically for malignancy requires significant skill and meticulous technique. Even so, it appears that port site metastases are significantly more common than metastases in large abdominal incisions. There are several theories to explain this, however, the important message here is that they do seem to occur with some frequency. Therefore it is prudent to counsel these patients preoperatively regarding the possibility and observe them diligently postoperatively to identify metastases early when they do occur.

INTRAOPERATIVE COMPLICATIONS

The two dimensional view, the limited visual field, and the lack of tactile sensation during laparoscopic surgery may be associated with several complications. Bowel injury may occur during adhesiolysis. The left ovary is frequently densely adherent to the sigmoid colon and the pelvic sidewall. Traction on the structures, intense dissection in a field with vision often limited by oozing and anatomic distortion and the use of various energy sources (laser, electrosurgery, ultrasound) may all cause injury to the bowel.

COMPLICATIONS OF ELECTRICAL ENERGY

You have to be very familiar with the energy forms that you are using during laparoscopic surgery. The surgeon must have an understanding of monopolar and bipolar electrosurgery, ultrasonic energy and laser energy in order to choose an appropriate technique and use it safely. If electrosurgical techniques are used be aware of the possibility of direct or indirect (capacitive) coupling, in order to avoid complications (Figures 12 and 13).

When using any kind of energy during laparoscopy keep in mind two simple rules: always keep the tips of your instruments in the center of the screen, while applying energy! Never use two different energy sources in the abdomen at the same time. It is very easy to get confused and to press a different pedal creating the potential disaster (Figure 14).

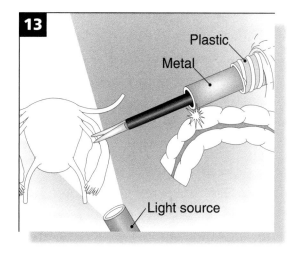

- KEEP THE TIPS OF YOUR INSTRUMENTS IN THE CENTER OF THE SCREEN, WHILE APPLYING ENERGY!

- NEVER USE TWO DIFFERENT ENERGY SOURCES IN THE ABDOMEN AT THE SAME TIME

Bowel perforations by scissors or tearing/shearing forces, if not recognized at the time of the surgical procedure, are likely to result in early and severe abdominal pain in the postoperative period. Many of these patients report extraordinary pain in the recovery room. Any patient with enough discomfort to require admission for pain management should be monitored with the suspicion for bowel perforation. Delayed perforation may occur in patients where adhesiolysis was accompanied by the use of energy techniques for hemostasis. Devascularization and coagulative necrosis may result in perforation several days after the procedure. Any patient who has a failure to thrive after laparoscopic surgery should be observed carefully. The surgeon must consider bowel perforation, incarcerated hernia and bladder or ureteral injuries in these patients. It is helpful to generate a

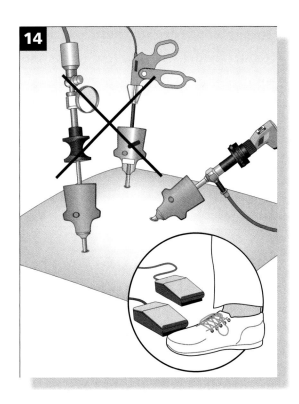

BOWEL INJURY

- Not from Veress needle

- Injury may not be apparent for 4–5 days

- Any symptoms of peritonitis (sharp abdominal pain, vomiting) must be considered as bowel injury unless proven otherwise!!!

- Use bowel prep

differential diagnosis during the period of observation. Choose laboratory and diagnostic studies to rule in or out each possibility, but remember that there is no substitute for good clinical judgment. Ileus, pelvic inflammatory disease and pneumonia are extraordinarily rare after laparoscopic surgery. If a patient returns with pain, fever and abdominal distention she has an intraperitoneal injury until proven otherwise. Delay in surgical intervention may be catastrophic.

If bowel injury is recognized during laparoscopic surgery, it can be fixed laparoscopically (Figure 15), or injured bowel may be pulled out through an expanded 10 mm incision and fixed. Sutured bowel may be carefully pushed back inside, avoiding laparotomy incision.

VASCULAR INJURY

Vascular injuries may occur in three different areas:

1. Pelvic sidewall

2. Intraperitoneal parenchymal bleeding

3. Retroperitoneal injury

Pelvic sidewall injury may occur during adhesiolysis, adnexal surgery, hysterectomy myomectomy, and lymphadenectomy. Careful anatomic dissection prior to initiating the surgical procedure may help to avoid some of

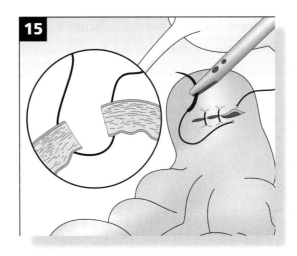

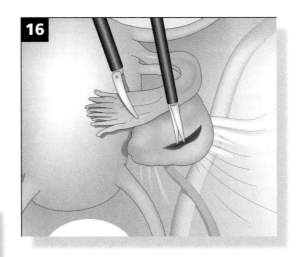

VASCULAR INJURY

ABDOMINAL WALL BLEEDING
- Inferior epigastric artery

INTRAPERITONEAL
    VESSEL INJURY
- Mesentery
- Ovarian artery
- Uterine artery

RETROPERITONEAL
    MAJOR VESSEL INJURY
- Iliac artery
- Vena cava
- Aorta

these injuries, however, at times the anatomic distortion is such that the injury may occur during the effort at dissection. The lack of tactile sensation and the limited operative field are particularly challenging for the surgeon under these circumstances. The external iliac artery and vein are at risk during adhesiolysis as well as adnexal surgery for ovarian cystectomies or ectopic pregnancy (Figure 16). Extreme caution is required when using energy sources in the pelvis, as the proximity of the pelvic sidewall vessels render them quite vulnerable to injury.

Whenever possible, the adnexa should be freed from the sidewall and surgical intervention carried out in the anterior cul-de-sac. If excessive bleeding is encountered, the external iliac artery must be dissected and inspected. Parenchymal bleeding can usually be treated laparoscopically. After irrigation with fluids and aspiration of blood, bleeding vessels are identified and hemostasis is established either with the help of laparoscopic suturing, endoloop, bipolar current, or simple mechanical pressure (Figures 17 and 18).

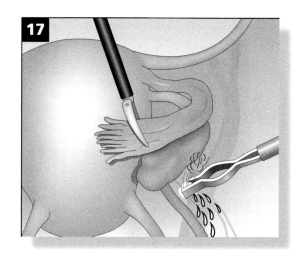

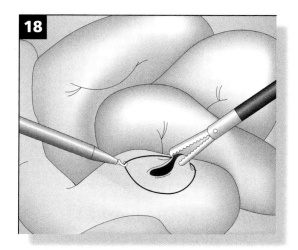

Remember that the pneumoperitoneum may collapse the veins. Injury to these structures may not become evident until the postoperative period. Before closure, release of the pneumoperitoneum and inspection of the pelvis under low pressure conditions, or under fluid, should help to identify these problems intraoperatively.

Retroperitoneal injuries are the most problematic complications of laparoscopic surgery. They usually occur as a result of Veress needle placement or primary trocar placement. Surgeons

RETROPERITONEAL INJURY

- Direct compression on aorta
- IV fluids
- Early recognition is the key to survival
- Do not open the peritoneum over a hematoma!
- Call a vascular or trauma surgeon

must be particularly careful with those procedures, and make sure that the operating table is in a flat position before Veress needle and trocar insertion. Always check visually with the laparoscope the area underneath the trocar for the absence of a retroperitoneal hematoma or bowel injury.

If retroperitoneal vessel injury is diagnosed, immediate laparotomy should be performed, and a vascular surgeon consulted. Manual pressure on the aorta underneath the renal arteries should be applied while the vascular surgeon is summoned. Additional IV access should be established to replace blood and fluids.

GENITOURINARY COMPLICATIONS

Bladder injury usually occurs as a result of the secondary trocar placement. The bladder is a very forgiving organ, and it can be fixed laparoscopically in two layers using absorbable sutures if an injury is detected during surgery (Figure 19).

The ureters may be injured up to ten times as frequently during laparoscopic surgery as they are during traditional abdominal procedures. At laparotomy we employ several techniques to protect the ureter. Traction on the uterus creates additional space between the ureter and the uterine artery during hysterec-

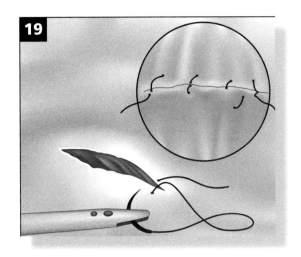

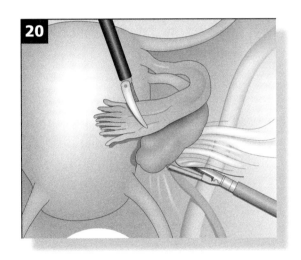

tomy. This usually permits safe control and division of the vessels as well as the cardinal and uterosacral ligaments without the need for complete ureteral dissection. At laparoscopy, it may be more difficult to deviate an enlarged, fibroid uterus enough to protect the ureter. In addition, we use some techniques for hemostasis much more often at laparoscopy. It is uncommon to use stapling devices, electrosurgery or lasers extensively during open surgery. These devices have all been associated with ureteral injury (Figure 20). The size of the stapling devices makes it difficult to see around them at times and any energy system, when used in proximity to the ureter, may cause thermal damage to the ureter itself or to its blood supply. This may result in delayed necrosis.

Once again, early recognition of ureteral injury requires vigilance and a high index of suspicion. The symptoms are often vague initially. Fever and pyelonephritis are rare after laparoscopic surgery. A patient presenting with flank pain and fever or abdominal distension should be evaluated for an

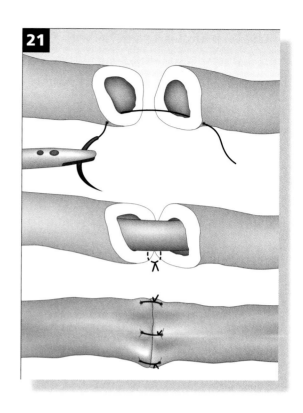

injury to the urinary tract. Early diagnosis via ultrasound or X-ray studies may enable the injury to be treated with stent placement rather than requiring re-exploration.

When in doubt that potential ureteral injury may have occurred during laparoscopic surgery, give the patient indigo carmine dye intravenously and perform cystoscopy to check ureteral function. It is much easier to perform cystoscopy and visualize ureteral orifices if using a video camera. You can also use a 5-mm diagnostic hysteroscope attached to the laparoscopic camera to perform cystoscopy. If ureteral injury is recognized during laparoscopic surgery,

BLADDER
      INDIGO CARMINE

- If < 1cm consider Foley catheter for 7–10 days

- If > 1cm laparoscopic 2 layer closure + Foley and Cystoscope

URETER
      TRACE FROM PELVIC BRIM

- Small non–electrical injury – primary repair over stent.

- Some injuries may heal with stent placement alone.

end-to-end anastomosis can be performed laparoscopically using 4.0 sutures at each quadrant over the ureteral stent. If a small ureteral injury or laceration is observed a ureteral stent should be passed and left in place without need for suturing (Figure 21).

CONCLUSION

While minimally invasive surgery has been a tremendous advance in the art and science of pelvic and abdominal surgery, it is not without its risks and complications. The only way to avoid these problems altogether is to avoid walking into the operating room. With careful attention to detail and a critical approach to patients who are at increased risk either by virtue of their anatomy or their history, complications may be anticipated in most instances and steps may be taken to minimize them. Thoughtful, reasoned and disciplined postoperative management of patients who are not recovering as expected will identify those with complications early.

BASIC LAPAROSCOPIC CONTRAINDICATIONS

ABSOLUTE

- Conditions, which mitigate against production of pneumoperitoneum

- Cardiovascular

- Pulmonary

RELATIVE

- Training and experience of a surgeon

- Availability of necessary instrumentation

- Diffuse peritonitis

- Shock or impending shock

- Obesity

SUGGESTED READING:

Hurd WW, et al. The relationship of the umbilicus to the aortic bifurcation: Implications for laparoscopic technique. Obstet Gynecol 1992;80:48-51

Boike GM, et al. Incisional bowel herniations after operative laparoscopy: a series of nineteen cases and review of the literature. Am J Obstet Gynecol 1995;172:1726-1733

Soderstrom RM. Bowel injury litigation after laparoscopy. Am Assoc Gynecol Laparosc 1993;1:74

Harkii-Siren P, Sjoberg J, et al. Finnish National Register of laparoscopic hysterectomies: A review and complications of 1165 operations. Am J Obstet Gynecol 1997;176:118-22

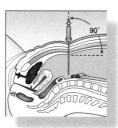

INDEX

salpingostomy 134

scalpel, harmonic 90–92

scissor dissection 30, 129–130, 141, 206

setup for laparoscopy 19–21

shoulder braces 56

sigmoid colectomy 292–294

soft coagulation 82

space of Retzius 15–16

specialty instruments 28, 34–35

square knot 103–104

sterilization, tubal by laparoscopy 107–114

steroid administration 151

stress urinary incontinence, laparoscopic treatment of 233–238

subcostal insufflation technique 62–63

subcutaneous emphysema 50, 62

subtotal hysterectomy 212

suction irrigators 133

superficial epigastric artery 8

superficial peritoneal anatomy 10–11

superior vesical artery 12

supracervical laparoscopic hysterectomy 211–222

surgery, pelvic floor 241–254

surgical management of ectopic pregnancy 162–168

suture in peritoneal cavity 98–99

sutures and adhesions 123

suturing

and gasless laparoscopy 311

endoscopic 96

laparoscopically 95–105

versus ligation 31

Swan-Ganz 42

T

termination of laparoscopic procedure 69–70

thermal coagulation 114

thermal damage 85

thin patients 64

thrombin 227

tissue

effects of electrosurgery 79–84

heating 77

removal 32

total hysterectomy 212

total laparoscopic hysterectomy 199

transesophageal echo 42

transumbilical insufflation 58–61

transuterine insufflation 65–66

treatment options for ectopic pregnancy 161–162

Trendelenburg position 2, 20, 38–40, 42–45, 58, 136, 258, 292, 332

trocar insertion techniques 55–70

trocar placement

and pneumoperitoneum 66–69

in hysterectomy 199–200

trocar, direct insertion of 64–65

tubal sterilization 44, 107–114

tumor seeding 336